RAISING A VACCINE

FREE CHILD

By

WENDY LYDALL

First published by AuthorHouse 01/27/05

ISBN: 1-4184-5017-0 (Paperback)

Library of Congress Control Number: 2003099849

This book is printed on acid-free paper.

Printed in the United States of America
Bloomington, IN

CONTENTS

"THE BENEFITS OF VACCINATION ARE WORTH THE RISKS"

~~~~~~

Vaccine Myth number One: Vaccination does sometimes have side effects, but these are much milder than the disease which the vaccine prevents.

~~~~~~

When parents try to decide which vaccines to accept for their children, they are not given accurate information by the authorities. It is impossible for parents to weigh up the risks of vaccination against the benefits, when they are not told what the risks from the vaccine are, nor how much chance there is that the vaccine will actually prevent the disease.

The myths of vaccination are so deeply entrenched in our minds that it comes as quite a surprise to learn that most of the claims made for vaccination are nothing more than fantasy. I was surprised when I learned that BCG, the vaccine for tuberculosis, does not prevent tuberculosis. I was even more surprised when I discovered that Edward Jenner's cowpox vaccine did not eliminate smallpox. It is a strange feeling when something you have believed for all of your life gets overturned in your mind.

My first baby was born in South Africa in 1982. I was well aware that the side effects of vaccination are far worse than the medical authorities admit, but I assumed that if I accepted the vaccine it would mean that my child would not be able to catch that disease. After weighing up the risk of the polio vaccine against the risk of getting polio, I decided to let baby Chandra have the oral polio vaccine. I knew that homoeopaths can cure

1

polio effectively and rapidly, but at that stage of our lives we spent a lot of time camping in the Drakensberg mountains of KwaZulu, where polio is endemic. If she had developed symptoms of polio it would have taken a long time for us to get from our camp site to a town with a homoeopath, so I felt that the risk from her possibly catching polio was greater than the risk of possible side effects from the vaccine.

I believed that oral vaccines have less side effects than injected ones, and I knew that being breast fed on demand reduced her chances of catching polio. What I did not know was that the vaccine would not make her immune to polio.

So in making the decision for Chandra, I had weighed up the risk of the vaccine against the risk of the disease, not realising that this was a faulty equation. As it happened, a polio epidemic did break out in South Africa while she was a baby, and I noticed some newspaper articles which said that the reason why vaccinated children were getting the disease must be because the cold chain must have been broken. When a vial of vaccine is not kept at a temperature below 4°C from the time it leaves the manufacturer until the time it is used, it is said that the cold chain has been broken, and the vaccine may have lost its virulence. I paid little attention to the issue, because it did not occur to me that anyone had a reason to lie.

The official literature that the health department had sent me said that three doses of oral polio vaccine would make my baby immune to polio. A few months after Chandra had had the third dose, a letter arrived from the city council informing me that it was time for her fourth dose. After a while the medical officer telephoned me to ask why I had not turned up for the fourth dose. She told me that Chandra was still in danger of catching polio, because three doses were not enough to create immunity. That was my first inkling of the fact that the polio vaccine does not work. Since then Chandra has never had any more doses of any type of vaccine.

My second baby was born at the beginning of the next polio epidemic in South Africa. By then we had moved to Cape Town, which is far away from the area where polio is endemic. My refusal to allow baby Kenneth to swallow any doses of oral polio vaccine caused a flurry in the medical bureaucracy in Cape Town. They even sent a top ranking doctor from Groote Schuur Hospital to my house. By then I knew from my research that the vaccine does not prevent polio, so all their dire warnings could not persuade me to conform. I had also realised by this time that vaccinationists are inclined to make statements which deviate from the truth, so I investigated the validity of the excuses given for the failure of the vaccine to prevent polio during that particular epidemic. The results of my investigation appear in vaccine myth number eight.

While Kenneth was still a baby we moved to New Zealand, and then eight years later we moved to Australia, so I have first hand experience of the behaviour of the vaccine bureaucracy in three countries. The officials who make up these bureaucracies take their cues from their mentors back in the USA.

When discussing the risks versus the benefits of vaccination, it is important to make a clear distinction between the two categories of infectious disease. These are childhood diseases and malevolent diseases. The issue of vaccination becomes muddled if the two categories of disease are lumped together, because childhood diseases are very different to malevolent infectious diseases.

Childhood diseases affect the immune system in a way that makes most people immune to the disease for the rest of their lives, but the malevolent infectious diseases do not do this. Vaccination is a partial copy of a natural infection, so when the germs of childhood diseases are injected into the blood stream, they create an artificial immunity that wears off and allows the person to catch the disease later on in life. There is a higher rate of complications with these diseases in older people.[1]

When the germs of malevolent diseases are used for vaccination, they do create antibodies, but that is not the same thing as creating immunity. Parents have a right to be given accurate information about the effectiveness of vaccines, but whenever vaccines are dramatically seen to fail, the establishment throws its energy into making excuses, instead of trying to understand the real significance of the available data.

To maintain the myth that the risk of side effects from vaccines is small, medical authorities say that most cases of vaccine damage are caused by something else. They also actively hinder scientists who wish to research the long term side effects of vaccination.

As I will show, the risk of death or brain damage from whooping cough vaccine is far greater than the risk of death or brain damage from whooping cough, yet glossy pamphlets tell parents that it is the other way round. Some deaths from measles vaccine are acknowledged,[2] but it is impossible to ascertain the risk of dying from measles vaccine when deaths are deliberately concealed.

Vaccinators do not tell parents what ingredients vaccines contain. Most vaccinators do not know that apart from the germs which are included to create antibodies, vaccines contain mercury, aluminium, formaldehyde, animal flesh, animal blood, human blood, human cells from aborted babies, potatoes, yeast, lactose, phenol, antibiotics, and unrelated species of germs which inadvertently get into the vaccine culture. How can parents work out the risk/benefit ratio of injecting these substances into their baby when they do not even know that they are included?

3

In all of my research, the only benefits which I have discovered to result from vaccinating a child, is that medical authorities do not harass the child's parents, and ignorant people do not accuse the parents of endangering vaccinated children.

Vaccination is a ritual which is held in awe by our modern society. Some people consider criticism of vaccination to be sacrilege. Many people hold the view that people who do not "believe" in vaccination are not only a danger to society, but that they are also crazy. Vaccination has the status of a holy cow, which makes some people consider it immoral to even question the claims made for vaccination.

Joseph Goebels was a master of propaganda, and he used a simple basic principle to convince people that Nazism was a good idea. The principle is that if people are told something often enough, they begin to believe that it is a fact and not an opinion. Repetition is the key to making a myth into a "fact."

The principle of repetition, combined with the suppression of factual data, is what the vaccine industry uses to keep millions of people around the world believing in the myths of vaccination. They constantly feed the media with half-truths and untruths aimed at promoting vaccination, and the media is reluctant to report negative facts about vaccination which are presented to them by parents or consumer activists.

Anti-vaccinationists face another problem which is similar to what the medieval astronomers faced when they tried to persuade people that the earth goes round the sun. The astronomers' claim sounded absurd at that time, because "everyone can see that the sun goes round the earth."

Nowadays the idea that vaccines are beneficial is regarded as a universal truth. It is considered quite "obvious," because everyone can see that smallpox and diphtheria are no longer with us, and the side effects of vaccination are not at all obvious because they are called by different names.

"SIDE EFFECTS ARE RARE"

Vaccine Myth number Two: Sometimes vaccination does have side effects like a rash, a fever, or a swelling at the site of injection. Serious side effects are extremely rare. The only long term side effect of vaccination is a scar on the skin from BCG vaccine.

The medical establishment has an effective way of ensuring that the official figures for vaccine reactions remain small. When confronted with a case of vaccine damage, they simply deny that there is a relationship between the vaccine and the symptoms. There are five ways that adverse reactions to vaccines develop;

*   Mild symptoms appear soon after vaccination, and then clear up after a few days. The child suffers no permanent effects.

*   Serious symptoms appear soon after vaccination, and they do not clear up after a few days. The child remains permanently damaged in some way.

*   Symptoms are mild at first, but slowly get worse, so that the full extent of the damage only shows up long after the date of vaccination. This is often how it happens when vaccination causes epilepsy and intellectual brain damage. A toddler has staring episodes the day after the injection, stops using language the next

day, becomes "clumsy" a week later, and has the first grand mal seizure five weeks after the injection. Intellectual disability is confirmed much, much later. The medical establishment gives the excuse that the epilepsy only started five weeks after vaccination, so therefore there is no connection between the vaccine, the epilepsy and the brain damage. When a tiny baby has this slowly developing type of reaction, it is very difficult to pinpoint the moment when the halt in development occurred, because it was not yet doing things like talking and walking at the time of vaccination.

* No symptoms appear at first, but a deep rooted problem, which takes a long time to surface, is set in motion by the vaccine. Auto-immune diseases are an example of this.

* A child is "not the same" after vaccination, with mild symptoms that persist for years, and lower the quality of health.

Vaccinators are happy to acknowledge the side effects that are not serious and go away after a while, like fever and swelling at the site of injection, but they are not keen to acknowledge side effects which alter a person's ability to enjoy life.

I used to assume that the incidence of side effects was researched before a vaccine was used on the public. Now I know that vaccines are approved for marketing without proper studies being conducted on their side effects. This situation has prevailed from the days of Edward Jenner up until the present. Once a vaccine is in use, the real incidence of serious side effects is not recorded.

Many countries rely on the American Food and Drug Administration (FDA) to ensure that the medical products which they buy are safe. The FDA is a taxpayer funded organisation in the USA which is supposed to protect the American consumer from dangerous substances, but as I will show further on, it fails to perform this function. The FDA should encourage research into the long term effects of vaccination, but instead it actively discourages long term research. For instance, Dr. Anthony Morris, a virologist and bacteriologist who was employed by the FDA in the 1970s, started some research into the long term effects of vaccination. This displeased his employers, and he was fired in 1976 for going to the press and warning the public not to accept the dangerous swine flu vaccine. The FDA took the opportunity to physically destroy the long term research in all his laboratories.[3]

Another example of obstruction of research by the medical establishment occurred when a professor at Otago University in New

Zealand applied for permission to study changes in the blood after vaccination. The research required a heel-prick to take a blood sample from each baby soon after birth, and then another heel-prick sample to be taken later on. Permission was denied on the grounds that it would be "too invasive." Heel-prick samples are taken from babies for all sorts of frivolous reasons, but it is not permitted when there is the possibility that the results may show that vaccination alters the immune system in undesirable ways.

Two professors at Florida University in the USA examined the blood of seven children who had been brain damaged by DPT vaccine. DPT vaccine is used to try and prevent whooping cough, tetanus and diphtheria. The professors found that six of the seven children had a particular tissue typing antigen. They applied for funding to research whether certain children are genetically predisposed to reacting to DPT vaccine. Funding was refused on the grounds that there is no evidence that DPT causes brain damage.[4]

There is a simple way to find out whether or not vaccines cause chronic diseases. You take a few thousand people who have had the vaccine, and a few thousand people from the same geographical area who have not had the vaccine, and you count what percentage of each group suffers from, or has died from, the diseases you are investigating.

So questions like, "Does hepatitis B vaccine cause diabetes?" "Does Hib vaccine cause brain damage?" "Does measles vaccine cause leukemia?" "Does the new DPT cause sudden infant death?" could easily be answered, if the medical establishment wanted to know the answers. It is remarkable that vaccination has been practiced on billions of people for more than two hundred years without these basic studies ever having been done.

The pharmaceutical industry and governments are the groups which have money to fund research. Governments have a moral responsibility to ensure that vaccines are properly tested for side effects before they foist them on their subjects, but all governments fail dismally in this duty. They prefer to take the easy option of just believing what the manufacturers say. In some countries, the government makes vaccines compulsory without having tested them for side effects, and does not pay compensation for the damage done. The way that the pharmaceutical industry conducts its "research" is discussed in vaccine myth number eleven.

There are individual doctors who not only care about the issue, they also have the opportunity, or make the opportunity, to do research. Dr. Michel Odent, the great French doctor who has done so much for birth and babies, founded an institution called the Primal Health Research Centre, to overcome the problem of pharmaceutical funding of research trials. This foundation is funded solely by donations from the public, so that no commercial bias is built into the results of the research. In their first study on the side effects of vaccination, they found, among other things, that DPT vaccine makes a person five times more likely to suffer from asthma.[5,6,7] The subjects had all consumed nothing other than breast milk for the first six months of their lives, and none had been weaned before their first birthday.

Their second study on vaccination confirmed the relationship between asthma and DPT vaccine, and showed that being born at home or in hospital made no difference to the risk.[8] The epidemic of asthma which afflicts children nowadays started with the use of DPT vaccine. The other side of the coin is that asthma is a huge money spinner for the pharmaceutical industry.

Another example of doctors within the medical establishment doing the right thing comes from the Inflammatory Bowel Disease Study Group at the Royal Free Hospital School of Medicine in London. This group is composed of three doctors who became suspicious that measles vaccine causes Crohn's disease. This is very strange because the symptoms of Crohn's disease are completely different to the symptoms of measles. Crohn's disease is a mysterious and horrible affliction of the intestines. The doctors' suspicions were aroused because measles virus persists in the tissue of the intestines of some people with Crohn's disease.[9,10] Measles vaccination started in Britain in 1968, and between 1968 and 1983 there was a three fold rise in Crohn's disease in Scotland.[11]

So with the help of a statistician from London University, these doctors did a study comparing the incidence of Crohn's disease in 2541 people who had not been vaccinated, with the incidence in 3545 people who had been vaccinated as toddlers thirty years earlier.[12] They also compared the rates of ulcerative colitis, coeliac disease, and stomach ulcers in the two groups.

The study revealed that measles vaccine makes a person 3 times more likely to get Crohn's disease, and 2.5 times more likely to get ulcerative colitis, but does not increase the risk of coeliac disease and stomach ulcers. So that means that two out of three of those people with Crohn's disease would not be suffering from it if they had not been injected with measles vaccine. Crohn's disease drastically reduces a person's quality of life. Health conscious parents can be grateful to this group of doctors for stepping out of line and doing this research. Another group of doctors have done a flawed study to try and prove this one wrong.[13]

Governments should fund scientifically sound research into the relationship between vaccination and all chronic diseases, instead of just adding more and more vaccines to their schedules. Governments should also start keeping accurate records of the occurrence of immediate reactions to vaccination.

The following are some of the reasons why the public is not aware of how common bad reactions to vaccination really are;

* When parents report a severe adverse reaction to a doctor, nurse, or government official, they are usually told that the vaccine was not the cause of the symptoms, and the event is not recorded.

* The victims are powerless because government agencies do not assist them, and the medical establishment will not help them. The people who made and marketed the vaccine are not accountable, and the media will not report on the victims' plight.

* Vaccines are perceived as something essential, the absence of which would cause widespread outbreaks of infectious diseases. There is psychological pressure on the medical fraternity to downplay the side effects that they observe. Journalists think that if they report cases of vaccine damage, readers and viewers will not vaccinate, and epidemics of disease will break out.

* When a doctor has the integrity to speak out about a case of vaccine damage, he or she is threatened and sometimes punished by a medical association or government officials.

* The link between the vaccine and the symptoms is not always obvious, even to the victim or the victim's family. Symptoms do not necessarily resemble the disease that the vaccine was supposed to prevent. Sometimes symptoms arise a few days or weeks after the injection, and the connection is not recognised.

* The diversity of symptoms caused by vaccines has made it easier for the medical authorities to deny claims that vaccines are harmful.

The eagerness of most doctors and nurses to brush aside the cases of vaccine damage that they personally encounter is the biggest problem. There is a conspiracy of silence which keeps vaccine damage out of the public eye. Some deaths from measles vaccine have been acknowledged,[2] but in most cases the parents are brow-beaten instead of being compensated.

It was only in 1991 that I became aware of just how common severe reactions to vaccination are. I was living in New Zealand, and my phone number was published in a health magazine at the end of an article about vaccination. In the following weeks I received scores of phone calls from people whose children had reacted badly to a vaccine, and who had been rejected and shunned by the medical establishment. Since being knee high to my mother I had known that there were cases of severe vaccine damage which were not being acknowledged nor recorded by the medical establishment, but this flood of phone calls jolted me into the realisation that vaccine damage is shockingly common.

The people who telephoned me were all relieved to be able to tell their story to someone who did not disparage them. The families of vaccine damaged children need emotional support as much as they need financial help. None of them had received any type of support from the official channels that are supposed to take responsibility. This was happening in a country that makes legal provision for vaccine damaged children to receive financial compensation, without any retribution to the doctor or nurse who administered the vaccine. Parents have no chance of getting compensation to help them cope with the financial costs of their child's disability when the doctors and nurses will not acknowledge their plight.

Now when I give talks or publish articles, I am no longer surprised by the number of terrible stories that I hear. Old people have stories to tell of what they saw the smallpox vaccine do when it was required for overseas travel from Australia and New Zealand, whereas younger people relate incidents about the other vaccines. In between talks and articles I receive a steady stream of phone calls from parents who have kept my phone number, but do not telephone me until someone is trying to jab another vaccine into their already damaged child, or into another child in the family. When a baby or child has died from vaccination, I find that it is never the mother who telephones me. It is someone further removed from the victim, like an aunt or a grandmother.

The only way we can stop the medical establishment from saying "side effects are rare," is by making the public aware of what is going on. Consumer groups around the world publish newsletters for parents, but the topic of side effects from vaccination is frozen out of the mainstream media. Because there is no discussion of the issue in the media, victims of vaccine damage are shut out of the public's consciousness. One of the consequences of this exclusion is that the families of vaccine damaged individuals are very isolated, and they do not realise how many other families there are suffering from the same problem.

There is a definite pattern of reactions from each vaccine, or combination of vaccines, but the most consistent thing which parents report to me is that doctors deny that the vaccine was responsible for the reaction. When parents move on to other doctors in the hopes of getting some help, they usually meet more denials that the vaccine could have been the cause. In rare cases doctors do admit it, but although they might say it verbally, they are not keen to put it in writing. Medical doctors cannot be expected to report side effects of vaccination which appear long after the vaccine has been administered, but if there were honest reporting of immediate side effects, a whole new picture would emerge.

In Australia, the 33 vaccines which are on the schedule for children under seven years are officially divided into 6 levels. Doctors are paid a bonus by the government each time they fill in a form saying that one of the levels has been completed for a child.[14] They are also paid a very large annual bonus if more than 80% of their child patients are vaccinated.[14] But they do not get paid anything for signing a conscientious objection form, nor for reporting side effects.[14] Unlike the situation in New Zealand, if parents want compensation for permanent disability caused by vaccination, they have to sue the drug company which manufactured the vaccine. The onus is on parents to prove that the vaccine caused the symptoms. The drug company does not have to prove that it supplied a safe vaccine.

To demonstrate the resistance which doctors have against acknowledging side effects of vaccination, I will describe four of the cases with which I was associated during my years as a campaigner in New Zealand, where, according to the law, compensation should automatically be paid, at taxpayers' expense. In theory all that has to happen is that the parents have to fill in form M46, and get it signed by any medical doctor. They then have to hand it in to the Accident Compensation Commission (ACC), which gets a panel of experts to investigate the case and decide whether or not compensation should be paid.

In 1991 I interviewed the father of a girl who was perfectly normal until a combination of the DPT and hepatitis B vaccines made her unable to sit up, unable to hold up her head, and unable to control her limbs. The only thing she could do was to make crying type noises when she was hungry. I could not tell whether or not her intellect had been damaged. Perhaps her mind was working normally and only the motor part of her brain had been destroyed. I saw a look in her eye that made me feel she was experiencing an emotional reaction to the conversation around her, but she could not speak nor control the direction in which her eyes looked. My interview with her father was filmed by a TV cameraman, but never shown on TV.

Auckland is the biggest city in New Zealand, and this family lived on an island close to the city. One day their doctor set off for the mainland saying that he was going to find out how they could obtain financial compensation. He returned to the island a frightened man, saying that the vaccine could not have been the cause.

When the family applied for compensation, the public health nurse said that she would support their claim. Then she was told that her job would be in jeopardy if she did that, because, "your action would make it appear that you are not supportive of immunisation policy." When I interviewed the father in front of the television camera, he related how the specialists who were supposed to be helping him submit his claim for compensation had treated him with suspicion, disrespect, and dishonesty. The thing that

11

amazed me about this interview was that despite all his experiences with the medical conspiracy, the father still believed that it was quite rare for a child to be affected in the way that his child had been. When I told him afterwards about the other cases we know about from the area, he was surprised to learn that his child was not "one in a million." If TV stations would allow that sort of footage to be aired, the public would become more aware of the extent of vaccine damage.

In another case, a girl was 15 months old when the measles, mumps and rubella vaccine (MMR) was injected into her hip. The hip and leg became swollen and painful, a lump of pus developed in the hip joint, and the cartilage disappeared from the joint. She also suffered a systemic reaction which put her in hospital for three weeks. Before the injection she had been toddling with free movements, but afterwards she could not put weight on that side.

The rubella component of MMR has a predilection for attacking the cartilage in joints,[15,16,17] but the lump of pus which was surgically removed seven days after the injection implies that the needle hit the bone. (Babies have very small hips and syringe needles are long). The surgeon who carried out the operation to remove the lump of pus met the girl's father and granny in the hospital corridor after the operation. He said to them, "That needle went in too far."

According to New Zealand law, the child is eligible for compensation for pain and suffering, for the travel costs to have her treated, for a plastic hip joint, for physiotherapy, and for whatever else she needs to cope with the consequences of the injection. The parents filled in form M46, but the doctor who administered the vaccine would not sign it, even though under New Zealand law he is immune from litigation if the finding is that he did put the needle in too far. No other general practitioner in the town in which they live would sign the form. The surgeon who said after removing the lump of pus that the needle had gone in too far would not sign the form, and no other doctor in the hospital would sign the form. The parents lived in a small town on the South Island of New Zealand, where all the medical people know each other, and they could not afford to travel to another town.

Even when parents have managed to get a doctor to sign the application form, they then have had to face the problem that the Accident Compensation Commission does not want to pay. ACC places the burden of proof on the victim, and then rejects whatever material the victim comes up with as being "insufficient evidence." The average young couple does not have the time nor the money to research the history of a vaccine and compile a scientific case proving that the vaccine was the cause of that specific set of symptoms. When they try, their effort is just brushed aside anyway.

A tiny proportion of vaccine damaged children do get financial compensation because of intervention by consumer activists. One of those was a child who was born 12 weeks prematurely. He spent six weeks in intensive care where he had to be vigorously stimulated more than a hundred times because he had stopped breathing. After he was moved into the regular prem unit the parents were told that he was thriving, so he could go home in a few days. They were also told that he must be vaccinated because he was very susceptible to disease. Although it was still six weeks before he should have been born, the parents naively gave permission for him to be injected with DPT.

After the jab in the morning he would not wake up for feeds. That night he was blue but the doctors told his mother not to worry. At 3 am a nurse walked past his cot and noticed that he was very blue. He was rushed back to intensive care and put on a respirator. At the time the doctors mentioned the vaccine as a possible cause of the relapse. He spent two weeks in intensive care and then went home to a life of "spastic quadriplegia" and "cerebral palsy."

It took a whole year for the parents to get the ACC form signed so that they could apply for accident compensation. The doctors were not keen to admit on paper that DPT vaccine was the cause of the child's condition, but they were in a quandary. The doctors who had assessed the baby before he was vaccinated had all put it in writing that the baby's prognosis was very good. When the baby's future turned to disaster, they were made to look stupid for giving such a good prognosis. So they wanted it known that their prognoses had been made before the baby had been injected with DPT. It seems that doctors are willing to tell the truth about DPT to protect their own reputations, but not when it is merely to help the victim get financial help in coping with their disability. The doctors' signatures made it possible for the family to apply to ACC.

The parents had two other things in their favour. One was that the reaction had occurred in hospital, under the eyes of lots of medical people. The other was that Hilary Butler, who is a voluntary worker with a huge knowledge base, spent eighty hours of her time combing the medical literature and putting together a written argument that it was in fact the vaccine which had caused the cerebral palsy, and the timing was not "just a coincidence."

The bigwigs at ACC were convinced by Hilary's evidence, and they ruled that compensation should be paid. However, a person lower down in the ACC hierarchy did not like this ruling, and sent a letter to the parents saying that compensation had been denied. It was only by chance that one of the bigwigs of ACC found out about this letter, and the lump sum compensation was paid three days later. None of the doctors who had agreed to admit that the vaccine was the cause of the little boy's disabilities reported the reaction to the Adverse Reactions Committee.

Another distressing case involved the death of a 32-year-old woman. She had developed an enlarged heart and an enlarged liver after giving birth in Auckland hospital. Many tests were done during the eight months of her illness, but her family did not receive an explanation for her condition. She was moved to Greenlane Hospital to have an operation in which they were to replace some swollen heart tissue with plastic. Before she was due to have the operation she was injected with a vaccine which contains the outer shells of 23 strains of germ that can cause pneumonia. She went into a coma, and her body swelled up and turned red. Then her skin became very painful to the touch, and it developed the appearance of a snow burn.

The doctors apologised profusely to the family for giving her the vaccine, because the official line on that vaccine is that it should not be given to anyone who is sick. But nothing was put on paper. Not only did the doctors fail to document the fact that she had reacted to the vaccine, they also failed to document that she had ever been given the vaccine. All they did was to write "operation cancelled" on the patient card, and send her back to Auckland Hospital.

The rash began to subside, and she came out of the coma. But the rash worsened when she had the heart operation ten days later. It was still there when she died of heart failure 25 days after the vaccination. This had been a very severe and painful rash; a sign that there was a serious disturbance within the body. The family believes that she would have survived the heart condition, had it not been for the vaccine. They are powerless against the medical establishment. What was a vaccine which is not supposed to be given to sick people doing in a fridge in intensive care? There is no accountability for what goes on in the name of "immunisation."

It is only when the public at large realises what is going on, and starts putting pressure on the politicians, that things will change. When the public knows that vaccination is largely responsible for the high incidence of behaviour problems, learning disabilities, chronic tonsillitis and ear infections, auto-immune diabetes (type 1 diabetes) and a host of other problems, they will stop being so compliant.

THE CRUCIAL DIFFERENCE BETWEEN CHILDHOOD ILLNESSES AND MALEVOLENT INFECTIOUS DISEASES

Discussion about the effectiveness of vaccination always becomes muddled unless a clear distinction is made between the two categories of infectious disease. Infectious diseases are usually classified according to the type of germ that causes them. So it is said that there are bacterial diseases, viral diseases, rickettsial diseases, protozoal diseases and so on. But that method of classification does not help us understand the effects that infectious diseases have on humans. From the point of view of prevention, treatment and immunity, it is more useful to divide them into two groups. This classification is based on how they interact with the human immune system, rather than on what type of germ causes them. One group is referred to in English as *childhood diseases.* The other group does not have a label in English, so I have labelled them *malevolent diseases.*

When childhood diseases are handled correctly, they have a beneficial effect on the child's long term health. When wrongly treated, they can develop complications which can harm and even kill the patient. The childhood diseases are the ones that you expect a child to get before the teenage years, like measles, mumps and chicken pox. There are eight of them. Few children get them all, but most children will get most of them. These diseases do not need any action to be taken to make them come to an end. They are self-resolving diseases which automatically come to an end by themselves. These diseases cannot be prevented by good nutrition, but the level of nutrition affects the way the child copes with the disease. One dose of the disease creates life-long immunity. The vaccines that are designed to prevent these diseases have a different effect on the immune system to the natural infection. Vaccines create a temporary immunity that wears off in time, so that vaccinated people get the childhood illnesses when they are teenagers or adults.

The malevolent diseases are the ones which we do not calmly "expect" our children to get. They are diseases which cause a panic, and rightfully so. Tetanus, tuberculosis (TB), polio, diphtheria, cholera, rabies, bubonic plague, typhoid, typhus and yellow fever are diseases that give absolutely no benefit to a person who gets them. Some of these diseases can be prevented by hygiene, but the germs of the airborne ones cannot be avoided during an outbreak. However, airborne germs will only be able to cause disease in a person who is susceptible, and good nutrition is an important protective factor.

A significant feature of the malevolent diseases is that catching one of them, and surviving, does not mean that the person cannot catch it again at a later date. When my son Kenneth was three he got measles. He did not like the spots because they spoiled his appearance. The sight of himself in the mirror made him upset. I consoled him by telling him that when it was all over he would never get measles again. A few months later he got gastric flu, and he felt terrible. With a sad look he said, "At least it means I'll never get it again." I had to tell him the bad news that gastric flu is not a childhood disease, so he would not get immune to it, and the germs which

Childhood Illnesses	Malevolent Infectious Diseases
infantum roseola	polio
rubella	TB (tuberculosis)
mumps (parotitis)	diphtheria
measles (rubeola)	tetanus
chicken pox (varicella)	cholera
whooping cough (pertussis)	typhoid
slapped cheek roseola	meningitis
scarlet fever	typhus
	hepatitis A
	hepatitis B
	hepatitis C
	rabies
	haemophilus
	smallpox
	yellow fever

Childhood Illnesses	Malevolent Infectious Diseases
Are self-resolving diseases which need proper care to prevent complications, but no intervention.	Are not self-resolving diseases and without intervention death is a possible outcome.
Cannot be prevented by good nutrition.	Good nutrition helps with prevention.
Cannot be prevented by hygiene.	Some can be prevented by hygiene.
Create life-long immunity to themselves.	Do not create immunity to themselves.
Vaccines create temporary artificial immunity.	Vaccines are either ineffective or have no proven efficacy.

cause it often come into the air, so he could get it again.

One can only get a disease when the germs for that particular disease are in the environment (except for TB, which is always in the environment). In some countries it is safer to assume that cholera and typhoid are always in the environment. Nutrition alone is not enough to protect you against those two horrors.

The germs that cause childhood diseases float in the air, and there is a concentration of them in the air space around a person who is brewing the disease, or who has the disease. The germs infect everybody, but not everyone gets the disease. Some people have already had it and are immune, while others are never going to get it, or are going to get it at a later date. Some children are repeatedly exposed to the germs by parents who are keen to get the childhood diseases behind them, but their bodies obstinately refuse to catch the disease.

A child's nutritional status has no bearing on whether or not he or she catches a childhood disease, but it does make a difference to how he or she handles the disease. It annoys me when anti-vaccinationists tell parents that a child who is breast fed and given only wholesome food will not get measles. That is not true.

Health-conscious communities have "measles parties" to give as many children as possible the opportunity of catching measles. This has to be done in a way that is sensitive to the needs of the sick child. Sometimes children who do not even like each other have to play together. But despite all this effort, there will be some children who just do not get it. This is very vexing, because if a person gets a childhood disease in adulthood, the risk of complications is much higher.[1] An exception to this is whooping cough. A young baby is vulnerable to the complications of whooping cough if it is not handled wisely, whereas complications seldom occur in older people, even with the worst medical treatments.

My mother-in-law had three brothers who all had mumps when they were children, but she did not get it. All seven of her children had mumps at one time or another, and she cared for them closely, but did not catch it. It would have been difficult for her if she had got it during her child caring years. Then, much to her amusement, she got it from one of her grandchildren when she was 62. She knew exactly what to do. She took herself off to bed and read books and caught up on her knitting until it was safe to get up again. She lived with a daughter who kept her well supplied with nourishing soup. People of any age with mumps need to be well cared for, but an adult with mumps who does not stay in bed is especially vulnerable to complications.

We have been conditioned to fear childhood illnesses, instead of being taught how to treat them. Once we know how to treat them safely, we do not need to fear them. However, we do need to have a healthy, well informed fear of the malevolent infectious diseases. These diseases need to be dealt with swiftly if they put in an appearance.

THE RISK FROM INFECTIOUS DISEASES

It is important for parents who want to make an informed decision about vaccination to understand the risk that infectious diseases pose to the health of their children. The vaccine industry would like us to believe that if it were not for the protection of vaccination, people would be accosted by deadly germs wherever they go.

As was shown in the previous section, there is a crucial difference between malevolent infectious diseases and childhood illnesses. Therefore they should be approached differently. Parents who fear childhood diseases wonder what the *risk* is of their child catching a childhood illness. Once liberated from the fear that has been cultivated by the vaccine industry, they change their thinking and wonder what the *likelihood* is of their child catching each particular disease.

Most vaccine free children are likely to get measles, rubella and chicken pox during childhood. Vaccinated children are likely to get them when they are teenagers or adults. When a mumps epidemic breaks out, it is advisable for little boys to play with infectious children to try and catch the disease and get it over with before puberty. However, exposure to the germ that causes mumps is unfortunately no guarantee that the disease will develop. A child who does not get infantum roseola during the first three years of life is not likely to get it later. Scarlet fever is so rare nowadays that there is very little likelihood of your child getting it. Slapped cheek roseola is a new disease that is becoming more common. Whooping cough has been undergoing a steady decline for more than a hundred years, but many children still get it. There is no known way of predicting which child will get it and which child will not, so therefore every caregiver should be equipped with the knowledge of how to treat whooping cough safely.

Whooping cough has a predictable cycle, and when it is in full swing it breaks out everywhere in the world at the same time. The other childhood illnesses have a random cycle, and they put in an appearance in different places at different times. Even cities as close as New York and Baltimore have measles epidemics at different times.[18] There is no risk of bad consequences from childhood illnesses in a child who;

* has been eating reasonably wholesome food with enough calories every day before catching the disease,
* is properly cared for while the disease is in progress, and
* has a reasonably healthy or perfectly healthy immune system.

Childhood illnesses cannot be prevented by a healthy lifestyle. Although these diseases are not the bogeys they are made out to be by the vaccine pushers, they should be treated with great respect. Childhood illnesses can have serious complications, and can even be fatal, if proper care is not given. Medical doctors and nurses are trained to treat these diseases by chilling the patient and suppressing the fever with drugs, and this causes complications and death. While good nutrition does not prevent a child from catching a childhood illness, it does make the child cope with the disease much better than a malnourished child does. Hygienic practices make no difference to the chances of catching a childhood disease. Vaccination against childhood diseases raises the age at which the disease occurs. The risk of complications from childhood diseases increases with age.[1]

The germs which cause malevolent infectious diseases come from three different sources; some live in water, some float in the air, and some can only be caught from another person's blood. For example, polio germs float in the air, cholera germs live in water, and hepatitis B can only be caught from another person's blood. There are actions which human beings can take to limit the impact of nasty germs, both on an individual basis and on a community basis. Since medieval times there have been three great improvements in the human response to infectious diseases. These are the chlorination of the water supply, directing sewage away from the water supply, and attention to personal hygiene. But the use of homoeopathy to treat infectious diseases has been blocked because the introduction of homoeopathy would damage the profits from patented drugs.

Germs that live in water can be avoided by drinking only water that has been chlorinated or boiled for 3 minutes. These germs can survive in very little water, so they may be present on a lettuce leaf on your plate in a restaurant if you are in a country that permits the use of unchlorinated water.

Germs that live in the air are not always present in the environment, but they cannot be avoided when they do put in an appearance. We can however protect ourselves and our children with good nutrition and a healthy lifestyle. In Australia the TV continually tells viewers that they will be healthy if they eat refined starch and avoid protein and oils. The opposite is true. We need well working immune systems in order to demolish any bad germs that might float our way. The germs enter through the nose and mouth and get zapped by immune system soldiers if the immune system is in good condition. People who have had their tonsils cut out need to take extra precautions to bolster the remaining parts of their immune system. Diphtheria is an airborne disease but there is very little risk of catching it these days because it has been undergoing a natural decline since long before the vaccine was invented. It does however sometimes break out in a limited geographical area.

AIDS and hepatitis B can only be caught if an infected person's blood makes contact with one's own blood stream. Schoolchildren who are carriers of the hepatitis B virus do not pass on the disease to other children in the playground.[19,20] Kissing people with AIDS is not dangerous unless you have open sores on your lips or oral mucous membranes. AIDS and hepatitis B are caught from dirty needles (acupuncture, tattooing, substance abuse, and medical injections in countries which do not practice medical hygiene), from contaminated blood products, or from sexual contact with an infected person. Some vaccines were contaminated with the HIV virus before the virus was identified, but hopefully none which are in use today are contaminated with that particularly nasty virus. Likewise vaccines are nowadays screened for hepatitis B and C, whereas in the past hundreds of thousands of people were infected through vaccination.

FEVER IS A FRIEND

Modern parents are taught to fear fever as if it were a disease, and to make it go away when it appears in a child. But suppressing fever, either by the use of drugs or by chilling the patient, is a dangerous practice, which sometimes causes the patient to die. Fever is part of nature's way of helping the body cope with invasion by a germ or by a toxin. If fever is suppressed during an infectious disease, the patient becomes more vulnerable to the germ that is the underlying cause of the sickness. Many parents believe that if they do not bring down the fever, their child will have a convulsion and suffer permanent brain damage. This idea is promoted even though it has been scientifically proven that it does not happen.

All non-Westernised cultures support fever as part of their care of a sick person, and Europeans did the same until very recently. The idea that fever is harmful started being promoted 150 years ago, because drugs which suppress fever were being commercially produced. It began in the world described by Mark Twain in *Tom Sawyer* and *Huckleberry Finn.* A tree that grows in this region of America contains aspirin in its bark, and it was noticed that chewing the bark reduced pain. Aspirin has the side effect of suppressing fever, so after isolating aspirin from the bark, and then synthetically reproducing and patenting it, the manufacturers promoted the idea that bringing down a fever is a good thing to do.

In up to date circles of modern medicine, aspirin is now frowned upon, and the fashion is to prescribe paracetamol or ibuprofen instead. Paracetamol is called acetaminophen in the Americas, but it is most commonly called by one of its two hundred trade names. Some trade names are Tylenol, Calpol, Panadol, Panado and Tempra. In this book I will refer to the drug as paracetamol. Now that science is beginning to discover how the immune system works, some of the reasons why a rise in temperature helps with the destruction of invading germs and toxins are becoming known.

Fever is not dangerous, but hyperthermia can be dangerous. Hyperthermia is where the body becomes too hot, while hypothermia is where it becomes too cold. When a person suffers from hyperthermia it is because their body has been made too warm by an outside influence, whereas fever is caused by the body deliberately making itself hotter than normal, usually as a reaction to an infection. When the body experiences hyperthermia, it tries to reduce its temperature, by, for example, sweating, or moving into the shade, or drinking cold liquid. (My children chew ice on hot days.) Young babies are unable to rectify the situation if they are too warmly wrapped up, and overheating is associated with sudden infant death syndrome.[21,22,23] When a fever occurs the temperature does not keep on rising until the body cooks itself. There is no danger from the increased temperature because it will stop rising when it reaches the right level to achieve what it needs to achieve.[24] With hypothermia the internal organs of the body heat up, and that is dangerous, but with fever, the internal organs do not get heated.[25]

Leukocytes are an assortment of cells in the immune system which fight unfriendly germs. They also fight the toxins which unfriendly bacteria make. Leukocytes move faster when the temperature goes up,[26,27] and they can eat invader germs at a faster rate.[28] When foreign germs invade the body, some leukocytes manufacture a protein called endogenous pyrogen.[29,30] There is disagreement about exactly how this protein stimulates fever, but the fact that it is the thing which provokes the fever is not disputed. Once the fever starts, the level of iron in the blood becomes reduced, so that foreign bacteria cannot feed on it.[31,32,33] The movement of iron out of the blood is not caused directly by the rise in temperature; it is a separate defence mechanism which works co-operatively with the fever to defeat germs.[34] The body also starts producing interferons,[35] which are substances that kill viruses and bacteria, and make leukocytes more active.[35,36] Interferon works faster at a higher temperature.[37] For instance, it is three times more effective at 40°C than it is at 39°C.[37] Antibiotics are more effective in the presence of fever.[38] Vitamin C helps leukocytes kill germs, and when the temperature is higher, the effect of vitamin C is greater.[39]

Leukocytes respond faster and more effectively when the temperature goes up to 40°C.[40] They also move to where they are needed faster and stay at the site where they are needed when the temperature is elevated.[35,41] T cells are an important type of leukocyte which are manufactured in the thymus gland in the head. When fever is present the thymus produces more

T cells.[42,43,44] Bacteria get weaker and are easier to kill at a higher temperature.[45,46]

Reptiles, very young mammals and debilitated mammals have something in common. That is that they all cannot raise their own temperature from within. When reptiles are infected with unfriendly germs, they move to a warm spot. If they are prevented from moving to a warm place, they die.[47] Very young mammals are instinctively kept warm by their mother, but if they become infected with harmful germs and are not kept warm by external means, they die.[24,28,48] Debilitated humans of any age who cannot produce a fever will die from infection.[38]

Drugs that reduce fever place both reptiles and mammals at a disadvantage. A study was done in which twelve iguanas were infected with a bad germ and kept in a warm environment, but they were also given aspirin. In 5 of these the aspirin did not work, and their temperatures went up, and they survived. In the other 7, the aspirin succeeded in preventing fever, and they all died.[49] Giving drugs to rabbits to reduce fever increases the death rate from infection.[50] Infected humans who experience fever have a better survival rate than infected humans who do not experience fever.[51,52,53,54]

By mindlessly reducing fever whenever they see it, the medical profession is sabotaging the body's attempt to defend itself. They are causing well fed affluent children to suffer one of the disadvantages which starving children suffer, as I will explain.

The immune system of a child who is severely malnourished cannot even begin to start fighting invader germs. That is why so many children in poor countries die from infectious diseases. Most children in affluent countries do not eat a wholesome diet of organically grown, unrefined, unprocessed food, but they do get *enough* food to make their immune systems work. As a result of eating the artificially fertilised, refined and highly processed foods, affluent children grow up to get the diseases which are now considered "normal" in people over 50, like sugar diabetes (type 2 diabetes), cancer, heart disease and arthritis. But at least they can fight off germs long enough to grow up and get the diseases of modern civilisation.

Children who have kwashiokor (severe malnutrition) cannot make pyrogen, and consequently they do not go into a fever when they get infected with germs.[55,56] "Infections in these circumstances are frequently fatal."[55] Dr. G. J. Ebrahim has worked extensively with these children, and he says,

> The child with malnutrition is very susceptible to infection. The body's defences are unable to mount an adequate response to microbal challenge so that the mildest infection tends to spread and

become life-threatening. In severe cases the clinical response to infection, like fever and phagocytosis, may be absent and the first sign of widespread infection may be sudden deterioration in the general condition, refusal to take food and hypothermia.[57]

Hypothermia means getting colder. So instead of getting a fever when something like measles starts, the body of a malnourished child gets colder. Measles without fever is a dangerous situation.

Most well fed children survive having the fever artificially reduced, but they do not all survive. Medical doctors and nurses are trained to give a fever suppressing drug other than aspirin to someone with an illness like measles or mumps.

One excuse given for reducing fever is, "It will make him more comfortable." A child in a high fever with measles is not uncomfortable. The child's behaviour is different to normal, mainly because he or she just lies there doing nothing. But the child feels okay. If pain or discomfort is present, it means that something is wrong. When something is wrong it is not the fever that needs to be dealt with. Reducing the fever will only make the child more vulnerable to whatever is wrong. Giving paracetamol to a child with chicken pox makes the spots more itchy, and makes the illness last longer.[58]

A child who is in a fever because of a childhood illness needs quiet surroundings, and needs to know that a parent or primary caregiver is nearby. A baby might want a parent present all the time while awake. A person with a fever needs to be given frequent drinks, and to be lying down and covered with warm bedding. The patient instinctively pulls the bedding up to the chin as the fever rises, and pushes it back when the fever recedes. Babies cannot adjust their covers, so they need adult help to ensure that they do not get too cold or too hot. Shivering is a sign that the fever is building up and warmth is needed. Sweating is a sign that the fever is over and the body is cooling itself down. Don't force a sweating child to stay under the covers, but also don't do anything that would make him or her cool down any faster than nature intends. The body will do it at the correct rate. When fever is achieved, the pyrogen shuts off its own production.[25] Then when fever is needed again, the pyrogen stimulates the production of fever again. That is why the fever comes and goes during the illness instead of remaining constant.

By recognising the role of fever in infectious diseases, we are better equipped to help the patient recover. There was a long standing tradition in Europe that, in certain circumstances, a disease could be cured by stimulating a fever. This ancient wisdom was misapplied when sick people were immersed in boiling water. The art of inducing fever to cure various conditions has not died out in German culture.

The Zulus also treated illness that was accompanied by fever by warming people up. Dr. Henry Francis Fynn described his experience of Zulu medicine in 1823.

> I discovered that their chief, Shaka, resided at too great a distance from there for me to reach him. Apart from this I became considerably indisposed, hence went back to where our vessel was, upon which I was immediately laid up with a severe attack of fever. During my absence, Maynard had sent for the schooner, hence I found myself left with only the sailor who had been with me the whole time. I obtained possession of a hut like those at Delagoa and there I lay for several days. I must have become delerious, for the first thing I remember was being taken from the hut by a native doctor and several women. On coming to an open space, they lifted me up and placed me in a pit they had dug and in which they had been making a large fire; grass and weeds had been placed therein to prevent my feet from being burnt. They put me in a standing position, then filled the pit with earth up to my neck. The women held a mat round my head. In this position they might have kept me for about half an hour. They then carried me back to the hut and gave me native medicine. I felt I was recovering. On the third day, I was able to communicate with the vessel.[59]

Zulu mothers still wrap up a feverish baby warmly, unless a white person intervenes and tells them to undress the baby and put it in a draught.

A similar story is told of Australian Aboriginals helping a sick white man whom they found wandering around in the bush.

> On seeing Buckley ill, they scooped out a depression in the ground, lit a fire all along it, later swept the fire out and laid Buckley in it, covering him with the warm soil. This method proved successful and he recovered fully.[60]

In the 1940s Dr. Benjamin Spock wrote a book on childcare which revolutionised the way children were brought up. In this book he devotes four and a half pages to telling parents how to take a child's temperature, then says, "on the other hand a dangerous illness may never have a temperature higher than 101 degrees. So don't be influenced too much, one way or the other, by the height of the fever." Then he goes on to advise giving aspirin and chilling the child with water, and then says, "remember the fever is not the disease. The fever is one of the methods the body uses to help overcome the infection."[61] Bring on the psychologists.

Measuring the temperature when a child has a fever does not provide information that helps to make decisions about care. The child's condition is what matters. It is normal for a child with fever to lie down, have glazed eyes, and not be talkative. Those symptoms are not a sign of danger. The symptoms that go with a childhood illness are also not signs of danger. But if there is pain, stiffness, seizures, vomiting, confusion, unresponsiveness, or a rash of tiny reddish purple dots, the cause of the symptom needs to be investigated. Also if there is a high fever which is not associated with a childhood illness, then the cause of the fever needs to be investigated.

There is no need for a parent to lose sleep if the fever is persistent at night. Fever often gets higher at night during a childhood illness because the child is at rest and the body can focus energy on doing what the fever has to do. Sleeping next to the child means that you will be woken if he or she needs anything. A baby with roseola needs frequent breast feeds or watery bottles during the night. If the fever is caused by a dangerous underlying condition, then emergency treatment is needed. It is not the fever that needs treating, it is the underlying condition that needs treating.

In this book we are primarily concerned with germs, but toxins, chills and emotional shock can also bring on a fever. After long term exposure to small amounts of environmental toxins, a fever appears when the body asserts itself and eliminates a batch of slowly acquired toxin. Short term exposure to a larger dose of poison can also provoke a fever. Sometimes one dose of a drug can bring on a fever. The latter shows that the body has a well functioning immune system, and is rapidly dealing with the toxin which has been introduced. The medical response to that situation is to give another drug to bring down the fever.

The way that catching a chill causes fever is still a mysterious process, and the fact that it can happen is vehemently denied by pharmaceutical medicine. Their attitude is that if you cannot put it in a test tube and look at it through a microscope, then it does not exist. To add to the credibility problem is the fact that many people have strong constitutions and never catch a chill, no matter what they do. Jane Bloggs can swim in cold water, then stand in a cold wind, then walk home barefoot on cold concrete paving, and not be affected in any way. Mary Bloggs would catch a cold from doing the same, while Fred Bloggs would catch double pneumonia. It is easy for hardy people like Jane Bloggs to scoff at the idea that getting chilled can bring on sickness. Those experiments that were done in England to see whether cold showers caused colds, were done on the type of people who do not catch chills. That is why they volunteered. People also have different levels of susceptibility to chills at different times. Having a fever is one situation that increases susceptibility.

When a child has frequent fevers which do not get very intense, it could mean that there is something seriously wrong, like glandular fever (infectious mononucleosis) or lupus. Giving drugs to suppress the fevers does not fix the problem. When recurrent fevers are treated homoeopathically, the objective should be to remove the underlying problem, not just to stop the fevers. This can only be done by choosing a remedy that is appropriate to all the symptoms present. Giving potentised *aconite* or potentised *belladonna* for every fever is almost as bad as giving aspirin or paracetamol. Malaria is a disease that is characterised by recurring fevers. It is easy to cure homoeopathically by giving homoeopathically potentised quinine. This makes the body kill the parasite that causes malaria. Non-homoeopathic quinine or one of its derivatives makes the fever temporarily subside, but it does not cure the underlying disease. It also causes serious side effects, including psychotic violence, whereas homoeopathic quinine has no side effects.

There are also herbs that boost the immune system, like golden seal and echinacea. Herbs can be used to help support a person with repeated low-grade fevers, but should not be used to abort acute fevers.

FEBRILE CONVULSIONS

There is a popular myth that if a child has a fever it is necessary to bring down the fever or else the fever could cause a febrile convulsion that would result in permanent brain damage. (Febrile means "from fever".) Febrile convulsions and febrile seizures are the same thing. A large-scale study, in which 54,000 children from a variety of backgrounds were studied from birth to the age of seven years, was published in 1978.[62] The study found that 4% of the children experienced febrile seizures before the age of seven, and none of the seizures resulted in death, brain damage nor epilepsy. One third of the children who had a febrile seizure, had at least one more febrile seizure before the age of seven.

The authors of the study offer a suggestion for why the myth that febrile convulsions cause brain damage has arisen. They suggest that it may have arisen because the only data that was in existence before their study was done, involved children who had neurological problems. Some of these children had had a febrile convulsion in their past, and this led to the wrong assumption that the convulsion had caused the neurological problems.

Twenty years later another large-scale study confirmed that children who have febrile convulsions do just as well academically, intellectually and behaviourally as other children.[63]

People who have a low seizure threshold are more likely to have a convulsion during fever than people with the usual threshold.[64,65] Febrile convulsions do not cause epilepsy,[66,67] but they are alarming to observe. Parents suffer shock and stress from seeing their child have a febrile convulsion. Some people hold the opinion that convulsions are sparked off not by the height of the fever, but by a rapid rise or a rapid fall in temperature. Some nurses and some ambulance officers believe that giving drugs for fever increases the likelihood of a convulsion, because when the drug takes effect it makes the fever drop very sharply, and when it wears off it makes the fever rise suddenly. The makers of fever suppressing drugs have not yet funded a study on the issue.

The pharmaceutical industry over-emphasises the danger from convulsions caused by natural fevers, while trivialising convulsions caused by vaccination. Many children are put on anti-epileptic drugs for years after just one febrile convulsion, even though the drugs make no difference to the child's long term neurological condition.[68] In 1997 it was officially confirmed in the USA that febrile seizures are harmless, that fever suppressing drugs do not prevent them, and that drugs to prevent epilepsy are not only useless, they are also harmful.[69] But the message has not been passed on to doctors, nurses and parents, because drugs are big money spinners.

DANGEROUS FEBRILE DISEASES

If a dangerous disease is brewing, suppressing the fever is not going to help the patient. The disease itself must be treated, not the symptom of fever. Some life threatening, fast acting diseases produce a fever if the person's immune system is working properly. For example, polio and meningococcal meningitis are diseases which usually produce a fever, and if a person who is suffering from one of these diseases takes paracetamol, the paracetamol helps the germ attack the body. On the other hand, lack of fever does not mean that there is no cause for alarm. Polio, meningococcal meningitis, typhoid, hepatitis A and many other life threatening diseases can progress quite far before the fever puts in an appearance. It is dangerous to think there is no problem when there is no fever.

There are many strains of virus and bacteria which can cause meningitis. The ones caused by bacteria can be successfully treated with antibiotics. Haemophilus, pneumonia, legionnaires' disease and some types of streptococcal infection can also be treated with antibiotics. But if the doctors give fever suppressing drugs as well, they are shooting their own treatment in the foot. As well as directly protecting the patient from the germs, fever helps antibiotics to be more effective.[38,45]

If a rash which looks like little reddish purple dots or like mottled bruising appears, it could be a symptom of meningococcal meningitis, which can kill a person in a matter of hours if it is not treated. Unfortunately meningococcal meningitis does not always produce a rash. There are many tragic stories of people with meningococcal meningitis going to hospital because they feel terrible and are almost collapsing, and being told by the overworked staff to go home, which they do, only to die a few hours later.

Meningitis occurs when there is infection and inflammation of the meninges. The meninges are the three layers of membrane which are around the brain and spinal cord. Encephalitis on the other hand is inflammation of the whole brain and spinal cord. Encephalitis usually starts suddenly, and the first symptoms are the same as meningitis. Symptoms of meningitis are a stiff neck and headache, the neck going rigid, pain all over which gets worse and worse, drowsiness, vomiting, fever, confusion and sensitivity to light. Some people get convulsions with meningitis, but convulsions are usually not present with meningitis. Sometimes the head goes backwards and the back begins to arch. This is a very bad sign. Some germs bring on meningitis really quickly, while others make it creep up slowly and insidiously. Bringing down the fever only makes it more difficult for the body to fight the germs.

Babies can be under attack from meningitis germs without showing any signs other than high fever, so a prolonged high fever in a baby with no obvious cause should be medically investigated, or treated by an experienced, properly qualified homoeopath. People who tell you to use potentised belladonna for every fever do not know what they are doing. If a baby's fontanel is not yet closed over, watch it for signs of trouble. If it sinks in, it is a sign of serious dehydration. If it sticks out, it could be meningitis.

CHILLING

Bringing down the fever with drugs knocks down the body's defences, and prevents the body from dealing with the underlying problem. Bringing down the fever by chilling the patient carries many more risks, the most obvious being pneumonia. However, this is not obvious to people brainwashed in the ways of modern medicine. Advice from them is to remove clothing and place the child in a draught. This advice is taken seriously by followers of modern medicine. I once heard a couple debating which was the draughtiest position in their house, so that they could put their baby who had roseola into it.

My husband's cousin's baby was admitted to the Red Cross Children's Hospital in Cape Town with croup, and was given a wild assortment of drugs which provoked a fever. He was then stripped to his nappy, and placed in front of an open window. Cape Town is notorious for wind, so at any window you can be sure of a good draught. He promptly developed pneumonia, and one of the nurses said to his mother, "Don't worry. It's normal for a baby in hospital to have pneumonia."

Bronchitis and ear infections are common consequences of the medical obsession with chilling. A person who is too hot from overheating, like from doing excessive exercise in hot weather, should be cooled down, but a person should not be chilled when the body is deliberately creating a fever.

"FEED A COLD AND STARVE A FEVER"

This wise old adage is dismissed today on the grounds that it is old fashioned. While experiencing a fever, children do not want solid food, they want, and need, liquid. During the fever they must take in lots of liquid, or else they will dehydrate and can die. At the height of the fever a child might be too floppy to ask for liquid, so offer a drink frequently. One of the consequences of too little liquid intake can be that the body fails to maintain the fever, so the invading germs can take over.

After the fever subsides in a childhood disease, the child begins to feel hungry. The more intense the fever has been, the more ravenous the hunger will be. This is the time to feed your child with loads of good wholesome food, not with ice cream and bread. Unpolished rice and mincemeat are a good starting point.

THE THEORY THAT CHILDHOOD DISEASES ARE BENEFICIAL

There is a small amount of evidence published in English which supports the theory that childhood diseases are beneficial, and there is empirical evidence that children benefit from a dose of measles or chicken pox. The concept that childhood illnesses are beneficial is more prevalent in Central European cultures than in Anglo-Saxon culture and all its offshoots. There is a theory that having one or more of the childhood illnesses makes a person less likely to get a chronic degenerative disease in later life. Women have a reduced incidence of cancer of the ovary if they have had mumps in childhood.[70,71]

People who have cancer are sometimes cured or put into temporary remission by catching measles,[72,73] and the same has happened with rubella.[72] It has also been observed that paediatric nephrotic syndrome can be cured or sent into remission by deliberately infecting children with measles.[74,75]

If you can get to a library that holds the *Lancet* of 1971, you can take a look at photos of a little boy who was rapidly cured of cancer when he caught measles in hospital. The first photo shows him with a tumour over and around his right eye. In the second photo he is spotty with measles rash and the tumour is already smaller. In the third photo the measles is over and the tumour is gone. Four months later when the article was written the boy was still "in complete remission," having had no cancer treatment.[76]

Some types of cancer are more amenable to being cured by measles than others. Not all people who have cancer react in the same way when they catch measles;

* Some survive the measles, although they die later from the cancer.
* Others die right away because the cancer, or the cancer treatment, makes them unable to cope with measles.
* Others are cured of cancer by having measles.

Some people believe that measles is a process of elimination. At present there is no research to support nor refute this idea. A child with measles begins to smell absolutely terrible when the rash appears. The putrid smell is strong enough to be noticeable from an adjacent room. Some people speculate that the smell is caused by something unwanted being eliminated from the child's body. After the measles virus enters the body through the mucous membranes, it travels around and multiplies in the lymph system.[77] When it moves from one cell to another it does so by breaking through the cell walls and temporarily making two cells into a big cell.[77] This phase lasts 10-14 days, and although it is not obvious that the child has measles, an observant parent will notice that the child's behaviour is different. Some of the measles viruses get broken up while others remain intact.[77] At the end of the incubation phase, the viruses move into the blood, Koplik spots appear in the mouth, and other types of spots also appear on the mucous membranes.[77] After 1 or 2 more days the typical measles rash appears on the skin.[77] Antibodies begin to appear in the blood at this time if they are going to appear at all,[77] and the measles viruses move from the blood to the skin, where they can be found in large numbers during the first 4 days of the rash.[78] The number of viruses in the skin decreases, and then they disappear completely before the rash fades.[78]

None of this explains the strong pong which comes out of the skin. So the issue of whether the process of measles actually benefits the cells of the human body remains unresolved until more research is conducted into what the virus is doing as it passes through the different types of cells.

Unless the patient was severely malnourished before the measles started, the measles virus is gone from the body 12 days after the rash first appeared.[79] In some well nourished individuals the measles virus is not eliminated from the body, and it goes on to cause chronic diseases like SSPE or Crohn's. When the measles virus is injected directly into the blood stream, as in the case of measles vaccination, it does not undergo that first 10-14 days of being processed by the immune system in the lymph glands. This is possibly why disintegrative disorders are more common after vaccination than after a natural dose of measles.

When the acute phase of measles is over, the child becomes ravenously hungry, with a particular need for protein. Lots of good wholesome food is needed to fuel the growth spurt that follows measles.

Children undergo a jump in maturation during the course of a childhood disease. There is a religious sect called anthroposophy which incorporates this phenomenon into their dogma. The fact that childhood diseases cannot be prevented by good nutrition strongly implies that nature considers childhood diseases to be beneficial.

Despite the lack of research, the idea that measles strengthens the immune system of an already healthy person is a widely held belief. The Pharmacy Guild of New Zealand said on a promotional flyer in 1989, "... common infections like measles and chicken pox are still around. These childhood illnesses help build up immunity to fight off infections in later life."[80] I was startled to see this opinion emanating from such a source, so I wrote to them and asked them how they knew. They backed off and said they had not meant it.

My daughter Chandra had measles when she was three years old. She baked with an intensive fever for two and a half days, but her temperature did not remain constant. It peaked and dipped, sometimes being very high, sometimes being low. I did not measure the level it reached at any stage, because I knew that the actual temperature was irrelevant to her well being. However, out of curiosity I now wish that I had measured how high it went when it peaked. When she emerged from the fever on day three she was markedly different. Her sense of humour had changed. It was still childish, but different. She no longer wanted to sleep in our bed, which was a great relief because she had been an awfully wriggly bedfellow. The sound of her cry had changed too, and it took me a while to become familiar with the new sound. Two weeks after the acute phase, while she was still recuperating, four mothers and their youngsters came round for morning tea. The children were playing in her room, and each time someone started crying, I would have to get up to see if it was Chandra. It is very strange for a mother not to recognise the sound of her own child's cry, but it took me a while to become familiar with the new sound. She also ate voraciously and she blossomed in many ways that are not easy to measure.

She had caught measles from her three-year-old friend Reuben. One day he asked his mother, "Was it Chandi's birthday?"

"No," said his mother.

"Then why did I give her measles?" he asked.

In a way, it really was a gift.

"BUT CHILDREN DIE OF MEASLES"

In some affluent countries the death rate from measles goes as high as 1 in 2000. This statistic is used to promote vaccination, but the public are not told the full facts. A child only dies of measles if he or she;

*   had a serious underlying condition before catching measles, or
*   suffers from severe calorie/protein deficiency, or
*   is accidentally or deliberately chilled while having measles, or
*   is given drugs to suppress the fever.

Doctors and nurses are taught during their training that a child with measles should be chilled and given drugs to suppress the fever. Parents of children with measles are advised to chill their offspring and administer fever suppressing drugs, or the chilling is done and the drugs given at hospital. Fever suppressing drugs seriously inhibit the work of the immune system.[81] I have explained above how fever is part of the body's defence mechanism. Modern medicine kills countless people by sabotaging the body's defences through chilling and giving drugs that suppress fever. It is not only people with measles who get killed by having their fever suppressed.

In poor countries the death rate from measles is higher than 1 in 2000. Severe malnutrition makes a child vulnerable to dying from measles. Susceptibility to death from measles is not genetically determined,[82] it is determined by poverty.[82] In severely malnourished children the symptoms of measles are different to the symptoms of classical measles, right from the start of the infection.

In 1984 the measles virus became virulent in New Zealand, and two children died during the ensuing epidemic. This was used to terrify parents in both New Zealand and Australia. The public was not told that both the children had terminal illnesses before they caught measles, and one of them was fully immunised.[83]

The next measles epidemic in New Zealand had been in progress for three months before a child died. As soon as the death happened, the propaganda machine swung into action. After the death toll reached 3, there was a correction, and the official number of deaths went back to 2. Then it rose again to 4. On the day that death number 3 was revoked, I spoke to a chiropractor who lived in the town where the death had occurred. He said that the child had been vaccinated against measles, and when the medics discovered this, they decided to change the cause of death. I was on the committee of a consumer group called the Immunisation Awareness Society (IAS), and we monitored the situation as closely as we could.

Although the health department's pre-planned propaganda campaign only lasted a week, for the next few months the media kept repeating that four babies had died of measles because not enough children were vaccinated.

While the epidemic was still in progress, a health magazine published an article[84] that I wrote about measles, in which I predicted that the authorities would never let the full facts about the measles deaths be published, as they had with the 1984-85 epidemic.[83] It was a safe prediction. The only thing that the official report let slip was that one of the "babies" that died was 12 years old. A member of IAS wrote to the 12-year-old's general practitioner and asked about the circumstances of the death. He replied, "My case was a very rare complication of measles and unlikely to happen again." He did not say whether or not the child had been vaccinated. A nurse who worked in the Wellington hospital where one of the babies died, told us that the baby had been hospitalised for pneumonia, and had caught measles in hospital. So that is two out of the four which we managed to confirm as not having just upped and died of measles. I am sure that if our spy network had been good enough, we would have learned similar facts about the other two.

IAS wrote to the Ministry of Health and asked;

*   whether the children who died of measles were old enough to have been vaccinated,
*   whether they had any underlying health problems prior to contracting measles,
*   and what their vaccination status was.

They refused to supply the information, although it is illegal for them to withhold it.

I sometimes have the opportunity to speak about vaccination to groups of Public Health nurses. When Chandra was ten years old I took her with me to one of these lectures, because she had the flu and was off school. The flu was well under control because she had already been in bed for a few days, and she had been having organic lemon and honey drinks and lots of vitamin C. I knew that taking her with me to the lecture would not cause a relapse, because she would go from a warm house to a warm car to a warm lecture theatre. She had caught flu by playing netball in the rain, then walking home in a cold wind, at a time when a nasty flu virus was felling people. If there had been a polio virus in the air, I would have been more conscientious and forbidden her to play netball, despite the negative social consequences of such an action.

When we got to the lecture theatre I settled her down at a desk in the front corner with her art gear. She got busy producing works of art, but her ears were listening to the goings on in the room. One of the nurses said she was not sick and she should be at school. Others nodded. They are clueless about how to prevent an infection from turning into a serious illness.

There were quite a few aggressive ladies in this group and they were angered by almost everything I said. When I said that TB is caused by wrong nutrition and damp housing, they all started barking that TB is caused by immigrants. This was in line with a campaign that was being waged against immigrants in the newspaper at the time.

When I said that suburban children do not die of measles unless there is something else wrong with them, one of the ladies tried to refute it by telling the story of a child she had nursed who had died of measles. "He was a perfectly healthy child. There was nothing wrong with him. And I so clearly remember, I was feeding him jelly and ice cream just before my shift ended. He had to be fed because he was on a ventilator because he had bronchitis. The next morning I heard on the radio that he had died."

A loud whisper came from the art factory in the corner, "Mommy, Mommy. Jelly and ice cream, jelly and ice cream." Chandra was concerned that I may not have noticed that the nurse had said that she had been force feeding the child with substances that are lethal for a child with measles and bronchitis. (Jelly is known as jello in North America.)

I am not a member of the anti-dairy products brigade. There are certain circumstances in which real milk, real cheese or real yogurt are health giving substances to consume. But there are also times when milk and its derivatives are not appropriate foods. Having measles which is complicated by bronchitis is one of those times. Milk encourages the production of mucous, which is not helpful for a child with bronchitis. It is staggering that nurses and doctors do not know that. Furthermore, jelly and ice cream contain sugar, artificial flavour and artificial colouring. Sugar irritates the mucous membranes and makes them produce more mucous, and sugar also suppresses the immune system. This nurse had been putting mucous producing, immune suppressing, toxic junk into the body of a child who was already struggling with a serious complication of measles.

A hubbub ensued and one nurse called out, "So are you saying that (name) caused the child's death by giving him jelly and ice cream?"

"Yes," I replied, "It certainly contributed to the death, and probably caused it." The hubbub turned into a near riot.

This gathering was Chandra's first experience of that type of mass hostility, and all the irrationality that goes with it. On the way home in the car she talked energetically about the nurses, and one of the questions she fired at me was, "Why do they think that someone with bronchitis is perfectly healthy?" I have to leave it to the psychologists to answer that, but I am grateful to the nurse for speaking up, because she proved my point beautifully.

SICK CHILDREN NEED CARE

The idea that a sick child needs bed rest and full time care has almost disappeared from Western culture. The new belief is that a child can be restored to health by a visit to a doctor. Often the child is dressed in flimsy clothing and driven to the doctor with the car windows open. The doctor writes out a prescription, which is then collected from a chemist, and the child is encouraged to carry on with his or her usual routine. Furthermore, society has changed in ways that make it more difficult for parents to stay at home and look after a sick child. A parent can lose a job or lose crucial income by staying at home with a sick child.

A child who has a fever because of flu or a childhood illness needs to stay at home, be lying down, and be kept warm. This is inconvenient for parents. Children are inconvenient things. If the fever is caused by a dangerous infectious disease then medical or homoeopathic intervention is needed, and the child must not catch a chill or become exhausted in the process of acquiring that intervention.

Even when parents are available to keep a sick child in bed, they often do not do it because they do not know how important it is. Health departments distribute pro-pharmaceutical propaganda to parents, instead of teaching them how to bring their children safely through colds, flu and the childhood illnesses. The people who work for health departments do not know how to treat childhood illnesses safely, because they have been trained in the pharmaceutical model.

The way that modern medicine treats childhood illnesses increases the risk of complications and death. Drugs are given to bring down the fever, and chilling is recommended when the child needs to be wrapped up warmly. The need for bed rest and a quiet environment is not emphasised, and food is forced on a child during the acute phase of the illness instead of waiting until the hungry phase of convalescence. The need for a period of convalescence is not even recognised. In short, they have got it all wrong. Some doctors have enough common sense not to do these things, but they are few and far between.

If a child with measles is not kept warm and in bed, it can result in things like bronchitis, pneumonia, ear infections or encephalitis developing. The last two can end up as deafness or brain damage. If the amount of light striking the eyes is not reduced, blindness can result. Mumps can also end up as brain damage and deafness if the child is allowed to run around, and it can damage the pancreas and cause sterility in a person past puberty. Scarlet fever can damage the kidneys and the heart, and chicken pox can end in brain damage if the patient is not kept quiet during the few days of acute disease.

If the patient with a childhood disease is a teenager or adult, the danger of complications is much greater. It can be very difficult to make a teenager or adult who feels driven by responsibility stay in bed during the acute phase, and to take it easy during convalescence. School and sporting commitments can put as much pressure on a teenager as earning a living or caring for children puts on an adult. They are at risk of wanting to get up and carry on with their usual routine, instead of resting.

During the winter months the radio and TV carry adverts for drugs which partially suppress the symptoms of colds and flu. The adverts advise people to take these drugs so that they can carry on with their family obligations and business affairs. If you die from following that advice don't bother suing the drug manufacturers. They are not legally accountable.

The concept of convalescence has almost disappeared from Western culture. Getting a child "right" in as short a time as possible is perceived as a great achievement, but it is not good for the child. A person with a fever needs to be wrapped up warmly. During convalescence he or she does not need so much help in staying warm, but still needs to be warmer than usual.

Sick children should not be bombarded with stimulation. If they are lolling about it does not mean that they are bored, it means that they need to rest. When they do become bored it shows they are approaching the end of the convalescence period. Teenagers who are normally addicted to pop music do not want it on when they have measles. When they start wanting the beat again, it shows they are getting better. A child should not be sent back to school as soon as he or she is "well enough to cope."

One day when I was helping at the afternoon session of a kindergarten there was a little boy flopping about instead of playing. The teacher telephoned his mother and told her to collect him. When the mother arrived she told us that the boy had had a fever in the morning, and she had given him paracetamol at lunch time so that he could come to kindergarten. Another mother expressed her anger to me afterwards, saying that the woman did not care about her child, and sent him to kindergarten to get rid of him for a few hours. I happen to know that that mother cares very much for her child, and it is just ignorance that made her do that. Fortunately the fever was not the beginning of anything serious, or the child would have been in trouble.

My best story is the one where the child with measles was taken out to see fireworks on a very cold night. He had a convulsion at 9 pm, allegedly from the coldness of the water he had been given to drink down his next dose of paracetamol. It flabbergasts me to think that parents will take a feverish child out into the open on a cold night, but I have to remember that if circumstances had not led me to research vaccination, I might have done the same.

A child with a fever does not interact with parents or caregivers in the usual way, but nevertheless is aware of the caregiver's presence. As well as providing a sense of security for the child, it is good to have someone keeping an eye on a patient with a childhood illness, so that if any symptoms that are not a normal part of the childhood illness show up, quick action can be taken. Things like polio and diphtheria and meningococcal meningitis can start off looking quite innocuous at first, and if they are allowed to progress too far before intervention begins, the outcome can be grim. Childhood diseases do not need intervention, they just need to be endured. However, they do need to be endured in the right way, or else they can develop complications. Complications need intervention, but the diseases themselves do not.

If someone is in danger of dying from an infectious disease, the first intervention should be injections of vitamin C.[85,86,87] Dr. Archie Kalokerinos has intervened with vitamin C injections to save the lives of children in Australia.[85,86,87] He has tried to educate the medical establishment, but they do not want to know. He has met with vilification and even persecution. One night I mentioned Archie's work to a group of nurses in Auckland, and one of them turned on me with a vicious character assassination of Archie. Why does a nurse in New Zealand feel so threatened by a doctor who is saving children's lives in the Australian outback?

Some people use megadoses of vitamin C to cut childhood illnesses short. It may be beneficial for the mother to be able to get back to work quickly, but is it beneficial for the child? There is no research to show whether or not cutting childhood diseases short with vitamin C is advisable, and I do not expect such matters will be researched for many a decade. In the absence of research, I consider the artificial shortening of childhood illnesses to be an unhealthy practice.

Vitamin C is appropriate for saving the life of a poverty-stricken child who is on the verge of dying from any type of infection. Even small doses would save lives, but the World Health Organisation does not use it because vitamin C cannot be patented and the drug companies cannot put a big profit margin on it. Megadoses of vitamin C are also appropriate for any child who is infected with the germs of a malevolent infectious disease. But I believe that megadoses of vitamin C are not appropriate for an adequately fed child who lives in a comfortable home and has uncomplicated measles, mumps, rubella, whooping cough, chicken pox, slapped cheek roseola or infantum roseola.

Some people use homoeopathic remedies to shorten childhood illnesses. I also do not approve of this. It is appropriate to use homoeopathy to treat the complications of a childhood illness, but not to stop the natural process of the self-resolving illness. Homoeopathy is also appropriate when a childhood illness does not finish off properly, for example when a child is chesty every winter after whooping cough, or when chicken pox turns to shingles.

CARING FOR A CHILD WITH :

INFANTUM ROSEOLA

This disease only happens during the first three years of life, and usually during the first year, if it happens at all. The symptoms are fever and a rash which looks like the measles rash.[88] Some people call it "baby measles," and some doctors misdiagnose it as measles, which makes the parents think the child is getting measles for a second time when he or she actually does get measles. The germ that causes roseola has not been isolated, so a vaccine for this disease has not yet been manufactured. As soon as a vaccine does exist, infantum roseola will be presented as a dangerous disease that needs to be prevented.

Some babies develop a high fever with roseola, while others experience a fever so low that roseola is not recognised until the rash appears. The baby needs to be kept warm and quiet for two or three days. It is preferable to stay indoors until a day after the fever has gone, but if you have to go out, wrap the baby very warmly for the excursion and protect the face from the wind. Frequent breast feeds or another source of liquid is all that is needed for nourishment. If the baby has already started on solids, give it a miss until the roseola is over.

If the world knows your baby has roseola the world will try to ply you with paracetamol and persuade you to dip the baby into cold water, so it is a good idea not to let the world know that your baby has roseola until the fever is over.

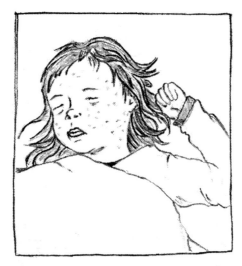

Chandra with measles.

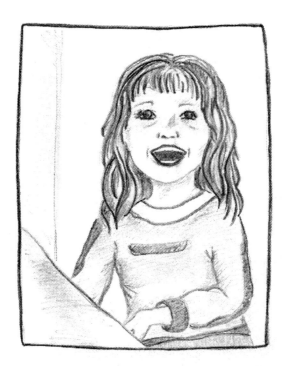

Chandra one month
after measles.

MEASLES

Measles (rubeola) is a disease that must be treated with respect. During the fever stage the child must be kept exceptionally warm, and while eye sensitivity lasts, must stay in semi-darkness. Complications like bronchitis, pneumonia, ear infections, blindness and death can occur when a child with measles is not properly cared for.

While it is wrong to try to prevent measles either by vaccination or by homoeopathic means, it is important to prevent complications. No medication is necessary for the prevention of complications. Proper care is enough. Certain homoeopathic remedies assist with the prevention of complications. However, they are not essential. Use of an inappropriate homoeopathic remedy can cause problems.

From the time that the child is infected with the virus, until the symptoms appear, he or she will grizzle and be difficult. An old rhyme says,

What's the matter Dolly Dumps?
Is it measles? Is it mumps?

While the child is still grumpy there will be a faint smell of putrefaction which often goes unnoticed. Then the nose becomes runny, there is a shallow but persistent cough, a red rim develops around the eyes, and the child is generally "watery." Most children are still miserable and clingy during this phase, but some become cheerful.

Usually the fever starts before the rash appears, but sometimes they start together. At first the rash consists of small red dots on the face and then the tummy. The whites of the eyes become reddish, the face becomes puffy and the eyelids swell. The eyes become sensitive to light, but in babies the sensitivity is usually milder than in children. White flecks called Koplik spots make a brief appearance inside the mouth.[89] The Koplik spots help to differentiate measles from rubella. The trouble with Koplik spots is that they are difficult to see if the child is not co-operative, and they vanish quickly. Their presence confirms measles, but their absence does not exclude it. With rubella, glands behind the ears and at the back of the neck swell up, which does not happen with measles. The rash of measles is darker than that of rubella. Measles rash spreads from the face downwards, and changes from small red spots to big mottled blotches. The spots on the feet are the last to fade.

The fever can become very high, and usually lasts for three days. It is crucial that the child be kept warm during the fever stage. Great care must be taken to ensure that the child does not catch a chill. A cold draught that lasts for three minutes can start the patient down the slippery slope of bronchitis, ear infections and pneumonia. It is often difficult for caregivers to focus attention on preventing draughts, because an adult who feels fit and well does not notice the movement of air.

Don't expose any part of the child's body to cold air while he or she is feverish. He or she must not walk barefoot over a cold floor to the bathroom. By this time the horrid smell of measles will have become strong, and parents feel tempted to wash the child. They often convince themselves that the child would be more comfortable if it were washed, when it is really the parents' hang up about the anti-social smell that motivates the bath. Many cultures consider it a social disgrace to skip bathing for three days, but there is no need to bath the child. The neighbours won't know, so don't run the risk of complications. The smell will go away of its own accord. When Chandra had measles I wanted to take a photo of her tummy because it looked so funny with the rash, but I did not, because I knew that if I uncovered her for long enough to get a picture, she would run the risk of catching a chill. Medical doctors and nurses are taught to scorn the concept of catching a chill. Chills lead to pneumonia, and pneumonia is the most common cause of death with measles.[90]

Once the child is well enough to get up, warm clothing is essential, and he or she must not play outside. Catching a chill is how a mild case of measles suddenly changes to bronchitis. During the three weeks after the rash appears, one type of germ fighting immune system cell becomes greatly reduced in number in the blood, and the few that remain become less active.[91] This might happen because the cells are more urgently needed elsewhere in the body.[91] The inactivity of these cells in the blood contributes to a person's increased susceptibility to bronchitis and pneumonia during measles. When this lowered immunity is combined with a deficiency of warmth somewhere in the body, the person becomes even more vulnerable to germs.

The intensity of light must be drastically reduced to protect the eyes. If the curtains are thin, pin a blanket or other dark cloth onto them so that more light is excluded. Another trick is to stick brown paper over the windowpanes as well as closing the curtains. When Kenneth had measles he was in our room, and we left the brown paper on the small side windows for long afterwards because it gave the room a nice hue.

The eyes remain very sensitive for about a week after the fever subsides, but sensitivity can last for up to 5 weeks. Children who are not inclined to complain are more difficult to protect, because you do not know when their eyes are uncomfortable. When eye damage occurs, the measles virus gets blamed, but the caregivers are really at fault. One of the big dangers of sending a child with measles to hospital is that they will shine bright lights in its face. The other big danger is that they will suppress the fever. Measles without fever is a dangerous situation. In affluent children the situation is created by drugs, while in poor children it is created by a protein/calorie deficiency.[55,57]

Measles is not a disease to be feared if it is properly treated. Watch how your child takes a jump in physical and emotional development after measles. Remember that the fever is part of the immune system's response to help fight the germs. Don't give any drug that will reduce the fever. Don't wipe the child down with cold water. Keep the child warm and cosy.

It is unwise to use a homoeopathic remedy to remove the symptoms of the measles. If you know your remedies well, or if you have someone who can prescribe for you, it is all right to use a remedy to prevent complications. For instance, in a child who tends to be chesty, *drosera* in the correct potency would prevent bronchitis, without aborting the measles. The famous Cape Town homoeopath, Dr. Jimmy Jones, told me that giving *morbillinum*, which is the potentised measles virus, to a child with measles, can cause seizures. Don't do it.

If the rash takes too long to appear, or does not develop into a proper measles rash, *bryonia* can help it blossom and get it over with. If chest, eye or ear complications develop, call in a homoeopath to rectify the situation. The homoeopath should visit the child at home. A homoeopath who expects a child with measles to be taken out of bed has little experience of measles. The same cannot be said for a pharmaceutical doctor who expects a child with measles to be taken to a clinic. Doctors have lots of experience of children with measles, but they consider it "normal" for a child with measles to have complications.

The only demands a child with a high fever will make will be for water, juice and fruit. Don't try and force the child to eat starch or protein. Keep offering liquid. Non-acidic tropical fruits are good if they are ripe, otherwise try tomatoes or cucumber, or just stick to water. Many children like to drink warm water with a teaspoon of honey dissolved in it. Preferably use honey from an organic source, which has not been filtered or heated before bottling. The child will instinctively know how much food to eat, so don't try and persuade him or her to eat more than necessary. Do keep offering a drink though, because often the child is too tired to ask for one.

Get stocks of protein and whole foods ready for the next phase. When the fever subsides the child starts to become hungry. This is because measles is always followed by a period of rapid growth. The level of hunger will be directly related to the intensity of the measles the child has experienced. The child will instinctively want to eat lots of animal protein. The human body does not know what is politically correct, it only knows what is good for it.

Measles causes a sudden halt in growth, which is followed by rapid catch up growth.[92] If the protein/calorie needs are not met during the post-fever stage, the child will never grow to the full size of its genetic potential. Children in impoverished countries who survive measles, but do not have sufficient food available, fail to grow in this phase, and they never catch up the height later.[93] Some children die in the weeks after measles because of insufficient food during this time of increased need.

Convalescence is a difficult stage to treat, because the child wants to get up and play, but must remain very warm and is still sensitive to light for a while. Parents must be vigilant that he or she does not catch a chill while playing out of bed. The child wants entertainment and food, but gets tired easily. He or she needs a quiet indoor lifestyle for 2 to 6 weeks.

When Chandra had moved out of the fever stage, my uncle showed her how to make a doily. That started an epidemic of doily making. We closed all the curtains so that she could move about the house, and in every room there grew a pyramid of doilies cut from discarded printout paper. She did not want us to throw away a single precious piece, not even the bits that had been cut out to make the patterns. Whenever I think of measles, I think of a pyramid of paper in every room. It was an ideal activity to keep her busy indoors. Her little brother is not so keen on art and crafts, so we had to entertain him during his convalescence.

The modern tendency is to send children back to kindergarten or school as soon as they can no longer infect other children. This is very unwise. The child is not given an opportunity to recuperate. Children remain sensitive to noise for about two weeks, and they suffer pain from sounds that are a normal part of a kindergarten or classroom. Remember that some germ fighting cells are very low in the blood for a whole three weeks after the rash appears.[91] A hundred years ago they did not know that immune system cells are deficient during this phase, but they did know that it was foolhardy to force children back into their usual routine before they had finished recuperating from measles.

Measles is inconvenient for parents, because the child needs a lot of attention during the acute phase, and needs surveillance for about two weeks afterwards. The glib solution is to vaccinate to prevent measles. But vaccination is no guarantee that measles will not occur during childhood, and it makes measles more likely to happen after childhood. The side effects of measles vaccine can result in a child needing special care for the rest of its life. That is far more inconvenient than having a child out of school for two or three weeks.

Teenagers and young adults with measles need the same intensity of care as a child with measles. We have yet to see what happens to middle aged people when vaccine induced immunity wears off.

It is helpful to clearly separate the symptoms of measles from the symptoms of measles complications. Classical measles in an unvaccinated person has the symptoms of fever, a putrid smell, red puffy eyes, a skin rash which starts as separate dots and then becomes mottled, a shallow cough, eye sensitivity and tiredness. Any other symptoms are either a separate disease, or a complication of measles.

If the person with measles has been vaccinated against measles, the symptoms will not be exactly the same as classical measles. This phenomenon is called "atypical measles." For instance, the rash might start on the hands and feet and move inwards and upwards, whereas in normal measles the spots start on the face and move downwards and outwards. Also the rash might be slightly raised, and there could be slight haemorrhaging.

MUMPS

Don't underestimate the potential of mumps to cause long term damage. A child must stay indoors and get a lot of rest to avoid complications. An adult with mumps is even more vulnerable to complications.

Mumps affects the salivary glands so that the jowls swell up and the person looks hilarious. The virus can also cause inflammation in the pancreas, the ovaries, the testicles, the brain and the ears. Sterility, brain damage or deafness can result from improper care of a person with mumps. By affecting the pancreas, the virus can cause diabetes. This was first documented in 1899.[94] The ovaries and testicles cannot be damaged in a person who has not yet reached puberty, which is one good reason for getting mumps over with in childhood.

An adult male is the most vulnerable to mumps, because men find it difficult to rest in bed for a few days. While trying to persuade me that vaccinating my children against mumps would be a good idea, a neighbour told me about a famous New Zealand athlete who developed encephalitis from mumps and was left partially paralysed. When I pressed him for details, it emerged that the athlete had run a race while the mumps was acute. Once upon a time people knew that they must not run a race when they have mumps. An old fashioned medical book states,

> The testicles are swollen, painful and very tender. When the inflammation subsides, it may be found that the patient has been made sterile. This is especially liable to happen if he has not taken proper care of himself during the acute stage of the inflammation.[95]

Vaccination increases the risk of sterility, because it makes people get mumps when they are older.

Much of the scaremongering about mumps these days focuses on deafness. I wish proper statistics were kept so that we could find out whether the use of paracetamol increases the risk of deafness, and whether there really has been an increase in this complication. The pamphlets also say that there is a high incidence of encephalitis with mumps, but they do not mention that this can be avoided with proper care. When MMR was introduced to New Zealand, a medical bigwig said on the TV that mumps needed to be prevented because it causes encephalitis in one in seven cases. We wrote to him repeatedly asking for the reference, and eventually he put it in writing that it was not true.

Although children with mumps do not look very sick once the fever is over, be careful. Keep them inside, keep them warm, and keep them quiet. Don't give starch or protein foods during the acute stage, and fruit and vegetables must be soft because chewing is painful.

The swelling can be very painful. This pain can be reduced by applying heat or cold to the swollen area. Trial and error will show whether a particular child is helped by cooling or warming of the jowls. A child with dramatic flair likes to have a medicated poultice held against the jaws with a scarf wrapped around the head, while a child who hates drama does not want a big silly thing flapping on his or her face. The tinctures or oils of *arnica*, *calendula* and *hypericum* (St John's Wort) reduce the pain of swollen jowls. These are extracted from European plants, and conveniently bottled for worldwide distribution, but nature has provided every continent with plants that can be used for the purpose. It is just a matter of knowing which they are. The tinctures and oils are for external application, not for swallowing. Any medication must be applied gently, as pressure will increase pain. If you use homoeopathic remedies during mumps, they should be chosen to make the child more comfortable, and not to abort the mumps.

RUBELLA

Rubella is usually less intense than measles or mumps. The fevers are usually not very high and do not last very long, but while fevers are coming and going, the child must be kept warm and in bed. After the fevers stop coming, the child needs to lead a quiet life for a few days. He or she can safely get out of bed for some of the day, and even play at another child's house if the mother is not pregnant. Going to the supermarket is a bad idea for the child's sake as well as the public's. The risk of complications is lower than with measles or mumps, but complications can happen, with sufficient provocation.

Chills are less dangerous to a child with rubella than to a child with measles. A mild chill would just cause a cold or flu, making the child feel sick and miserable, but it would not cause bronchitis or death like it can during measles.

Playing quietly does not include activities like jumping on a trampoline. Chandra's little friend Sarah felt so well with rubella that she forgot she had it. After a few minutes of jumping she developed a bad headache which lasted the rest of the day. Too much activity can bring on convulsions and vomiting. The symptom of sore joints often accompanies rubella, and this can progress to arthritis if the patient does not take care.

The rash looks like the measles rash but it is fainter. It also moves from the face downwards, but it moves and disappears more quickly. The way to differentiate rubella from measles is by the swollen glands at the back of the neck. Rubella often goes undiagnosed in children with dark skin because the rash can be too faint to show up. The parents of a dark skinned child notice that the child is tired and listless and a bit feverish, but unless they look at the glands at the back of the neck, they might not realise it is rubella.

Because rubella is such a mild disease, the vaccine was introduced with the excuse that it was needed to prevent congenital rubella syndrome. Congenital rubella syndrome is the name given to a variety of problems that a baby can be born with if the mother gets rubella during the first three months of pregnancy. The virus that causes rubella can damage the heart, ears, eyes and brain during the first three months of a person's development. Having a high level of antibodies to rubella before becoming pregnant, does not mean that a woman will not give birth to a baby who is deformed by congenital rubella syndrome.[96,97,98,99,100,101] It is best for a girl to have rubella when she is a child, so that she can develop natural immunity to the disease, and will be far less likely to get it when she is pregnant. Mass vaccination of pre-adolescent girls did not eliminate congenital rubella syndrome, and mass vaccination of infant boys and girls, followed by re-vaccination of boys and girls during childhood, has also failed to prevent congenital rubella syndrome. There are now calls for adult women to be re-vaccinated.[102] Rubella vaccine causes acute and chronic arthritis in some adults.[17,103,104] The call for re-vaccination of women does not include a call for women to be informed of possible side effects, nor for women to be informed that the vaccine is made from aborted baby. Rubella vaccine was one of the first to be made with the flesh of an aborted baby.[105,106]

WHOOPING COUGH

The incidence of whooping cough has been decreasing for more than a hundred years, which means that very few children get it nowadays. Your child might be the one who gets it, so you need to know what to do to keep a child with whooping cough comfortable and safe.

The first two weeks of whooping cough seem like a bad cold with mild fever and occasional fits of coughing. Suddenly the cough becomes more intense, and the child starts waking at night with spasms of coughing. When you hear that first "whoop" you know that whooping cough has arrived and it cannot be ignored. It is time to batten down the hatches and get ready for broken nights and long days.

Two things make whooping cough more bearable; a firm resolve and a plastic bowl. The first few whoops are alarming to observe, but you soon get used to them. If you panic you make the child tighten up and gasp all the more. Whooping cough is far worse for the parents than for the child. The sooner you settle into a happy routine of throwing up and cleaning up, the easier it will be for the family. (The child does the throwing up, you do the cleaning up.)

The coughing spasms are not glamorous affairs. The eyes bulge and the breath is pulled in through a constricted throat, causing that awful whoop sound. At the end of each spasm the child vomits up thick mucous, and sometimes food. Between spasms he or she sleeps soundly, or is cheerful and chirpy. Whooping cough does not cause the grumpiness that measles and mumps cause. The whoop sound is not always present in babies under six months of age, but the tongue will protrude and the eyes will bulge, and the cough will bring up mucous and food. There are some bad coughs which are not whooping cough, and in babies they are commonly misdiagnosed as whooping cough. This leads the parents to believe that the child has acquired immunity to whooping cough.

The two worst problems with whooping cough are that the parents become exhausted because they are woken frequently at night, and the child can become malnourished because of repeatedly throwing up. The secret of nutrition is to feed the child immediately after he or she throws up. Don't wait 10 minutes, do it immediately. Then the food will stay down.

Avoid foods with crumbs, because they irritate the throat and cause vomiting. Things like nuts which get bitty after chewing also cause vomiting. Just a little food after each spasm will keep up the child's calorie intake and prevent too much loss of weight. Observe which type of food suits the child most. Some prefer fatty foods, some starchy. At night give a sip of water after each spasm. If he or she can swallow vitamin supplements without discomfort, that is all to the good.

Make sure the child sits up every time the coughing starts so that he or she cannot choke on vomitus. The father of a child who is severely damaged by whooping cough vaccine told me that the brain damage made it really difficult to convince the child to stay sitting up during each whoop, although she was four years old when she got whooping cough.

Sleeping near the child makes things easier, and means you get the child upright quickly when coughing starts. Keep a plastic bowl at hand so that bedding does not get soiled. When Chandra had whooping cough I did not wash the plastic bowl at night. I just put it beside the bed after every whoop, and went back to sleep as soon as she was settled. Then in the morning I would hurl the contents under a bush and wash the bowl.

At the beginning the spasms occur every half-hour, then they become less frequent. They can go on for 6 weeks or 6 months, but usually it is all over in 10 weeks. A family in Australia had three of their four children come down with whooping cough at the same time. All four children had been fully immunised before getting whooping cough. Granny and an aunt flew in from New Zealand to do night shifts, so that the parents could function properly during the day. If all families were that supportive, whooping cough would have a less detrimental effect on parents' health.

Excitement or physical exertion will bring on a coughing spasm. Visitors are usually greeted by the sight of a red-faced child gasping for breath with bulging eyes, and then retching up large globs of revolting mucous. The parents smilingly explain that this is all happening because the child is pleased to see them.

Don't let anyone pollute the air with tobacco smoke near a child with whooping cough. That would increase the number of spasms. Some parents give their children an electrolyte solution to drink to prevent dehydration. It is a good idea, although not essential. Electrolyte solution can be bought from the chemist, and it tastes nice. Followers of anthroposophical medicine give their children *Pertudoron 1* and *Pertudoron 2*, which are taken alternately. They are composites of homoeopathic remedies, and are not designed to abort the process of whooping cough. *Pertudoron 1* is to soothe the coughing reflex, and *Pertudoron 2* is to relieve the coughing spasms in the lungs.

Antibiotics shorten the length of time which coughing lasts if they are given at the beginning, but they make no difference if given once the cough has set in.[107] Sometimes antibiotics are given to "prevent a secondary infection." Antibiotics kill the good bacteria in the intestines which help digestion. Killing these bacteria does not strike me as a sensible idea when there is a need for optimum uptake of nutrients from a limited amount of food. Sometimes the tongue gets sore from friction. If you know of a solution to that problem please tell me what it is.

There is no need for the child to stay in bed all day after the first week of whooping. Lack of warmth is not as dangerous with whooping cough as it is with measles, but a child with whooping cough is far more vulnerable to getting bronchitis, ear infections and pneumonia from a chill, than a child who does not have whooping cough. Some doctors think it is normal for a baby with whooping cough to have the symptoms of a cold, because they are accustomed to seeing babies that have not been kept warm enough. A friend of mine had the bad luck of her baby and one other of her four children getting whooping cough during the pre-Christmas preparation period. She was distracted from the baby for a few minutes and it caught a cold. She found the cold far more of a nuisance than the whooping cough. Pneumonia will not set in from the mild type of chill that results from a minute's distraction, but consistently being cold makes a baby or child vulnerable to pneumonia. Sometimes parents do not realise that their child is not dressed warmly enough. 90% of deaths from whooping cough are caused by pneumonia.[108]

Vaccinated children with whooping cough are sometimes officially diagnosed as "croup" to hide the failure of the vaccine, but the symptoms are quite different. Croup is a serious condition that can be caused by a variety of bacteria and viruses. Susceptibility lies within the individual. The throat swells so that air cannot get through. Homoeopathy can cure the acute condition, and it can convert a child who is prone to getting croup to one who does not experience this horrible and life threatening condition. Medical doctors can treat the acute condition by inserting a tube into the throat to allow air to pass through, but all they can do about the susceptibility is to wait for the child to outgrow the tendency. Croup is not a childhood illness and it is quite different to whooping cough. The throat closure in whooping cough comes in a spasm and then it opens up again. In croup the lips can turn blue and death can result from asphyxiation. As far back as 1860 the difference between whooping cough and croup was clearly understood, but now the difference is being fudged to obscure vaccine failures.

A child with whooping cough does not enjoy going out until the disease is almost over. He or she is especially bothered by moving air. What feels like a mild breeze to an adult feels like a gale to a child with whooping cough. Even a child who is normally discontented and bored without social contact will play happily at home when he or she has whooping cough. After six weeks we thought Chandra was ready for a treat, and as there was no wind that day, we took her to a nearby beach for a change of scene. She was not happy. It seems unthinkable that a four-year-old could be unhappy on Boulders Beach on the Cape Peninsula, but she hated it. We beat a hasty retreat back home.

If a baby who cannot sit up gets whooping cough, the parents are in for a very tiring time. Babies are very prone to ear infections when they have whooping cough. The biggest danger is that the child might choke if he or she vomits while lying down. When my elderly neighbour heard Chandra whooping, I expected her to lean over the fence and give me a blast for not having her "immunised." But instead she told me about how she had suffered when her son Johnathan got whooping cough at the age of three weeks. "We had just moved to Joh'burg. I was feeling weak from the birth, Ted had to go away on business, and I had to hold Johnathan upright on my shoulder all through the night. Sometimes I sat in a chair and dozed between whoops, and sometimes I walked up and down patting his back. It was terrible. I'll never forget it." I was amazed to hear this, because at that stage of my life I thought that young babies were supposed to die from whooping cough. The baby she was describing was by then a man whom I often saw visiting his parents with his wife and children.

I have since learned that in previous generations parents used to know that they must hold a baby with whooping cough upright at night. Millions of children have enjoyed the books about Noddy, The Famous Five and The Secret Seven, which were all written by Enid Blyton. Enid Blyton got whooping cough when she was three months old, and her father stayed up at night to keep her upright and warm during the acute phase of the disease.[109] He believed that she would have died if he had not.[109]

In 1992 the New Zealand Immunisation Awareness Society held its first international symposium on vaccination. While we were organising it, committee member Judy Gilbert telephoned a paediatrician at Auckland hospital and told him it was his duty to attend the symposium. He shouted into the phone, "I'll come to your symposium if you'll come to my hospital and see all the children with whooping cough." We were very keen to go to the hospital to see the children with whooping cough. We wanted to know what medication they were being given, whether they were being held upright during whoops, why the parents had sent them to hospital, and to find out how many doses of DPT each child had had prior to getting whooping cough. But the visit never materialised because there were no children in the hospital with whooping cough. He still refused to come to our symposium.

Medical textbooks recommend some treatments that are harmful and useless, like immune serum globulin, and some treatments which are helpful, like a constant warm room temperature. Some deaths from whooping cough in the early days of modern medicine were caused by the dreadful treatments that were used, like injections of ether. Nowadays chilling is the biggest cause of death.[108]

The vaccine industry tries to frighten parents into believing that whooping cough carries a high risk of death. In many countries vaccine promoting pamphlets say that one out of 200 babies under six months of age with whooping cough will die. This sounds very frightening, as it is designed to do. The wording fails to point out that most children will not get whooping cough, because of the natural decline in whooping cough that has been happening for more than a hundred years. Some parents are told that the risk of brain damage from vaccinating is one in a million, while the risk of death from not vaccinating is one in 200. When doctors and nurses say this, they are re-interpreting the statistic in a deceitful way.

That figure of "one in 200" is used consistently in many countries, so I thought it must be based on something, not just made up, like some official figures are. I found it difficult to track down the source because most people who were using it were just repeating it from other unreferenced sources. Eventually I found that it came from a report on whooping cough in the USA during the years 1986 to 1988.[110] The report does not tell the reader how many of the babies that died during those years had been vaccinated. It does, however, tell the reader that 66% of the cases in children aged between 3 months and 4 years had had at least one dose of the vaccine, but it does not tell us what proportion of those in this age group who died had been vaccinated. It tells us that 85% of the total cases were given an antibiotic, but it does not tell us whether those who died were given antibiotics, nor does it mention fever suppressing drugs and chilling. It also does not say whether the children actually died of whooping cough, or of bronchitis or pneumonia. The report admits that 90% of cases of whooping cough in the USA are not reported.

It is deceptive to say that every baby has a one in 200 chance of dying if it is not vaccinated. It is also dishonest to say that every baby who gets whooping cough has a one in 200 chance of dying. The risk of death is affected by the type of care provided, and by other factors. In Sweden there were 19,000 cases of whooping cough in an epidemic that ran from 1977 to 1979, with no deaths.[111] If I were to use this statistic to print a pamphlet saying that young babies with whooping cough have no chance of dying, I would be behaving as dishonestly as the vaccinators behave.

Most of the children who died in the 1974 and 1977 outbreaks of whooping cough in England were already chronically ill when they developed whooping cough.[112] People trying to encourage vaccination often repeat the claim that when the vaccination rate fell in Britain in 1976, it caused a big epidemic of whooping cough and lots of deaths. This is a lie which I have dealt with in the section on herd immunity.

Droplets of saliva are infectious to other children for six weeks from the time the mucousy symptoms start. A child with whooping cough should be kept away from babies and severely malnourished children, whether or not the latter two have been vaccinated.

When Chandra was no longer infectious and had recovered enough to want to go out, I always took the plastic bowl with me. She kept it on the seat beside her in the car, and once she had thrown up we knew we had time to do some shopping before the next spasm. One day she threw up during her violin lesson, and the teacher shouted at me for not having her "immunised." Thanks to the plastic bowl, no harm was done to the carpet.

After 11 weeks we travelled from Cape Town to Johannesburg by car. We drove at night so that she could sleep while travelling and would not moan about boredom. We stopped for petrol in a desolate Karroo town, and she woke up when the motion of the car stopped. She then whooped, and the petrol attendant got a terrible fright. He probably thought she was choking to death. He did not understand English, so we could not explain that it was only the tail end of whooping cough. He was disturbed by our casual attitude and looked very worried as we drove off into the night.

Her very last whoop was 13 weeks after the first. As we arrived at a minitown, the minitrain was about to set off, so we ran to catch it. The excitement and exertion brought on a whoop. There was no plastic bowl as she had not needed it for ages, so I cupped my hands and she threw up into them. She then forgot all about me and enjoyed the thrill of rattling along in a minitrain through a minitown, while I sat there wondering what to do with this handful of yuk. As we crossed a minicreek I dumped it, and then I used my one and only paper handkerchief to clean my hands. These are the tribulations of parenthood I would far rather endure than coping with a brain damaged child, or grieving for a life cut short by DPT.

CHICKEN POX

Caring for a child with chicken pox involves spending a lot of time dabbing liquid or ointment onto the spots to stop the itch. The spots which chicken pox causes are quite different to the rash caused by measles or rubella. Each spot starts off looking like a little pimple, then it forms a yellow watery blister on top. This top changes to a crust which must not be knocked off. The spots are usually itchy, and the patient feels tempted to scratch them. If the spots become infected from scratching they will form scars. There are lots of things that can be applied to stop or soothe the itch. Best of all is rhus tox ointment or rhus tox tincture. Many other remedies from the health shop reduce itching without harming the skin or suppressing the elimination process. From the chemist there is calamine lotion and gentian violet, which are harmless and effective. (Gentian violet has been changed from an over-the-counter remedy into a prescription only medicine in Australia and New Zealand, because it competed for sales against patented drugs.) Whatever you use will only have a temporary effect, and it has to be dabbed onto each spot over and over again. Sometimes it has to be repeated after only half an hour. There are liquids and ointments that stop the itching that is caused by things like urticaria or flea bites, but do not stop the itch of chicken pox. If a substance you are using does not stop the itch, don't persevere with it - try something else. On some children the spots get very big and leave scars when they burst. When the skin has healed over, you can apply vitamin E oil or hydrogenated lanolin to help the scar tissue convert to normal tissue.

Chicken pox varies in intensity. A child who has it mildly can play with a playmate between fevers, but a child who has high peaks of fever needs continual bed rest and warmth. The fever comes and goes as each new batch of spots appears.

Sometimes the chicken pox does not finish off properly and the virus lingers on in the body. Later it reactivates and causes a horrible skin condition called shingles. Homoeopathy can cure shingles.

Adults who get chicken pox usually suffer horribly for a few days, but when it is over they feel wonderful. They can describe the feeling of being cleansed and renewed, whereas children do not stop to tell you. Of course an adult who dies from chicken pox or whose brain is damaged from the encephalitis does not speak well of chicken pox afterwards. As with all spotty childhood diseases, adults are more vulnerable to complications than children if the disease is not properly managed. An adult who does not stay in bed when he or she has chicken pox is asking for trouble, and will probably get it.

Doctors, nurses, chemists, glossy magazines and neighbours tell parents to give paracetamol to children with chicken pox. Like most medical practices, this treatment became dogma without being tested. In April 1984 a year long study was commenced to investigate whether paracetamol affects the duration or severity of chicken pox.[58] This was the very first time that the use of paracetamol during chicken pox had been studied. The study found that the drug made the itching a little bit worse, it made the illness last one day longer, and it made absolutely no difference to vomiting, insomnia, headaches, abdominal pain or fussiness. The results were published in 1989, and this would have been a good time for the medical establishment to inform everyone that it is not a good idea to give paracetamol to a child with chicken pox.

In some countries the chicken pox vaccine is being introduced with scaremongering that chicken pox is a "killer disease," while in other countries the authorities are being more coy and saying that the vaccine is necessary because it is bad for the economy when caregivers take time off work to look after a child. The chicken pox vaccine is manufactured on aborted babies.[113,114]

Before the introduction of the vaccine, the death rate from chicken pox in the USA was 22 times higher among adults than among children.[115,116] When the vaccine has been in use for some time, we will see the disease shift to adolescents and young adults, despite the inevitable introduction of more and more doses. The death rate from chicken pox will then become higher.

SLAPPED CHEEK ROSEOLA

This disease is becoming more common. It seems to be replacing scarlet fever, but so far it is not very intense and does not pose as much of a risk as scarlet fever used to. It is caused by a virus called parvovirus B19. It comes in epidemics and when it spreads through schools and preschool centres it causes quite some comment. It gives children a rather hilarious appearance, but does not make them feel very sick. The most striking feature is that the cheeks and side of the jaw become bright red. They do not really look as if they have been slapped, because the redness is too solid and extensive. My little boy called it "slap-cheek-roll-me-over." The rash on the body is mottled and lacy, and is very peculiar because it comes and goes. The rash itches some of the time, and having a shower makes it itch more. It does not get as itchy as chicken pox. The fever is not very high and the tiredness is not a complete wipe out. Nevertheless children should not be given paracetamol and expected to meet their sporting commitments.

It will be interesting to see whether this disease becomes more intense as well as becoming more common over the next few decades. When laboratory workers manage to make the virus grow on some kind of animal or human protein, they will market it as a vaccine, and parents will be told that they are irresponsible if they do not have it injected into their children.

"WHEN VACCINATED CHILDREN GET THE DISEASE THAT THE VACCINE WAS SUPPOSED TO PREVENT, THEY GET IT LESS BADLY"

Vaccine Myth number Three: Vaccinated children sometimes get the disease that the vaccine was supposed to prevent, but when they do, the severity of the disease is greatly diminished.

Whenever I hear an apologist for vaccine failure say the above, I am tempted to ask if death from measles is less severe in the vaccinated than in the unvaccinated.

A vaccinated child with measles does not experience the typical symptoms of classical measles, but gets what is called "atypical measles." Unvaccinated children with measles have a more comfortable time than those who experience atypical measles. The rash in a vaccinated child is often paler than a normal measles rash. That is not a reason for celebration. A Danish researcher has found that a lack of rash in people with measles antibodies is associated with cancer and degenerative diseases later on in life.[117] The subjects in his study averaged 38 years of age, and none of them had been vaccinated. Those who had not had measles, but had antibodies to measles, either from being infected with the wild virus without developing symptoms, or from being injected with immune serum globulin, had a much higher rate of a wide range of degenerative diseases than those who had had measles with a proper rash.

The first measles vaccine contained a killed measles virus instead of a live measles virus. When people who were injected with the first vaccine catch measles, the symptoms can be so different to ordinary measles that it is often difficult for a doctor to diagnose what is wrong. The rash does not look like a measles rash, and it does not start on the face and move downwards. It starts on the hands and feet and moves inwards. It can look like a severe allergic reaction, or like chicken pox, and it itches and stings.

It is sometimes mistaken for meningitis, scarlet fever, Rocky Mountain spotted fever, an allergic reaction to drugs, pleurisy or lung cancer. The greatest danger from having atypical measles after the killed virus vaccine is that doctors might do harmful invasive tests to try and find out what is wrong. If left alone, the sickness will heal itself spontaneously, although it can persist for months before it suddenly clears up.

I am intrigued by the fact that a person who has been injected with a dead virus gets a worse form of atypical measles than a person who has been injected with a live virus. There is speculation about possible reasons for this in the medical literature.

Figures from Zambia showed that the death rate from measles during an epidemic was higher among the vaccinated than among the unvaccinated.[118] In the USA the vaccine has made measles start occurring in infants and adults instead of in children, and the death rate is more than three times higher.[119]

When diphtheria was still prevalent, parents whose children got the disease despite vaccination were fobbed off with the claim that the disease was less severe because the child was vaccinated, unless of course the child had died. In vaccine myth number seven I discuss a study done by the British Medical Research Council which sought an explanation for the failure of the vaccine to prevent diphtheria. The study doctors were expecting to find that vaccinated patients with diphtheria who had a high level of antibodies would have a less severe form of the disease than vaccinated people with a low level of antibodies. But they did not. "... there was no significant association, however, between severity and antitoxin content."[120]

"DIPHTHERIA DECLINED BECAUSE OF MASS VACCINATION"

Vaccine Myth number Four: Diphtheria disappeared when mass immunisation of babies was introduced. Before then many children died from the disease. Nowadays it is still necessary to vaccinate all children against diphtheria, because if the vaccination rate falls below 95%, herd immunity will no longer protect the unimmunised.

Diphtheria has not disappeared, but it has become very rare. When singing the praises of the diphtheria vaccine, vaccinationists fail to mention that diphtheria declined far more before the vaccine was introduced than it did after the vaccine was introduced. Its rarity nowadays has nothing at all to do with the vaccine, because the vaccine does not work. During the decades when diphtheria was still common, roughly half of the victims were adults, and half were children.[121] Britain started using diphtheria vaccine in 1913,[122] but mass vaccination was not commenced until 1940.[123] The British Medical Research Council did a study on antibody levels which started in 1939 and was published in 1950.[124] The aim of the study was to see whether the reason why vaccinated people got the disease was because they had failed to make enough antibodies. This study is discussed in vaccine myth number seven.

Britain is one of the few countries in the world that has kept a record of infectious diseases for a long time. Deaths from diphtheria in England and Wales were recorded from 1866. The British Department of Health has this to say in a booklet that is aimed at promoting vaccination,

The introduction of immunisation against diphtheria on a national scale in 1940 resulted in a dramatic fall in the number of notified cases and deaths from the disease. In 1940, 46,281 cases with 2,480 deaths were notified, compared with 37 cases and 6 deaths in 1957. From 1979 to 1986, 26 cases were notified with only one death.[123]

If you look at a graph of the drop that occurred after 1940, it appears that the vaccine was very effective at eliminating deaths from diphtheria. That is why health departments around the world use graphs of the British experience since 1940 to promote vaccination. The difference between their graphs and mine is that mine looks less posh because it is hand drawn.

Deaths from diphtheria since vaccine introduced

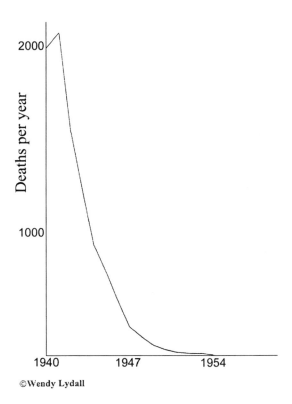

©Wendy Lydall

But the graph becomes a lot less impressive when you look at the history of the drop that occurred after 1902.

Deaths from diphtheria since 1902

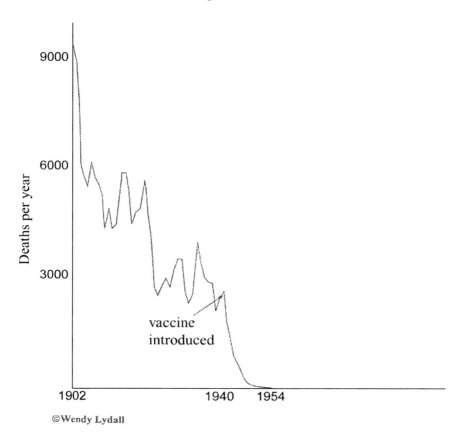

©Wendy Lydall

But this too, does not tell the whole story. From 1866 to 1893 there had been a huge increase in the number of deaths from diphtheria. It rose to a peak during the last decade of the 19th century, and then began to decline. The number of deaths from diphtheria in 1899 was three times as high as it was in 1869, while the population was only two fifths greater.

Deaths from diphtheria since 1866

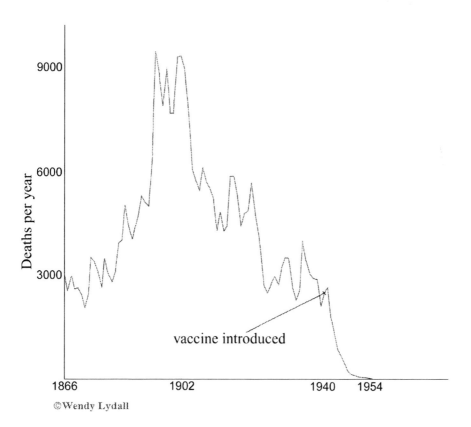

©Wendy Lydall

Should we give the people who compiled the British Department of Health's book on "Immunisation" the benefit of the doubt, and suggest that perhaps they did not know the history of diphtheria in their country? But if they did not know something as fundamental as that, then why was the British taxpayer paying them a salary? I believe that they deliberately tried to mislead the reader.

The idea that nutrition and hygiene made diphtheria decline is also without foundation. A look at the history of infectious diseases shows that nutrition and hygiene are irrelevant to the coming and going of germs. A hygienic lifestyle protects from waterborne diseases like cholera and typhoid, but it offers no protection against an airborne disease like diphtheria. Being malnourished does make a person more susceptible to a germ if the germ comes along, but what a person eats, and how much each person eats, does not make germs enter or leave the environment.

If the hygienists were correct, then the rise in diphtheria in Britain during the last century would have been caused by poverty and unsanitary living conditions. Living conditions in the cities had been very bad from the time of the industrial revolution, and the importation of wheat from North America caused more country folk to become destitute and to head for the cities. So there was a rise in the number of severely malnourished and unhoused people during the last part of the 19th century. Before declaring that this was the reason why the incidence of diphtheria rose at that time, we should ask ourselves why deaths from whooping cough and from scarlet fever were dropping sharply at the same time. Sometimes there is a coincidental correlation between the rise and fall of airborne infectious diseases and the worsening or improvement of human living conditions, but overall there is no correlation.

In Victorian England most of the population lived in dire poverty, and the corrupt Relieving Officers and Guardians and cruel Taskmasters intended to keep it that way. A woman named Charlotte Despard decided to get the workhouses, and other institutions which entrenched poverty, abolished.[125] She realised that lack of nourishment caused ill health in poor children, so she forced the government to start school feeding schemes.[126]

Rickets is a disease of the bones that is caused solely by the socio-economic factors of malnutrition and lack of sunlight. It has no life cycle of its own because it is not caused by germs. In central London there was a permanent thick smog which blocked out the sun, and the impoverished people who lived there had deformed bones because of the smoke and the lack of food. Rich people chose to believe that poor people had rickets because they were inferior. The wealthy Charlotte Despard was considered to be extraordinarily stupid by her friends and relations for saying that rickets was caused by poverty.

Charlotte Despard also initiated the concept of officialdom checking up on the health of babies,[127] which has now degenerated into another way of selling pharmaceuticals. She was powerful because she was wealthy, and she brought about social reforms that triggered the elimination of rickets and the end of some causes of child mortality. However, these reforms are not the reason for the decline of airborne diseases like diphtheria and scarlet fever. The virulence of those germs is not affected by housing and plumbing conditions. Like English sweating sickness and bubonic plague, they have dwindled because of natural forces which we do not understand and which no-one is researching. In 1963 Ethel Douglas Hume wrote,

> During the four years 1941-1944 the Ministry of Health and the Department of Health for Scotland admitted almost 23,000 cases of diphtheria in immunised children and more than 180 that proved fatal.

In regard to the decline of diphtheria in Great Britain during 1943 and 1944, we are reminded that fifty-eight British physicians, who signed a memorial in 1938 against compulsory immunisation in Guernsey, were able to point to the virtual disappearance of diphtheria in Sweden without any immunisation. On the other hand, if we turn to Germany we find that, after Dr. Frick's order in April 1940 for the compulsory mass immunisation of children, this country in 1945 had come to be regarded as the storm-centre of diphtheria in Europe. From some 40,000 there had been an increase to 250,000 cases.

An article in the number for March 1944 of a publication called *Pour La Famille* points out the rise in cases of diphtheria after compulsory immunisation. For instance, the increase in Paris was as much as thirty per cent; and in Lyons the diphtheria cases rose from 162 in 1942 to 239 in 1943. In Hungary, where immunisation has been compulsory since 1938, the rise in cases was thirty-five per cent in two years. In the canton of Geneva, where immunisation has been enforced since 1933, the number of cases was trebled from 1941 to 1943.[128]

Although diphtheria has become a rare disease, there still are sporadic outbreaks. When an outbreak does occur, people who have been vaccinated are not immune. In 1969 there was an outbreak of diphtheria in Chicago. According to the official statistics, 25% of the cases had been fully immunised, 18% had been partly immunised, and another 12% had been partly immunised and had made enough antibodies to make them "immune."[129] The world would not have been told about this little epidemic and the failure of the vaccine if the ever vigilant Dr. Mendelson had not reported it in his newsletter, *The People's Doctor*. How many more outbreaks have there been in which the vaccine has failed, but the failure has been kept under wraps by the medicrats?

When the germs that cause diphtheria become virulent in an area, most of the people who live in that area breathe in diphtheria germs. Some of the people who have diphtheria germs residing in their throats remain lively and healthy, while others get sick with the symptoms of diphtheria. This is because the immune systems of the former group are able to keep the germs under control. The ability of their immune systems to do this does not depend on whether or not they have been vaccinated, nor whether or not they have a lot of antibodies.[124] People who have diphtheria germs living in their throats but have no symptoms of sickness are called "carriers." Finding diphtheria germs in the throat of a person who is suffering the symptoms of

67

diphtheria confirms that diphtheria germs are the cause of the sickness, while finding diphtheria germs in the throat of a person without symptoms confirms that diphtheria germs are present in the air at that time.

There was a time when carriers were considered a danger to others. *The Evening News* of 4th June 1920 reported that the medical authorities in a town called Alperton in Middlesex, England, took throat cultures from 700 children and examined them for diphtheria germs. They found that the germs were present in 200 of the children, so these children were accused of being "carriers," and were put in quarantine.[130] It appears that the authorities learned their lesson and did not continue to round up and imprison "carriers." They realised that there are far too many "carriers" for them to lock up, and it is better not to seek them out.

In June 1992 a teenage girl who was in one of Hilary Butler's gym classes in a town south of Auckland got diphtheria. At first it seemed to be just a nasty cough. She did not take a break even though she was overworking both academically and physically. When her condition became serious, she was admitted to hospital, where her aunt came to visit her. Her aunt had nursed diphtheria cases in Britain in the 1950s, and she said that her niece had the typical symptoms of diphtheria. The girl was flown by helicopter to a bigger hospital in Auckland, where they took a swab from her throat and confirmed diphtheria. When they learned that the girl was fully immunised, one of the doctors said to the mother, "Then it can't be diphtheria." They changed the diagnosis to bacterial tracheitis.

Many of the children in the same town had the same nasty cough, but only one other girl went on to get full-blown diphtheria. When she was hospitalised with the same classical symptoms of diphtheria, they took a swab which confirmed that she had diphtheria. Again they refused to call it diphtheria because the girl was up to date with her jabs. This case was labelled epiglottitis and infected asthma.

We do not know how many other cases like this happened in New Zealand at that time. We only know about these two because they happened so close to Hilary. The medical people did not want to put it on paper that the two girls had diphtheria, because then there would have been an official record that vaccination had failed. Hilary asked the medical authorities to take swabs from all the children in the region who showed mild symptoms of diphtheria, but they refused. It is probable that many of the children who were suffering from a "nasty cough" were actually battling against diphtheria germs. It is also probable that many of the people who lived in that area and had no symptoms at all had diphtheria germs in their throats too.

The dishonest behaviour of the medical people involved in these two cases in New Zealand is probably replicated all over the world when diphtheria germs become active in the environment. Hilary said to me, "Just imagine if it had been my child that had come down with the symptoms. It would have been front-page news that I had caused an outbreak of diphtheria. But of course my children wouldn't get diphtheria because I give them enough vitamin C."

At the same time as this small outbreak occurred in New Zealand, there was quite a big outbreak happening in Russia. The vaccine industry used the outbreak in Russia as an excuse for selling millions more doses of diphtheria vaccine. They persuaded their lackeys in health departments around the world to make it policy for diphtheria vaccine to be injected into teenagers and adults at intervals varying from 5 years to 15 years. They have combined diphtheria toxin with tetanus toxin, and most recipients think they are just getting a tetanus shot.

The vaccine industry claimed that the rear guard diphtheria outbreak in Russia in the early nineties was caused by a drop in the vaccination rate. However, there was no drop in the vaccination rate, and when the rate was increased in response to the epidemic, it made no difference.[131,132] The World Health Organisation said the reason for the epidemic was that the vaccine does not give life-long immunity like the disease does.[132] If that were the case, there would have been epidemics everywhere else too, because every other country in the world which used diphtheria vaccine had been giving it to babies only, and not to anyone who was older. Anyway, a natural dose of diphtheria does not give life-long immunity like a natural dose of measles does, because it is not a childhood disease. Hygienists say that the epidemic was caused by the poverty that resulted from the break up of the Soviet Union. It is true that widespread malnutrition will provide more victims for the virulent germ, but malnutrition does not make the germ become virulent.

Because the history of the disease has only been recorded for 150 years, we cannot predict what it is going to do next. It is possible that diphtheria is going to come back in a big way. We cannot assume that it is going to disappear entirely just because English sweating sickness disappeared.

If the diphtheria germ decides to become virulent again, vaccinated people will get diphtheria, and the whole scenario of excuses and accusations will start up. If diphtheria does not break out again, they will continue to claim that their vaccine is the reason for the absence of diphtheria.

The history of scarlet fever in England and Wales gives some insight into the natural rise and fall of virulent diseases. In 1870 scarlet fever killed twelve times as many people in England and Wales as diphtheria did. A vaccine was sporadically used in some parts of Britain,[122] but it never became one of the routine vaccines on the schedule for children. Yet scarlet fever declined so dramatically that it ceased to be listed in the British statistics from 1950.

Deaths from scarlet fever since 1866

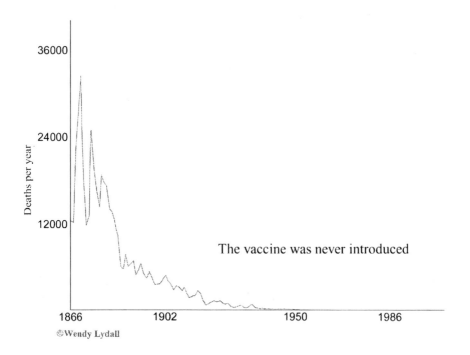

© Wendy Lydall

On the next page I have superimposed the histories of the two diseases onto each other. Scarlet fever was so much more of a killer than diphtheria that I have had to squash down the diphtheria line.

Scarlet fever and diphtheria

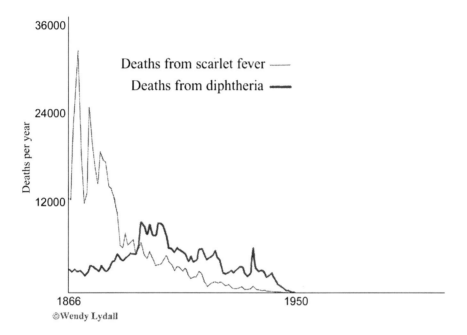

Deaths from scarlet fever ——
Deaths from diphtheria ▬▬

©Wendy Lydall

During the 1930s and 1940s a number of articles which sung the praises of various scarlet fever vaccines were published in the medical literature. Despite the efforts of the manufacturers, no vaccine was ever introduced as part of any country's schedule. If it had become one of the routine shots which babies are nowadays given, the vaccine industry and their lackeys in the media would constantly be telling us that it is because of vaccination that the world was saved from scarlet fever. Parents who refuse to accept the vaccine would be told that they are irresponsible and a danger to society.

Like diphtheria, scarlet fever has not entirely disappeared. Outbreaks are very rare, but they still happen. In 1989, when we were living in New Zealand, some cases of scarlet fever occurred in our suburb. In the IAS newsletter I asked if any readers knew of other cases, and people wrote in from all over New Zealand and told me that their children had had it. The 1989 flare up of scarlet fever might have shown itself in other parts of the world too. Perhaps scarlet fever is going to come back, or perhaps it was just having a rear guard action.

If vaccination against scarlet fever were routinely practiced, the cases which occurred would have either been explained away with the excuse, "the vaccine is only 99% effective," or the disease would have been labelled as something else, just like the diphtheria cases which Hilary witnessed. But because there is no vaccine for scarlet fever, the health department just kept quiet about the outbreak. If a vaccine had existed, they would have been telling parents that their children needed extra shots, and they would have accused parents of unvaccinated children of being the villains who caused the outbreak.

"WITHOUT VACCINATION THERE WOULD BE EPIDEMICS"

Vaccine Myth number Five: Epidemics of killer diseases used to sweep across the land until vaccination put an end to them. If vaccination were to cease, these epidemics would start again.

No-one knows what causes epidemics to start and end, nor why some remain in a certain locality, while others spread. Epidemics are an interesting phenomenon, and if someone would spend as much time and money on researching them as is spent on researching what causes earthquakes, we might begin to understand the natural forces behind them.

Some epidemics rise fast and then disappear suddenly, while others start slowly, stay at a peak for a long time, and then fade away slowly. Within the general rise and fall there are highs and lows which make the history of a disease look spiky on a graph. When an epidemic spreads across a large part of the world, it is called a pandemic.

The germs that cause TB (tuberculosis) are an exception. They do not come and go. They are always there, ready to cause disease when an individual is susceptible. The rise and fall of TB in any community is determined by socio-economic conditions, not by changes in the virulence of the germ. Human activity can make a difference to the number of people who get a disease during an epidemic, but humans have no power over the coming and going of the germ. The vaccine establishment wants people to think that if it were not for their intervention, we would constantly be threatened by terrible diseases. When there is an epidemic, they say that their vaccine can make the epidemic go away. When there is no epidemic, they say that the reason there is no epidemic is because some people have been vaccinated. When a vaccine is introduced during an epidemic, or an intensified campaign is conducted during an epidemic, the vaccinators claim credit for ending the epidemic. They do this even if the epidemic ends years after mass vaccination begins.

I have a dog who thinks she defeats thunderstorms. If she barks long and loud enough, the thunder goes away, and she has an air of satisfaction at her victory. She believes she has successfully defended home and family from the threat. It suits the vaccine industry very well that medical bureaucrats choose to think the same way as my dog does.

Nutrition is not a factor in the spread of epidemics. During epidemics of non-childhood diseases, good nutrition is a crucial defence mechanism for the individual, but it does not affect the duration of an outbreak, nor the locality. During epidemics of childhood diseases, good nutrition makes no difference to the incidence of the disease, but it does affect the death rate.

It is trendy among anti-vaccinationists to claim that modern hygienic measures have made some diseases go away, but airborne diseases are not affected by hygiene, and while waterborne diseases need a lack of hygiene to flourish, vast areas of the world do not practice hygiene, yet are free of those diseases.

Human beings have many quaint ideas about what causes epidemics to start and end. Bubonic plague broke out in China in the 12th century, and there happened to be a lot of earthquakes occurring at that time. Many people thought that the earthquakes caused the bubonic plague. In 1665 London suffered from a bad epidemic of bubonic plague, and then in 1666 it suffered a terrible fire. Because the fire occurred in the year after the plague, many people believe that it was the Great Fire of London that made the plague dwindle in the whole of Europe. The rationale behind this theory is that the fire killed all the rats that carry bubonic plague. Yet eyewitness accounts describe how the rats ran away from the flames faster than the humans did. The fire destroyed 136 acres of London, which was much less than half of the area of London. More than 100,000 people were made homeless, but less than 50 people lost their lives, because the fire spread slowly from building to building over three days and nights. The fire occurred only on the north side of the Thames, so all of the rats on the south side lived to a ripe old age. The fire could not possibly have made the plague disappear from the rest of England and Europe, yet children's books and computer resources for children say that the Great Fire of London put an end to the plague. In the new millennium there is still a lot of unscientific thinking about infectious diseases.

The scourge of sweating sickness was at one time a bigger killer than smallpox, yet it disappeared without a trace before microscopes were invented. Knowing the history of epidemics helps us to see that the claims of the vaccine industry are not valid. I have focused on the history of bubonic plague and cholera because they are the most dramatic examples of virulent diseases coming and going of their own accord. Don't forget that the less dramatic diseases also come and go of their own accord.

BUBONIC PLAGUE

The earliest recorded pandemic of bubonic plague started in Arabia and reached Egypt in the year 542. It moved across Europe to England, and devastated Ireland in 664.

The pandemic of bubonic plague which has the greatest impact on modern thinking is the one referred to as the Black Death. The title "Black Death" is not a description of the symptoms, it was only given to the pandemic 300 years after it was over, and was the result of a mistranslation. The plague started in central Asia, and moved eastwards into China, southwards into India and westwards towards Europe. It took a jump from the Black Sea to Italy by ship, where it arrived in 1348.

Bubonic plague is characterised by buboes. Buboes are lumps that grow on the body, and burst open when they are as big as eggs. The first symptom of the plague is red spots in the groin and armpits. The spots swell and grow together forming buboes, and the victim either dies within five days, or recovers. Death usually occurs on day 5, but in some cases the lungs are attacked, and then the victim spits blood and dies on the third day. A less common form of the disease occurs when the bacteria proliferate so quickly in the blood that the victim dies in a few hours or even minutes. There is still a widespread belief that the Black Death was caused by three different germs travelling together at the same time, but it was only one species of bacterium that affected each victim in one of the three ways.

It must have been alarming to see friends and relatives keeling over, spewing blood, oozing gore, smelling repulsive, and then becoming a hideous gnarled corpse, especially when you had no idea what was causing it, nor how to avoid being the next victim.

The bacterium that causes bubonic plague lives in the stomach of a type of flea which usually resides in the fur of rodents. The bacterium is found on rodents even when there is no epidemic. At least 38 species of rodent harbour the plague, but most rodents stay in one place. Rats are an exception. They are by nature travellers, and sometimes they migrate en masse, transporting the fleas over great distances. The presence of the rat is not necessary for the survival of the fleas, so bubonic plague can be transported on cargo and on humans. Other species of fleas can transfer the bacteria during an epidemic. There is no need for a flea to bite a human, it just has to alight on the skin, and the bacterium can burrow its way into the blood stream. Today a lot is known about this bacterium, but it is not known why it suddenly spreads among humans. Rats migrate all the time, and humans in Europe lived in filthy conditions for hundreds of years without being subjected to plagues.

During the Black Death most doctors refused to attend the sick, because they knew that going near a victim increased the likelihood of catching the disease. Lack of medical attention made no difference to the victim, because medieval medicine could not alter the course of the disease.

The homoeopathic cure for bubonic plague is potentised *baptisia*, but there were no homoeopaths 500 years ago. Cases of bubonic plague were still occurring in Europe after homoeopathy was discovered, and as part of the homoeopathic treatment, the bedding of plague patients was burned. This was done because Dr. Samuel Hahnemann, the doctor who discovered homoeopathy, believed that the disease was caused by tiny little animals that were too small to be seen. People who did not have the advantage of knowing about homoeopathy tried to prevent the plague with frequent bloodletting, the burning of aromatic plants, avoiding exercise, and the swallowing of all sorts of useless potions.

Attacking defenceless minority groups was also regarded as a worthwhile form of prevention. Arabs, Jews, the deformed, widows and lepers were killed to try and stop the plague. The Cypriots murdered all their Arab slaves before heading for the hills, where the plague overtook them. The persecution of the Jews reached a peak during the Black Death that was not to be equalled until the time of the Nazis. The Jews did not drink sewer water like the gentiles did, but collected water from clean streams. This was regarded as evidence that they had poisoned the wells in the towns and had caused the plague. The Jews died of the plague in the same numbers as everybody else, because hygiene does not prevent plague, but the high death rate among Jews made no difference to the thinking of the persecutors.

"Confessions" were acquired from some Jews who were tortured on the rack in a town in France, and the torturers sent notification of the "confessions" to neighbouring towns. This sparked off widespread massacres, and the persecution spread throughout Europe. Travelling bands called the Flagellants roamed from town to town, dressed in peculiar clothing, singing and wailing that the Jews were causing the plague.

In some towns the massacres were carried out before the plague arrived. In Basle and in Freiburg special wooden buildings were built, and all the Jews were penned in and burned. In other towns huge wooden scaffolds were built and Jews were thrown on while the flames roared. Any that escaped were set on by the mob and murdered. At Mainz the fires were so large that they melted the lead in between the pieces of stained glass in the church windows. Any Christians and other gentiles who opposed the burnings, (and there were many,) were also thrown into the flames. There are still in existence some of the documents that proclaim their guilt by association. After the burnings, Christians and gentiles who were suspected of sympathising with the Jews were tortured on the rack.

The pope and many political leaders tried to halt the persecution, but they lacked the military strength to enforce their will. Even the threat of excommunication did not deter the mobs. The King of Spain tried to punish those responsible, but officials sabotaged his attempts. He personally recompensed the Jews who had survived attacks, and established an armed guard around one ghetto to prevent further violence. A German prince gave the Jews sanctuary in his castle, but the mob ransacked his castle and killed all the Jews. The leader of Poland was the only one who was completely successful at preventing the murders, and many Jews fled Western Europe and took refuge there, if they were not murdered by peasants on the way.

No-one knows exactly what percentage of the total population died during the Black Death. In places that kept records, the death rate from the disease varied between 12% and 66%, with the figures being higher near the sea. In an isolated community in Sweden, it killed everyone except for one young girl. She was found years later, living alone in the wild. She inherited all the land in that area, and it remained in the possession of her descendants for centuries. Historians estimate that roughly one third of the population of Europe died.

Pandemics of bubonic plague spread rapidly, and kill most of their victims in the first few months, but they do not end abruptly. They linger on, and flourish sporadically. The "Plague of London" in 1665 was one of the Black Death's last encores. During this revival of the plague, a tailor in an English village ordered a cloth from London. This cloth was contaminated with plague, and he died soon after it was delivered. Then 267 of the 350 people who lived in his village died too.

The most recent pandemic started in China in 1892, and killed millions of people in India before travelling by ship to numerous ports on other continents. It did not take hold in any of the ports, not even in the cities with terrible slums. Bubonic plague continues to break out sporadically, but it does not affect great numbers. It killed a few people in Britain in 1910, and there was a very small outbreak in South Africa in 1982. A relatively large outbreak in India in 1994 caused international hysteria before it petered out of its own accord.

Although orthodox medicine does not claim direct credit for the disappearance of the Black Death, it uses the Black Death for general fear mongering about infectious diseases. For example, a British made "educational" TV program, which is repeatedly shown in Australia and New Zealand, tells the story of the village community that was devastated by the cloth that brought the plague from London, and then it tells the mythical story of how Edward Jenner invented a vaccine which wiped out smallpox, and then it shows schoolgirls lining up for their rubella jabs in order to be protected from germs. This is a classic case of manipulation by association. It conditions people to accept vaccination.

When Chandra was a baby, someone told me that in the old days one in every seven people died of the plague, and if it were not for vaccinations, that situation would arise again. "Just imagine what it would be like if one out of every seven of us died," she said, as part of her reason for why I should vaccinate Chandra against whooping cough.

During the New Zealand measles epidemic of 1991, the Health Department tried to create a plague mentality by whipping up hysteria against non-vaccinating families. The vaccinationists portray health conscious families as pariahs who threaten society. They will continue to be able to do that until the general public learns the facts about herd immunity, vaccination, and epidemiology.

CHOLERA

Cholera originated in the delta of the Ganges River, where it had been in existence since the 7th century. In 1817 it suddenly took off and spread. It travelled westwards across Europe, and eastwards across Asia. It killed large numbers of people in Europe, and it aroused fear and superstition. News of the epidemic travelled ahead of it into Europe, and people became utterly paranoid in advance of its arrival. Cholera caused a lower death rate in China than in Europe, because hygiene was more widely practiced there.

Cholera is caused by a bacterium that survives very well in water. Some of the people who drink water that is contaminated with these bacteria do not come down with the disease. The explanation for this is not simple, and it is not safe to assume that being well nourished and strong and fit renders one immune to cholera. The bacteria pass from the human body into the sewage, and if the water supply is contaminated with sewage, more people become infected with the bacteria.

Cholera is a severe, fast acting disease that makes the victim lose water very quickly. Death occurs from dehydration unless the disease is stopped by homoeopathy, or the patient is continually rehydrated for five to seven days. Without treatment death can occur within 24 hours of infection. The victim suffers violent vomiting and writhes in agony because of terrible cramps. There is massive diarrhoea that involves mostly yellowish water.

From 1817 to 1902 there were eight pandemics in which cholera spread like waves across large parts of the world. The first wave started in India and stopped its westward movement at Turkey. The next one, which started in 1826, enveloped Russia, Europe and North America. In each place it struck suddenly and with devastating results. In 1840 another wave started in India, and it also reached North America. The next pandemic followed a different course; it went from the Mediterranean to Russia, instead of the other way round, and it did not reach America. The fifth one started in China and travelled westwards across Europe, and then across the sea to America. America suffered badly in this one. The sixth one started in 1870, and spread more quickly than the others. The seventh wave started in 1891. It must have seemed to the inhabitants of Europe that cholera epidemics were going to pass over the land from east to west every few years for the rest of time. The eighth wave started in 1902, but it did not spread beyond southern Europe, and it claimed fewer victims as it went. In less than a hundred years, cholera had almost played itself out.

In 1972 there was another pandemic, and epidemiologists were dismayed that none of their interventions could stop it from spreading into Western Europe. Nowadays cholera occurs in some localities, but it does not spread. In many countries sanitary plumbing has been installed, so that the people no longer drink their sewage. This means that cholera cannot break out in those places, even when the bacteria exist in the environment. Political upheavals or earthquakes that result in the loss of the clean water supply make cholera break out in areas where the bacteria are present. However, there are still areas of the world in which people routinely drink their sewage, but because the bacteria are not present in the environment, they remain cholera free. When cholera bacteria move into these areas, the disease breaks out.

During the cholera epidemics, orthodox medicine used all the usual remedies; mercury, bloodletting, opium and laudanum. Arguments raged between those who believed cholera came from the air, and those who believed it was passed from person to person. In Oxford, a lecturer in anatomy recognised the value of nutrition in protecting people from cholera, and he arranged that mutton broth be distributed to the poor. He insisted that the broth have a high density of meat.

Five years after the London homoeopathic hospital opened, it had its first opportunity to treat cholera. Sixteen percent of its cholera patients died, while in Middlesex hospital nearby, which used conventional treatments, fifty three percent of the patients died. The doctor who compiled the parliamentary report on cholera intentionally excluded the homoeopathic hospital's success, but the truth was published after the chairman of the hospital board made a great fuss.[133]

It took an awfully long time for anyone to work out that cholera epidemics are caused by people drinking water that is contaminated with sewage. When the people who discovered the connection between cholera epidemics and contaminated water published their findings, they were ridiculed and condemned. The most compelling evidence came from an investigation done by Dr. John Snow, who lived and worked in Soho, London. In those days Soho was an appalling slum. Dr. Snow observed that there were no cases of cholera among the people who got their water from the Lambeth Water Company. The Lambeth drew its water from the Thames upstream of London, while the others drew water after it was contaminated with London sewage. His suspicions about the water led him to investigate where each household obtained its water, and how many cases of cholera there had been in each household. The data he collected showed that cholera is spread by water contaminated with sewage. He published his findings in 1855, and within weeks he was attacked by the traditionalists as an enemy of progress. He had previously been considered a weirdo by the medical establishment because he refused to do cruel experiments on animals. (Nowadays people who refuse to vivisect are not allowed to become doctors.) Dr. Snow's evidence did not explain the few isolated cases which occurred in distant spots. He suggested that flies could transmit cholera by walking on sewage and then flying long distances. His guess was later proved correct. If Dr. Snow had done his research in the orthodox manner, which is by torturing animals in a laboratory, he would never have discovered how people can avoid catching cholera.

At the same time as Dr. Snow's study was published, a doctor in Bristol also published the theory that cholera was transmitted by contaminated sewage. He produced less evidence, but it was enough to convince anyone with common sense that his theory was right. Nowadays it is regarded as self-evident that cholera can be prevented by keeping the water supply free of sewage.

The Red Cross and other aid organisations are becoming increasingly successful at getting clean water to people who have lost their water supply, and this saves lives. If they used homoeopathy as well they could save even more lives in these circumstances.

When refugees fled from Rwanda in 1994, they had no choice but to drink water contaminated with cholera, so those of us who watch TV were subjected to the spectacle of lorry loads of bodies being dumped into pits.

How different it would have been if the international drug conspiracy had allowed homoeopaths to come to the scene and save those people's lives. If the doctors who belong to *Medicin Sans Frontiers* understood the principles of homoeopathy, they would be able to cure cholera, typhoid, typhus, E coli and every other infectious disease that ravages poor communities. The medicine required to cure each patient would cost only a few cents, which is the main reason why the drug companies do not want homoeopathy to happen.

"IF ENOUGH PEOPLE ARE VACCINATED, THE DISEASE WILL DIE OUT"

Vaccine Myth number Six: When enough people are vaccinated, the unvaccinated people are protected and will not get the disease. If the infectious agent has no animal reservoir, the disease can be eliminated from this planet by vaccinating a high enough percentage of the human population. When enough people are immune to the disease, it cannot be passed on, and the germ dies out. This state of herd immunity is created when 55% of people have been vaccinated. Er, whoops that should be 75%. We now know that 95% have to be vaccinated to create herd immunity. Actually, 98% isn't a high enough percentage, so we'll have to vaccinate everybody, and we'll have to give them booster shots every ten years. No, that will have to be every five years. Perhaps every three years will be more effective.

The health department in the city of Baltimore, USA, kept a record of every case of measles from 1900 to 1931. Dr. A.W. Hedrich, who lived in Baltimore, studied these statistics on measles because he wanted to find out what proportion of children had already had measles at any one time. He laboriously analysed the figures, month by month, to find out how many children under the age of 15 years there were in Baltimore each month from 1900 to 1931, and how many of them had already had measles. His analysis showed that the proportion of children under 15 who had already had measles never went above 53%, and never dropped below 32%, during those thirty two years.[18] This means that every time an outbreak came to an end, at least 47% of the children in Baltimore had not yet had measles.

The vaccine industry has misrepresented Dr. Hedrich's research to come up with the claim that when 55% of children are immune to measles, either through having had measles or through having been vaccinated against measles, epidemics cannot develop.[134,135]

Since then the vaccination rate which is supposed to create herd immunity has steadily crept upwards from 55% to 95%. The measles virus has still not read the instructions. It becomes virulent whenever nature intends it to, and epidemics occur even when there is a 98% or 100% vaccination rate.[136,137,138,139,140,141,142,143] During these epidemics, both vaccinated and unvaccinated people get measles.

A lot of claptrap has been written about herd immunity,[135,144] but in the real world it does not exist. According to the theory of herd immunity, when the vaccination rate is high enough, unvaccinated people will be protected from the disease by the fact that so many are vaccinated. In real life that does not happen. When there is no outbreak of infectious disease, they say that herd immunity is working very well, but when an infectious germ becomes virulent in the environment, and herd immunity is seen to fail, they make the excuse that a different mathematical formula should have been used for that type of population group.

Measles belongs in the category of childhood diseases, so people who have been vaccinated get the disease at an age older than the natural age for the disease. This phenomenon leads to delusions about the possibility of eliminating measles. When the measles vaccine was introduced, it was with the promise that one shot would provide life-long immunity. But within the first year it was obvious that this was not so. Then they discovered that during pregnancy, the mother passes antibodies through the placenta to the baby, and in most babies these antibodies stay in the blood until the age of nine months. They thought that these maternal antibodies must interfere with the baby's production of its own immunity. So they declared that if a child were to be injected with the measles vaccine at the age of 10 months, it would build its own antibodies, and therefore have life-long immunity. But the vaccine still did not work. So they decided that at ten months a baby's immune system was not mature enough to develop enough antibodies, and they changed the dogma to say that the vaccine must be injected at 12 months.

When that did not work, the correct age for injection went up to 15 months. In most people this has the effect of postponing measles until the teenage years or later. When epidemics started breaking out among previously vaccinated teenagers, they decided that it was necessary for children to have a booster jab at the age of 11 years. These changes to the dogma are described as "fine tuning."

A 1977 study in Los Angeles showed that a booster dose of vaccine gave only a slight boost in antibody levels, and that after a year the level dropped back to where it had been before the booster.[134] As they believe that antibody levels represent "immunity," the Los Angeles result meant that, according to their dogma, booster doses were going to be useless. At this point they should have stopped spending the taxpayers' money on measles vaccination, and started spending it on pamphlets informing parents on how to care for a child with measles.

Because the vaccine postpones measles in each individual, there is always a period after mass vaccination is introduced in which it looks as though the vaccine is winning against measles. In the USA the vaccine was introduced in 1963.[134] The government said that its aim was to eradicate the measles virus from the USA by 1982.[134] They thought that 20 years of compulsory vaccination would make it impossible for the wild virus to survive. Mass vaccination at the age of 15 months caused a huge decline in the incidence of measles in the USA - at first. When the artificially induced immunity started wearing off, the graphs started going upwards again. The medicrats have a deceptive way of making it look like less of a failure. In some discourses, any person with measles who was vaccinated under the age of one, or who did not receive the booster jab at the age of 11 years, is classified as "unimmunised."

New Zealand is running a decade behind the USA, but following exactly the same path of changes to policy as each policy is seen to fail. Australia gives the second dose of measles vaccine at the age of four years, and they claim this will give life-long immunity.

The history of measles in Hungary shows that there is no such thing as "herd immunity." What happened in Hungary also shows that it will not be possible for humans to eliminate the measles virus. When Hungary was under communist rule, the medicrats there maintained a vaccination rate of 98% for 14 years, and they gave booster doses. But measles epidemics continued to occur.

The vaccine was introduced to Hungary in 1969. Although the "correct age" for vaccination was said to be 10 months, all children from 9 to 27 months were vaccinated during mass vaccination campaigns. In 1974 the vaccine became part of routine childhood vaccination, and mass vaccination campaigns were stopped. After that they kept up a vaccination rate of 98%. In 1978 the "correct age" for vaccination was changed from 10 months to 14 months. Five years after the vaccine was introduced, the virus became virulent, and it was mainly unvaccinated 6-9 year-olds who caught measles. Six years later an epidemic occurred in which it was mainly 7-10 year-olds who caught measles. After this experience, they decided that as ten months had been the wrong age to give the vaccine, all children who had been jabbed at the age of ten months needed a booster shot.

In 1988 the measles virus became virulent again in Hungary, and an epidemic which lasted six months followed. During this epidemic the oldest people who had had the vaccine were 21 years old. Children who were 11-16 years old had had the booster shot. Seventy five percent of the cases for whom ages were recorded were aged 16 to 22 years. The age-specific attack rates were highest in 17-year-olds and second highest in 18-year-olds. From these figures it is obvious that the booster shot adds an extra postponement onto the original postponement, in some individuals.

The Hungarian statistics are published in a report[145] from the Centers for Disease Control (CDC) which is based in Atlanta, USA. The compilers of this report comment, "Assessing waning immunity may be difficult because virtually all persons 17-21 years of age were vaccinated approximately the same number of years before the epidemic." This is a really strange statement. Do they think that artificial immunity will wane at the same rate in each individual, and do they really believe that measles virus is present in the environment all the time?

In 1971 the World Health Organisation thought that measles had been eliminated from the African country of Gambia, because 96% of the population was vaccinated in 1967.[146] In 1972 measles was back in a big way, but they still thought that the strong faith that mothers have in modern medicine was going to help them in "the struggle to attain global control and eradication of measles by the year 2000."[146]

In the years before vaccine induced immunity wears off, measles vaccination does succeed in decreasing the number of cases of measles which occur, but it does not succeed in preventing measles in unvaccinated individuals. In 1984 an outbreak of measles in a Gambian village clearly showed that the background vaccination rate of 90% did not prevent unvaccinated children from getting the disease.[147] 30.1% of the unvaccinated children in the village got measles, while only 3.6% of the vaccinated children got it.[147] This shows that the vaccine prevents or postpones measles in the vaccinated, and that herd immunity does not exist. If there were a totalitarian state strong enough to force 100% of its population to be vaccinated against measles, they still would not be able to wipe out the virus. Dictators can regulate people, but they cannot bully the measles virus.

A typical opinion about measles is, "Measles is an eradicable disease. … humans are the only natural host and the epidemic spread … can only be maintained as a chain of serial direct transmissions of virus, involving acutely affected individuals."[148] This is errant nonsense. The measles virus is caught by humans in one of two ways. It is either caught from a person who has measles, or it is caught from the air. It does not need to be living in a human in order to survive. From time to time the virus becomes virulent and causes an outbreak of measles. In between these times it goes dormant, but it is still alive and well. Some outbreaks of measles are caused by an infected traveller coming into the region, while other outbreaks are caused by the virus coming out of its dormancy.

There are many schools and colleges in the USA in which 100% of the students have been "fully immunised." But this does not prevent measles from breaking out in them.[119] The medicrats usually make the excuse that the infection must have entered the school from an unvaccinated person in the community. Sometimes they try to find out who was the unvaccinated contact who started the epidemic.

The medical authorities decided to investigate the origins of an outbreak in Sangamon County, Illinois, in 1983.[136] Twenty-one cases of measles occurred. Sixteen of them were high school students, one was a college student, and four were preschool children. The high school and college students had all been vaccinated after the age of 15 months, which is currently regarded as the "correct age." Two of the preschoolers were too young to be vaccinated, and two were old enough to be vaccinated, but had not been vaccinated. According to medical mythology, the latter two should have been the ones who started the outbreak, but they were not.

The person who gets measles first during an outbreak is called the "index patient." In this case the index patient was a 17 year old boy who was fully immunised. He sat in the classroom and coughed for 3 days before the rash appeared. Nine students developed the measles rash 10-14 days after being exposed to the index patient. The rest of the cases all occurred within 34 days of the first case, and then the epidemic died out. Referring to the index patient, they say, "the source of his infection was not identified."[136]

I can tell them the source of his infection. It came from a virus that had recently entered a virulent phase, and was floating in the air. Simple. But they want to believe that measles can only be caught from another person with acute measles. Their point of view requires a traveller who is brewing an acute case of measles to enter the community before an epidemic can start. It negates the possibility that the virus goes dormant at times, and then gets virulent again. What happened here is that the 17 year old boy who was the index patient, was the first susceptible person to breathe in the virus when it changed from being dormant to being virulent.

The writers admit that the outbreak died out without any human intervention. "No vaccinations were given as part of the outbreak control program ... The outbreak subsided spontaneously, and active surveillance for illnesses with rash in the community did not identify any additional cases of measles during the 4 weeks before or after the outbreak."[136] Often when the first few cases of measles occur, the medical authorities swing into action to vaccinate and re-vaccinate everybody in the region. The outbreak then subsides of its own accord, but the medical authorities claim that it was their vaccination campaign which made it end.

The editorial note says, "This outbreak demonstrates that transmission of measles can occur within a school population with a documented immunization level of 100%. This level was validated during the outbreak investigation."[136] Not only does it demonstrate that measles can be transmitted within a fully vaccinated school, it also shows that measles can *originate* within such a school population.

When the Centers for Disease Control surveyed 93 outbreaks of measles in the USA, they found that 20 of the outbreaks had an index patient who came from overseas, while 73 of the index patients were local people, and no source of infection could be found. This shows that most outbreaks of measles are caused by the dormant virus becoming virulent. In these outbreaks 47% of the index patients were fully immunised.[149]

I can understand why the concept of a virus going into hibernation is foreign to mainstream thinking, because these days so many people live their entire lives separated from nature. I was fortunate enough to grow up on the African veld, where I witnessed the phenomenon of life resurging out of "nothing" in so many ways. For instance, a patch of land that is a dust bowl in the winter, turns into a big pond teeming with aquatic insects, eating each other mercilessly, when the summer rains come. When cattle walk across the spot in the winter, their hooves kick up the dust, and I wonder how the eggs of the insects can survive.

There are some parts of Australia where it does not rain for years at a time, and the creatures that live in these areas have to survive for long periods without water. There are frogs living in these regions even though they need constant moisture to stay alive. When rain falls, puddles and billabongs form on the ground, and frogs abound. After a while the water dries up, so the frogs burrow 30cm down into the ground, where they slough off skin cells to form a watertight cocoon around themselves. They live inside these cocoons for several years, until it rains again. As soon as the next rain season begins, they scramble to the surface and start shouting for a mate.[150]

I suspect that germs that are not in evidence for fairly long periods of time, and then suddenly make their presence known, are able to go into some type of hibernation which is very hard for us to imagine. No-one knows what the measles virus does between epidemics. Perhaps the technology needed to trace the measles virus between epidemics already exists. It is also not known what stimulates the virus to become virulent at the end of the dormant stage. The health status of the human host is not the trigger, nor is the movement of people, nor the size and density of communities. There is no space for a dormant measles virus in the thinking of people who want to sell measles vaccine. If research money were committed to exploring the matter, it might be discovered that measles viruses use epidemics to strengthen their DNA. Perhaps the virus can replicate itself while in the dormant state, but gains something extra when it causes measles cases in humans.

According to the theory of herd immunity, unvaccinated children are being protected by the vaccinated children. This is also errant nonsense. When an epidemic breaks out, the vaccine neither protects the vaccinated nor the unvaccinated.

In South Africa in 1980 I heard a doctor say that the Blacks were protected from disease because the Whites were all vaccinated. In effect he was claiming that a 20% vaccination rate is sufficient to create herd immunity. Even more ridiculous is the claim that Edward Jenner's cowpox vaccine made smallpox decline in Britain at the end of the 18th century. The vaccine supposedly did this with a vaccination rate of less than 1%.

People who want to bully health conscious families into vaccinating continually harp on the point that the unvaccinated are protected because the vaccinated create herd immunity. They want to influence public opinion to make people think that non-vaccinating parents are selfish people who exploit those who are vaccinated. In March 1992 the vaccinationists in New Zealand started feeding the media with the idea that polio and diphtheria epidemics were going to occur because too many parents were not vaccinating. They could not seem to make up their minds exactly what percentage of people needed to be vaccinated to create herd immunity, but it wobbled around in the 80s and 90s. What they were careful not to tell the public is that the vaccination rate had been "too low" to prevent epidemics for ages, without any epidemics occurring. The existence of the vaccine is not the reason for the general absence of diphtheria.

Before the 1993 New Zealand general election, some candidates tried to win votes by saying they would save the country from infectious diseases by promoting vaccination. This started the media and the medicrats into a frenzy of scaremongering about diseases, and the lie that the measles epidemic of 1991 was caused by unvaccinated children was repeated over and over again. By then they had made up their minds what percentage created "herd immunity," because they kept on saying that a 95% vaccination rate is necessary to prevent further outbreaks.

The date for the elimination of measles has been set at 2007.[151] The vaccinationists hope to achieve elimination by vaccinating nearly everyone on the planet at least twice. The myth of herd immunity is great ammunition for vaccinationists, because families who do not "co-operate" immediately become cast as the villains of the piece.

People who think that they can control nature by large-scale interference, without causing side effects, always end up doing more harm than good. People with this mentality do not learn from the mistakes of others. A typical example of the results of this type of thinking happened in China during the rule of the megalomaniac named Mao Tse Tung. He introduced communist economic policies to China which caused terrible hardship for the people. From time to time he staged "improvement" campaigns to distract his subjects from their real problems, and to boost levels of patriotism. One of these was an anti-sparrow campaign in which he persuaded the populace to use every means at their disposal to kill sparrows. The alleged reason why this was necessary was that sparrows eat crops, and consequently are a threat to human food supplies. The nation swung into action. Schools and villages vied with one another to see who could kill the most sparrows. Truck loads of dead sparrows were paraded up and down the streets. Dead sparrows were strung up on display, and the number of sparrows in China decreased drastically. The resultant imbalance in nature meant that insects ravaged the crops, and food shortages worsened. Of course the people did not manage to kill every last sparrow, and sparrow numbers have now returned to normal in China.

In June 1992 the New Zealand Health Department launched a mass vaccination campaign in schools which targeted 11-year-olds for MMR vaccine. The Immunisation Awareness Society (IAS) circulated a fact sheet about MMR vaccine in some schools. This incensed the Health Department. The medicrats in Wellington issued a press release saying that New Zealand has a chance of being the first in the world to eliminate measles, but the efforts of the health authorities are being undermined by IAS, which is circulating information that is "misleading" and "quite wrong." "New Zealand has been the first in a number of fields, and there's no reason why we shouldn't be the first with measles," they complained. They said that measles was likely to be the next disease eliminated worldwide, after smallpox and polio. They were deluding themselves that they were on the verge of eliminating polio because at that time the date for eliminating polio was set at the year 2000.[152]

The World Health Organisation still claims it is going to eliminate polio from the planet, even though the date for elimination has been passed.[152] Although polio is in a relatively dormant phase at present (having run from the 1880s until the 1960s), accounts of it having occurred in ancient and medieval times suggest that it will come back. If the polio pandemic which is still petering out does come to a complete end, the vaccinationists will say that it was vaccination that made it happen. On the other hand, if the polio virus has a resurgence of virulence, they will say it is because people did not have enough doses of the vaccine.

The last case of polio in Fiji occurred in 1959. Polio vaccination was introduced to Fiji in 1963, and it is credited with ended the epidemic.[153]

In 1991-92 there was a polio outbreak in Vellore, India, which had a 98% vaccination rate, and an 80% vaccination rate in the rural areas surrounding it.[154] What happened to herd immunity? A letter in the *Lancet* says that this shows it is not going to be possible to eradicate polio with a four dose schedule. They therefore recommend a seven dose schedule.

There was an outbreak of polio in the country of Oman on the Arabian Peninsula in 1988-89 which worried some officials from the CDC, UNICEF and WHO because it showed that it is not going to be possible to eliminate polio. The title of the CDC/UNICEF/WHO report was, *Outbreak of paralytic poliomyelitis in Oman: evidence for widespread transmission among fully vaccinated children.*[155] They want to believe that vaccinated children cannot pass on the disease, so evidence that this is not true makes them uneasy.

The polio outbreak started five months after an intensive vaccination campaign had increased the vaccination rate of twelve-month-old children from 67% to 88%. They believe that 67% is too low to create herd immunity, while 88% means that polio cannot break out, not even in the unvaccinated. The report says, "Among the most disturbing features of the outbreak was that it occurred in the face of a model immunisation programme and that widespread transmission had occurred in a sparsely populated, predominantly rural setting, ... [and] a substantial proportion of fully vaccinated children may have been involved in the chain of transmission." This happens all the time. Vaccinated children pass on the disease because vaccination does not work. In 1996 four babies died of whooping cough in New South Wales. Three of the four had caught whooping cough from a vaccinated person, and one from a person of unknown vaccination status.[156]

The belief in herd immunity leads to many delusions. One of them is that when the number of immune people in a community drops below a certain point, it will make the next epidemic come sooner. In 1976 in Britain the vaccination rate for whooping cough dropped from 76% to 42%, because there had been publicity of bad side effects from the vaccine. The medicrats expected that the drop in the vaccination rate would make the next whooping cough epidemic come sooner, as well as expecting it to be worse. The whooping cough bacteria paid no attention to human theories, and the disease followed the usual timing of its natural cycle of virulence. Medicrats expressed surprise that the epidemic did not come sooner.[157] There were also fewer cases and fewer deaths during this epidemic. The much lower vaccination rate of 42% made no difference to the long term decline of whooping cough, which had been happening for a hundred years.

In the process of trying to bully parents into ignoring the danger from whooping cough vaccine, the vaccinationists in many countries claim that this drop in the British vaccination rate caused an epidemic of whooping cough, with many deaths. But the epidemic was not caused by the drop in vaccination, and there were fewer deaths than in the previous epidemic.[158] Dr. Gordon Stewart says,

> The epidemics of 1977 - 1979 and 1981 - 1982 were in fact the expected cyclical recurrence of whooping cough every 44 months.[159]

The Central Public Health Laboratory in London compiled a report on the difference between the epidemic that happened before the vaccination rate fell (1974 to 1975), and the one which happened after it fell (1977 to 1979). It says,

> Since the decline in pertussis immunisation there has been an unexpected fall in whooping cough admission and death rates - a fall that has affected children of all ages and vaccination status.[112]

If they had looked at the long term history of whooping cough, they would have seen that the fall which occurred at that time was not unexpected. Officials who make the statement that a drop in vaccination in Britain caused a deadly outbreak of whooping cough are not telling the truth.

The natural decline in the incidence of whooping cough has become a rallying point for the vaccinationists. They say that the fact that the incidence of whooping cough is declining in the unvaccinated as well as in the vaccinated shows that herd immunity is working.[160,161] Whooping cough is declining in the unvaccinated because whooping cough has been naturally declining for over a hundred years, and it is still undergoing that decline. When a disease is undergoing a natural decline in incidence, it can be made to look as though herd immunity is the reason for decreased exposure. The vaccinationists are turning the natural decline in whooping cough to their propaganda advantage, by claiming that they are eliminating the disease from the planet.

When reading the following excerpt about the decline of whooping cough in the USA, bear in mind that the writer is a person who is very keen on promoting vaccines.

There is little question that the natural history of some infectious diseases has changed spontaneously over the years, for reasons not entirely clear. An example of such a disease is pertussis [whooping cough], which exhibited a mortality rate of 12.2 per 100,000 population in the United States in 1900. By the late 1930's, prior to widespread immunization against pertussis, the mortality rate had decreased to approximately two per 100,000. In 1975 only eight deaths due to whooping cough were recorded in the United States. Whether this reduction prior to the development of widespread immunization (and even the change subsequent to immunization) is due to variations in the organism, changes in the host, or other undetermined factors is unclear.[162]

Look at the way that whooping cough declined in England and Wales from 1866.

Deaths from whooping cough

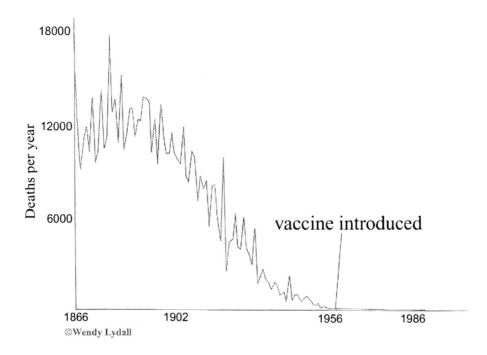

©Wendy Lydall

As you can see, whooping cough has become very rare in Britain. This has not happened because of the vaccine. It has happened because of a natural decline that was in full swing for 80 years before the vaccine was introduced. The same decline in whooping cough has happened in other countries which have kept statistics for a long time, and it has probably also happened in countries which did not keep statistics. Accurate figures were not collected in Australia, New Zealand nor South Africa.

Whooping cough has small cycles within the big overall cycle. On the small cycle it peaks every forty four months, which is why the line wiggles so much. The regularity of the mini cycle is not so obvious from the graph, because the mini cycle is chopped up by the human calendar year. No-one can predict whether whooping cough is going to disappear entirely, like English sweating sickness did, or whether it will reach a very low level, and then make a comeback. The natural decline in whooping cough has been strong and steady, and it appears that some medicrats believe that it is going to disappear. They seem to have the intention of claiming that it has been "eliminated" by the vaccine. As I have described below, vaccinated children with whooping cough are often recorded as having something else, to hide the fact that the vaccine failed, but now there is a new development. Some doctors and some laboratories will not test a child with the symptoms of whooping cough for whooping cough, because the disease "no longer exists."[163] They feel quite comfortable about calling a case of whooping cough by another name, even if the child has not been vaccinated.

In 1991 there was an outbreak of whooping cough in Cape Town, South Africa, which showed clearly that herd immunity does not exist. Apartheid was collapsing, and resources were being directed at vaccinating black children. The outbreak occurred against a very high background vaccination rate, and the published commentary was refreshingly honest.

> [Vaccination] does not eliminate the circulating disease agents. As long as this is the case, the unvaccinated will remain susceptible even in the face of high or even very high vaccination levels.[164]

That type of admission has now become politically incorrect. If whooping cough does actually disappear, they will probably claim that they wiped it out, just like they claim they wiped out smallpox.

"IMMUNITY CAN BE MEASURED BY THE DENSITY OF ANTIBODIES IN THE BLOOD"

Vaccine Myth number Seven: When the germs which cause a particular disease are weakened and then injected into the human body, the immune system builds antibodies, which are defences against that particular disease. If antibodies are present in the blood in sufficient quantities, the person will be immune to the disease. The number of antibodies that are present in each cc of blood reflects the level of immunity. A person who does not have antibodies will get the disease when exposed to the germ.

The idea that the density of antibodies represents immunity is treated as a scientific fact because it is the marketing base for selling vaccines. The vaccine industry promotes the myth that antibodies are the most important part of the immune system, because vaccines create antibodies. The technology involved in counting antibodies has become increasingly sophisticated since antibodies were discovered, but the theory behind counting antibodies has never been scientifically sound.

When a natural infection occurs, the formation of antibodies is only a part of the immune system's response. As I will show, people with lots of antibodies can still get the disease, and people who lack antibodies can remain fit and well despite being exposed to the germs. The level of antibodies in the blood that is supposed to prevent a person from catching a disease is not determined by scientific investigation; it is just arbitrarily chosen. The history of the discovery of antibodies explains why the antibody threshold theory came to be accepted by the medical establishment.

Elie Metchnikoff was a Russian born zoologist[165] who discovered that there are cells within the bodies of humans and animals which fight invaders, and that these cells travel all around in the body, even in animals which do not have blood. He called these cells phagocytes. He went to work for the Pasteur Institute in Paris, and he postulated the theory that phagocytes were the means by which the human body defended itself from germs. He experimented with a variety of bacteria, and published many papers and a book promoting his phagocyte theory.

This theory was not well received by the German scientists who believed that immunity was caused by something in the blood. Although Metchnikoff had been born in Russia, he had become a patriotic Frenchman, and at that time the Germans and the French were antagonistic towards one another, because it was not long after the Franco Prussian War.

German scientists had evidence that there was something in the blood that killed germs, and they saw it as their patriotic duty to prove Metchnikoff's phagocyte theory wrong. A heated and not very polite debate carried on for many years. One side said that it was mobile cells that killed germs, and the other said that it was something in the blood which killed germs.

The Germans produced evidence that phagocytes do not always consume germs, and that the presence of blood makes phagocytes more effective, and that sometimes germs could be killed by the blood without phagocytes being present. The French on the other hand produced evidence that no matter how effectively blood could kill bacteria in a test tube, that did not necessarily mean that the owner of the blood would be able to resist the disease.

The Germans and the French were both right of course, but the war of words did not end with them realising that their respective discoveries were equally important. The war of words ended with the Germans winning, because their theory was commercially profitable. The great breakthrough for the "something in the blood" theory came when Emil von Behring and Shibasaburo Kitasato discovered that blood can make antibodies to diphtheria toxin and tetanus toxin. They claimed that antibodies to diphtheria were the only thing that a human needed in order to be immune to diphtheria. The year after antibodies were discovered, Robert Koch made a public announcement that the phagocyte theory was dead. Paul Ehrlich published diagrams of how he thought antibodies operated, and these pictures captured the imagination of laboratory workers around the world. His theory of how antibodies function is now known to be wrong, but the pictures had a profound impact at the time.

Although scientists continued to talk about phagocytes, research work focused on antibodies. Antibodies were much easier to study than phagocytes, and they were also more exciting because the blood can make antibodies in response to any substance. It can make antibodies to all naturally occurring substances, like germs or rabbit flesh or yeast, and it can make antibodies to man-made substances like plastic and neomycin. All that has to happen is that the substance be injected into the blood stream, and the blood will make antibodies to it. The substance that is injected is called an "antigen." The most important reason why antibodies became regarded as the way to measure immunity is that human beings can cause antibodies to be made. There is no commercial benefit to be gained from saying that phagocytes are of supreme importance to immunity when you cannot make phagocytes.

Because the phagocyte theory became unfashionable in 1891, research into phagocytes was neglected for 60 years, although the technology to do this research already existed in the 19th century. In the 1960s research into phagocytes started in earnest again,[165] and now there is consensus that phagocytes and antibodies are of equal importance to immunity. But the vaccine industry is not about to abandon the antibody theory.

Diphtheria is caused by the toxins that diphtheria germs produce, not directly by the germs themselves. When a person is infected with diphtheria, their blood begins to make antibodies to this toxin. The young vaccine industry called those antibodies "antitoxin," and they claimed that having antitoxin in the blood was the same thing as being immune to diphtheria. When clinical experience showed that having antibodies in the blood does not necessarily make a person immune to a disease, Bela Schick came up with an idea to make the antibody theory sound plausible. Bela Schick was a Hungarian scientist who became an American citizen in 1923. He said that a person had to have a certain density of antibodies in the blood in order to be able to fight germs successfully. If the number of antibodies in a millilitre of blood was below that critical threshold, then the person would contract the disease. If the number of antibodies in a millilitre of blood was above that critical threshold, then the person would not get the disease. He even went so far as to declare that the critical threshold for diphtheria was one thirtieth of a unit of antitoxin. So now instead of the antibody theory, we have the antibody threshold theory.

In 1924 a vaccine for diphtheria was introduced to Britain. The new vaccine was made from diphtheria toxin, and the idea was that the person who was injected with it would make antibodies to the toxin, and consequently be immune to diphtheria. Vaccinationists wrongly claim that the existence of this vaccine is the reason why diphtheria is rare nowadays. As the graphs in vaccine myth number four clearly demonstrate, vaccination has been irrelevant to the decline of diphtheria. When outbreaks of diphtheria do occur nowadays, it can be seen that vaccinated people are not protected. The ineffectiveness of the vaccine was more obvious in the early years of its existence, because diphtheria was still virulent in the environment.

In 1950 the Medical Research Council in Britain published the results of a ten year study that had been conducted by nine doctors to see if they could find an explanation for why vaccinated people get diphtheria.[124] The authors of the Medical Research Council study had expected to find that the vaccinated people who were suffering from diphtheria had low levels of antibody, and their contacts who did not catch diphtheria had high levels of antibody. They were hoping that they could explain to the public that the vaccinated people who got diphtheria were the ones who had failed to make enough antibodies when vaccinated.

> With a view to advancing the schemes for active immunisation then being initiated, and in order to encourage the more detailed investigation of cases of diphtheria which were being reported as occurring in inoculated persons, the Sub-committee offered to carry out certain examinations of pathological material from such cases. It was arranged that this service should consist of the examination of the bacterial flora of the nose and throat of the patient and the estimation of the circulating antitoxin of the serum separated from blood samples taken at the same time or, in any case, before diphtheria antitoxin had been administered as a therapeutic measure.[166]

The idea that there was an antibody threshold above which a person became immune to diphtheria had been accepted without question, and had become part of the medical dogma. In the preface to the Medical Research Council report, the authors state,

> Contrary to expectation it was found that quite a considerable proportion of cases of diphtheria occurred in inoculated persons who, judged by the antitoxin content of their serum, would normally be expected to be safe from attack.

They began the study by looking at the level of antitoxin in blood samples of 62 vaccinated people who were suffering from diphtheria in England and Wales. When the results were "paradoxical," they halted the investigation and reviewed their method.

The paradox was this: on repeated occasions it was found that a sample of serum, taken from a patient with a clear history of inoculation, who had yielded diphtheria bacilli from nose or throat swabs, and who according to the clinical history exhibited some or other of the classical symptoms of true diphtheria, was found to contain quite large quantities of diphtheria antitoxin. Now according to Schick, persons whose serum contains not less than one-thirtieth of a unit of antitoxin per ml. or, according to workers in this and other countries, persons whose serum contains not less than one-hundredth of a unit of antitoxin per ml., should not contract diphtheria. Yet of 62 of the patients investigated prior to April 1942 no less than 25 (40%) were found to contain one-tenth of a unit, or more, of diphtheria antitoxin per ml. of serum; and of these, 5 contained 10 units or more, 7 contained 1 to 4 units, and 13 contained 0.1 to 0.8 units per ml. of serum; there was no significant association, however, between severity and antitoxin content.[120]

So not only had they found that high levels of antibody did not prevent diphtheria, they also found that it did not make the disease milder. The table they provide shows that according to the dogma of the "workers in this and other countries," 69.3% had enough antibodies to make them immune to diphtheria, and 8% had more than a thousand times the density of antibody that is supposed to confer immunity. So instead of being able to explain away vaccine failures to the public, the authors found themselves in the possession of evidence that the antibody threshold theory is a load of hooey.

They decided that there must be some mistake in their method. They thought that perhaps the glass syringes that were used to draw the blood samples still had antitoxin clinging to them from the horse blood or human blood that had been in them during previous use. So they decided to set up a second investigation in which they would be sure that the syringe had been properly cleaned before the blood sample was taken from the diphtheria patient. The second part of the study focused on the geographical region of Newcastle and Gateshead, and they took great care to ensure that none of the equipment was contaminated with other blood.

The primary object of the second part of these investigations was to determine whether it is a fact that true clinical diphtheria occurs in patients whose serum contains a concentration of antitoxin in excess of the level originally laid down by Schick as providing adequate protection against the disease, viz. one-thirtieth of a unit of antitoxin per ml. It was considered that an answer to this question could be obtained if rigid adherence to certain conditions relating to the selection of patients and the collection of pathological material and its examination was observed.[167]

Well an answer to that question was obtained, and the answer was that true clinical diphtheria does occur in people who have more antitoxin in their blood than the cut off level "laid down" by Schick. They decided to keep the results from Gateshead and Newcastle separate, so that they would know there was a problem with their method if the results from the two regions were very different. The results from the two areas were the same. So this was really two studies, and they both proved the same thing. They both proved that being vaccinated, and having a high level of antibodies in the blood, does not protect a person from getting diphtheria. Some of these victims had one hundred and twenty times the density of antibody in the blood than that which should have protected them.[168]

Another thing which perplexed the researchers was that they found that many of the nurses and family members who were in close contact with the diphtheria patients, and had very low levels of antibody in their blood, and also had live diphtheria germs living in their throats, did not catch diphtheria.[169]

On page 154 of the Medical Research Council report they give the results of a study done in Copenhagen. The Danish study was more thorough than the British one because it used controls. They measured the antibody levels of four groups of people;

* the vaccinated with diphtheria,
* the vaccinated without diphtheria,
* the unvaccinated with diphtheria,
* and the unvaccinated without diphtheria.

They found that vaccinated people who had diphtheria had the same spread of levels of antibody as vaccinated people who did not have diphtheria, and both of these groups had much higher levels of antibody than the third and fourth groups. So this study proved conclusively that vaccination does produce antibodies, but it does not produce immunity.

They also refer to earlier studies which showed that the antibody threshold theory was wrong.

As long ago as 1920 Solis-Cohen et al. showed that the blood of some persons destroyed diphtheria bacilli whereas that of others did not and that the result was independent of the antitoxin content; others (Bloomfield, 1924; Arnold, Ostram and Singer, 1928) have emphasised the importance of the mucous membrane of the nose and throat in removing micro-organisms deliberately applied thereto, and Digby (1923) ascribed an important role to the tonsils and the subepithelial lymphoid tissue in effecting a similar clearance and destruction of micro-organisms.[170]

So as early as 1950 there already existed a weighty body of evidence which showed that vaccination against diphtheria is a useless procedure, and that the antibody threshold theory is baloney. Yet diphtheria vaccination is still forced on babies today. The Medical Research Council study of 1950 was done by nine doctors in a prestigious institution of orthodox medicine, yet it has been steadfastly ignored by the medical establishment. The lesson the medical establishment learned from this study is that they must not do studies on the relationship between antibodies and immunity, because maintaining the myth of the antibody threshold theory is essential for the promotion of vaccines. Subsequent evidence that the antibody threshold theory is false has emerged in anecdotal comments in reports on vaccine failure during epidemics.

In 1980 a vaccine promoter who was reviewing the history of measles vaccination in the USA, and making recommendations about future policy, had this to say,

> We must also acknowledge that questions remain about measles serology - for example, what titer shall we agree upon as the cutoff indicator of immunity?[134]

(Serology means study of the blood, and titer, in this context, means density of antibody.) If achieving a certain density of antibody in the blood actually means that the germs of that disease cannot replicate in the owner of the blood, then it should be possible, by doing research, to find out what that critical density is.

There is a book entitled *Antibodies and Immunity*,[171] which, judging by the title, I expected to discuss the relationship between antibodies and immunity. To my surprise I found that the book does not broach the issue of whether having a lot of antibodies prevents the disease. That is an assumption made by the writer before the book is written, and the validity of the assumption is not even considered in the book. On page 123 the author says,

> ... the progressive rise and fall of the level of antibodies in the serum after the injection of a powerful vaccine ... has fascinated students of immunology for 50 years, and ever more detailed

analysis has given us deep and precise insights into the cellular events of antibody production.[171]

Quite true. They love those graphs of the rise and fall of antibodies. They produce them at every opportunity to show how wonderful vaccines are. A great deal is now known about the way that cells make antibodies, but they have forgotten to consider whether the graphs represent anything of relevance to human health. There is still no evidence that the *number* of antibodies that are created reflects the level of immunity.

Antibodies can do many different things. They can cover an invading germ to make it easier for the scavenger cells of the immune system to eat it. They can attract complement proteins towards a spot on the surface of a bacteria, and the complement proteins then punch a hole in the bacteria and make it explode. They can also immobilise a virus by grabbing hold of certain points on the virus and making it impossible for it to reproduce.[171] All of this is very useful, but the fact that antibodies can do these and other things does not automatically mean that having a certain number of antibodies in the blood will prevent the clinical symptoms of disease from developing in any particular human being.

There is a genetically inherited condition which makes a person unable to manufacture antibodies of any kind. Children who have this condition can have measles in the normal way, and acquire immunity despite not manufacturing any antibodies.[172,173] This shows that something else is providing the immunity.

When a person's blood makes antibodies, the medical jargon used to describe the event is "seroconversion." Another phrase that crops up in vaccination talk is "immunogenic efficacy." This is medical jargon for "effectiveness at causing immunity." Before a new vaccine is marketed, it is tested to see whether it makes "enough" antibodies. The density of antibodies that is going to be accepted as "enough" is not decided by clinical experimentation. If the vaccine creates "enough" antibodies in 80% of the test people, then they say, "The immunogenic efficacy of the vaccine is 80%."

The idea that antibodies are all that has to be considered in immunity has become so ingrained in the thinking of vaccinationists, that they consider the words "antibodies" and "immunity" to be interchangeable. In many articles in medical journals they use the word "immunity," when they are really talking about the level of antibodies. This skewed thinking leads to mental confusion in the bureaucrats who administer orthodox medicine.

An example of this skewed thinking occurred after the Immunisation Awareness Society compiled a fact sheet about the MMR vaccine for distribution in New Zealand schools. The Chief Medical Advisor to the

Health Department wrote a rebuttal of our fact sheet which tried to convince parents that they should not believe what we had written. One of the points our fact sheet made is that the measles vaccine does not prevent measles, it merely postpones measles till the person is older than the usual age for measles. The way that the medical advisor tried to refute that point was by saying that the vaccine "has been shown to produce antibodies in over 90-95 percent of those who are vaccinated." This indicates that he believes that manufacturing antibodies is the same thing as acquiring life-long immunity. What was especially amazing about this clumsy rebuttal was that it was made soon after an epidemic of measles in New Zealand had demonstrated that vaccinated children got measles as adolescents, while unvaccinated children got measles as preschoolers, or in the early years of school.

Shortly before the measles epidemic started, I gave a talk about the wrongs of vaccination to a group of nurses. This was followed by a talk on the virtues of vaccination, given by a doctor. Instead of trying to refute the information I had presented, the doctor spent her part of the talk drawing graphs on a blackboard showing what antibody levels do in the majority of people after the injections. She explained that live viral vaccines are given once only because they create "enough" antibodies at the first shot, while other vaccines are given three times because a first sensitisation gives only a few antibodies, but subsequent doses create sufficient antibodies.

I was entertained by the body language of the audience while she spoke. My supporters from the Immunisation Awareness Society flopped with despondency. The young nurses who doubted the wisdom of vaccination looked bored because they had heard all this claptrap before, but the nurses who loved vaccination sat bolt upright, with their ears perked up and their eyes bright. They lapped it up because it justifies what they do all day.

On each of the graphs the doctor drew a line at the level at which immunity is supposed to be achieved. When she was discussing the polio graph, I asked her if she knew of any studies which confirmed that that particular level of polio antibodies really does cause clinical immunity. She replied that she did not. I commented that I had been looking for such a study and had not been able to find one. She was completely unperturbed by the lack of evidence to support the dogma. I suppose that she thinks that because so many people in the medical profession believe the dogma, there must be some evidence to support it somewhere.

During the measles epidemic that started a few weeks after this gathering, half the reported cases occurred in vaccinated children. This made the Health Department change its policy to saying that two doses of measles vaccine are necessary. So the dogma that says that live viral vaccine is needed once only was thrown out of the window, but they still love the graphs.

There are accounts of women with high levels of antibody getting rubella during pregnancy and the baby being born with congenital rubella syndrome.[96,97,98,99,100,101] The myth that antibody levels reflect immunity will continue to be accepted by the government officials who buy vaccines from the manufacturers until the consumer brings about a change.

Before antitoxin and antibodies were discovered, the medical profession used a different, but just as unscientific, theory to decide whether or not a vaccine had caused immunity. If scratching smallpox pus into the skin caused a flare up around the scratch, then it was said that the vaccine had "taken," and the vaccinator could be satisfied with his handiwork. If there was no reaction on the skin, then it meant that the vaccine had not taken, and it needed to be done again. They never had any scientific basis for this theory, they just made it up. Perhaps it originated as a way of pacifying people who were unhappy about the pain that the flare-up caused.

Some enlightening figures were collected during an outbreak of smallpox in Italy that ran from 1887 to 1889. Before the outbreak started, 98.5% of the general population had been vaccinated at least once, and many had been vaccinated more than once. All soldiers were vaccinated every six months. The Italian army kept a record of whose vaccinations had "taken" and whose had not. During the epidemic, 47,772 people died of smallpox.[174] Among the soldiers, the rate of smallpox was greater in those whose vaccinations had "taken," and out of those who got the disease, the death rate was twice as high in those whose vaccinations had "taken."[174] So we can see that it is not true that a bad reaction to smallpox vaccination means that the vaccination has created immunity.

"THE VACCINE FAILED BECAUSE ....."

Vaccine Myth number Eight: The vaccine failed because the person had not had enough doses. We now know that you need two/four/five doses of that vaccine to become immune. The vaccine could not have been properly stored if it failed after so many doses. The vaccine did not work because it was given at the wrong age. The strain that made the disease break out must be different to the strain in the vaccine.

The vaccine industry claims that the reason why most people are not suffering from infectious diseases is because of vaccination, when in fact most of the time there is no virulent naturally occurring germ in the environment to test whether or not people are immune. A vaccine only gets an opportunity to fail when the disease comes into the environment. Very few people ever experience an infectious disease other than flu and the childhood illnesses. When an epidemic of one of the less common infectious diseases breaks out, only a tiny proportion of people actually come down with the prevailing malady. The exception to this is bubonic plague, which at the peak of its wave affected a high proportion of the population.

When a germ does become virulent, and an outbreak of the disease occurs, vaccinated people get the disease. In some circumstances the medical authorities feel compelled to make excuses for the failure of the vaccine. I have encountered thirteen excuses to which vaccinationists resort when they are confronted with evidence that vaccination does not work. During epidemics they often use more than one excuse at a time.

Excuse number 1: "The cold chain must have been broken."

This is an excellent excuse because it is hard to prove that the cold chain was not broken. They say that each vial of vaccine must be kept at a temperature below 4°C from the time it leaves the manufacturer until the time it is used, or else it will lose its virulence. In the absence of any investigation it is easy to say that someone in the transport line must have left the vial of vaccine out of the fridge for a while, and hence the cold chain got broken.

During the 1982 polio epidemic in South Africa, the medicrats said that polio was affecting the immunised because "the cold chain must have been broken." They collected 17 vials of vaccine from remote outposts, and brought them back to Johannesburg, making sure that the cold chain was not broken on the way back.[175] These were tested for virulence by seeing how much virus could be grown from the vaccine, and by being injected into children who had no antibodies to polio at all. The virus colonies grown from half of the vials were not dense enough to meet the internationally accepted "titre," but all of the children manufactured a satisfactory level of antibodies, so a conclusion about whether the cold chain had been broken could not be made. They then took strong measures to protect the cold chain, so this particular excuse was not available to explain away the failure of the vaccine during the next polio epidemic, which occurred in 1987 (see below).

One of the excuses for the failure of measles vaccination in New Zealand in 1991 was that the vaccine gets warm when it travels by ship from Europe. If that is so, then according to their dogma, there is no point in importing the vaccine. They might as well stop subjecting the children of New Zealand to the risk of side effects.

Excuse number 2: "It must be a different strain."

This one amuses me because vaccination started off with the claim that cowpox could cause immunity to smallpox, but when it suits them they do a complete turn around and say that in order to create antibodies which will be effective, the surface antigen of the germ in the vaccine has to be exactly the same as the surface antigen of the invading germ. In other words, the germ that happens to come along years later and tries to cause disease, has to be the same strain as the germ which was in the vaccine, or else the antibodies will not work.

The "different strain" excuse is frequently used for whooping cough in immunised children, and now they are even beginning to use it for measles. It is not a popular excuse with the makers of measles vaccine, because they stand to gain financially from the introduction of repeated doses of vaccine. So they tend to support the "waning-immunity-which-needs-a-booster-shot" line.

The whooping cough vaccine contains a bacterium called bordatella pertussis. Whooping cough can be caused by bordatella pertussis, by bordatella parapertussis, or by an adenovirus. A natural dose of whooping cough creates life-long immunity, no matter which of the three strains sparked off the disease. The vaccinationists choose to forget this when they blame a "different strain" for causing whooping cough in a vaccinated child.

A natural dose of measles is caused by only one strain, yet it confers life-long immunity to all the strains of measles virus. The reason why vaccines for childhood illnesses do not confer life-long immunity, while a natural infection with the disease does, is not known. One theory is that an injected vaccine bypasses the mucous membranes, and therefore does not go through the initial processing which a natural infection does. The lining of the nasal passages, throat, and digestive tract contain different aspects of the immune system to what the blood contains. For example, there is Immunoglobulin A in the mucous membranes, but Immunoglobulin G and Immunoglobulin M in the blood.

All the childhood illnesses are caused by germs that float in the air. They enter the human body via the mouth and nose, so they meet the immune system in the mucous membranes, and the germs spend a few days in this area before they move on to meet the different features of the immune system in the blood. It is theorised that something happens in those few days which makes the immune system able to mount life-long immunity after the encounter with the blood. The significance of different types of antibodies and different types of immunoglobulin is beginning to attract research.

Another theory as to why a natural infection causes life-long immunity is that the process which creates the symptoms of each childhood disease also causes something else to happen which has not yet been detected. The vaccine industry has little incentive for researching how life-long immunity is generated, nor why vaccines for childhood illnesses do succeed in creating temporary immunity.

Medical dogma says that a person who swallows the oral polio vaccine, which contains three strains of polio virus, can only make antibodies to one strain at a time. They also say that having antibodies to that particular strain does not make a person immune to the other two strains. They say that is why a person has to have three doses of vaccine, and cannot be considered "immune to polio" after swallowing only one or two doses. This is a useful excuse when children who have had one or two doses of vaccine get polio, but it becomes obsolete when children who have had three, four or five doses of vaccine get polio.

When I first heard the claim that the human immune system can only make antibodies to one strain of polio at a time, I naively believed it, although I thought it was strange because the body can make antibodies to nine different diseases at the same time. This anomaly niggled in my mind until I read the official report of the 1982 polio epidemic in Gazankulu, South Africa, in which the authors describe the tests they did to see whether vials of vaccine had lost their virulence. Thirty percent of the children who had no antibodies at all before vaccination, developed antibodies to all three strains after one dose. The report comments that this was consistent with previous observations made by the professor.[175] So we see that this excuse is not valid.

Excuse number 3: "Too few doses of vaccine were given."

For each vaccine there is a certain number of doses which is regarded as "scientifically correct." A plausible sounding reason is given for declaring that that particular number of doses creates immunity to that particular disease. But the number changes when the real world intervenes and demonstrates that the alleged magic number of doses does not cause immunity. When they change the number they also change the reason.

At the beginning of 1991, the dogma in New Zealand was that one dose of measles vaccine was sufficient to create life-long immunity, because it is a live virus vaccine. This was old fashioned dogma which had already been discarded in the USA. When the 1991 measles epidemic showed the vaccine to be useless, the dogma was changed to say that a second dose had to be given. Now some governments are adamantly claiming that two doses of measles vaccine will give lifelong immunity. But it has already been seen that children who have had three doses of measles vaccine get measles.[176]

As mentioned above, the theory behind giving three doses of polio vaccine is that human blood can only make antibodies to one of the three strains of polio virus at a time, which sounds plausible enough until you know that this is not true and that blood can make antibodies to all three strains at the same time. When an epidemic of polio breaks out, and people who have had three doses of vaccine start getting polio, they increase the number of doses needed to cause immunity to polio to four. As they have then run out of strains to blame, they stick to talking about "doses" and avoid mentioning strains.

The rationale behind giving whooping cough and diphtheria vaccine three times was that the first shot only creates a small number of antibodies, while the second and third shots greatly increase the density of antibodies in the blood. But now they give the vaccine four times, and five times in some countries, because three doses does not work. When the whooping cough vaccine was first introduced, it was given to babies of six months. At that age the first dose does make a lot of antibodies. When the age for the first shot was brought down to six weeks, it was found that such young babies could not make antibodies, hence the introduction of a second and then a third dose. Running alongside all this unscientific claptrap about antibody levels and doses is a complete disregard for the fact that the vaccine causes far more cases of brain damage at six weeks of age than it does at six months of age.

Excuse number 4: "The victims did not create enough antibodies when they were vaccinated."

The antibody threshold theory is the commercial backbone of the vaccine industry, which is why I devoted considerable space in vaccine myth number seven to tracing its historical origins and exposing the myth. This excuse is not valid, because the level of antibodies in the blood is not a reflection of the level of immunity.

Excuse number 5: "It was given at the wrong age."

This excuse lasts until children who were vaccinated at the latest "correct age" get the disease. Then they have to change the "correct age" yet again, or revert to other excuses.

I have described how after the measles vaccine had been used for a year in the USA, the "correct age" for vaccination was set at 10 months. Then it was moved to 12 months, then it was moved to 15 months, but children still got measles. Then they realised they would be making good and proper fools of themselves if they raised it to 18 months, so they opted for a booster dose at the age of 11 years, instead of altering the "correct age" yet again.

New Zealand went through almost the same scenario. When the vaccine was first introduced it was given at ten months, but then they changed the "correct age" to 12 months. Then it was changed to 15 months, and then to 15 months plus a booster at 11 years. They lagged a decade behind the USA with each policy change. If a child is vaccinated at 15 months, then gets measles at the age of eight years, they recommend that he or she should still have the booster dose at 11 years. Some children get measles before the age of 15 months, and the Health Department recommends that they should still be vaccinated.

Some countries say that eleven years is the "wrong age" for the second dose, and giving the second dose when children are much younger will solve the problem. They are combining the "incorrect age" excuse with the "too few doses" excuse. Australia has introduced the second dose at the age of 4 years, and is claiming that this will give life-long immunity. They are saying in their promotional literature that having the second dose at 4 years means the recipients will not need another dose when they are young adults. We will have to wait to see what they say when these 4-year-olds become young adults.

It is not ideal for babies to get measles during the first year of life,[1] and when a woman has a baby before she has had measles, the baby is vulnerable to getting measles during the first year.[177] Now that the measles vaccine has existed for more than a generation, a new scenario is happening. Babies of vaccinated mothers who have not yet had measles are getting measles very early on, and suffering from a high rate of complications and death.[119,178]

Excuse number 6: "The vaccine was improperly handled."

This is a great excuse because it does not mean anything. It is used surprisingly often. People who are impressed by medical qualifications might think this statement has great import when it emanates from medically dignified vocal cords.

Excuse number 7: "The vaccine must have been overdiluted."

Do they mean that the total amount of the original substance was used but too much liquid was added, or that less than the total amount of the original was used before it was diluted? In the case of a live viral vaccine it is of no consequence anyway, because the virus starts to replicate once it gets into the body, and you end up with an unpredictable "dose."

With killed vaccines, dilution is also irrelevant, because the vaccine industry has never bothered to work out a "correct dose" per body weight. A six-week-old baby gets injected with the same amount as a five-year-old child.

In every instance where I have seen this excuse used, there has been no mention of any investigation into whether or not the vaccine really was diluted.

Excuse number 8: "The vaccination rate in the community was too low to create herd immunity."

The brilliant logic of this excuse is that the unvaccinated children caused the vaccinated children to get the disease, whereas if there had only been a few unvaccinated children, they would not have been able to cause the vaccinated children to get the disease.

The myth of herd immunity is used as a weapon against health conscious families. Therefore I have discussed it in detail in vaccine myth number six.

Excuse number 9: "It must have been a bad batch."

This is usually an excuse made for bad side effects, but it is sometimes used for vaccine failures. I have never seen this excuse used in conjunction with an investigation into whether or not all the people who caught the disease when the germ became virulent were injected with the same batch.

Excuse number 10: "He had not had time to develop immunity yet."

This excuse was introduced to explain away the failure of Louis Pasteur's rabies vaccine,[179] and it has been used ever since to reduce the figure of vaccine failures. An arbitrary length of time is chosen in which "immunity" is said to develop, and anyone who gets the disease within that time period after vaccination is not counted as a vaccine failure.

This is a particularly good excuse for them to use when a mass vaccination campaign is started up during an epidemic. Most of the vaccine failures can be excused away, because most of the vaccinated people who got the disease had been vaccinated "too recently." Epidemics always come to an end, and then they say that those who were vaccinated during the campaign, and did not get the disease, were protected by the vaccine, while at the same time saying that those who were vaccinated during the campaign, and did get the disease, were not protected because they had not had time to develop immunity.

This excuse is also used when the vaccine causes the disease it was supposed to prevent. A natural infection takes a while to incubate, so they say that the person must have been exposed before they were vaccinated. The germs in the vaccine go straight into the blood, so in a person who is susceptible to getting the disease from the vaccine, the symptoms show up quickly. When this happens, the vaccinators say that the injected germs did not cause the symptoms. They say it was just that the person "had not yet had time to develop immunity." Doctors even sometimes say this when it happens in the absence of an epidemic.

Excuse number 11: "The wrong type of vaccine was used."

This is a useful excuse for those cases of measles that occur in the now older age group who were injected with killed virus measles vaccine, before live viral vaccine was invented. The converse does not happen. When a person who was injected with live virus vaccine gets measles, they do not make the excuse that killed virus vaccine should have been used, because killed virus vaccine is definitely out of favour.

The makers of oral polio vaccine and the makers of injected polio vaccine accuse each other of providing "the wrong type of vaccine." Although injected polio vaccine was ditched in most countries 40 years ago, it has made a comeback in some affluent countries, and is being used in impoverished countries where infections of the digestive tract are common. The given reason for the latter is that when a person has diarrhoea, the oral vaccine passes out of the body too quickly for antibodies to be formed. So with each epidemic, the manufacturers of the type of vaccine that was not used in the affected area, can claim that the other type of vaccine is no good.

Excuse number 12: "The parents might have falsified vaccination certificates."

I have only seen this excuse used once, in a letter to the editor of a medical journal.[180] He was referring to a previous article about an outbreak in a high school with a 100% vaccination rate. His argument was that he had once come across a group of parents who opposed vaccination for non-religious reasons, and he had "reason to believe" that some of them had falsified vaccination certificates. He apparently realises that this is a rather feeble excuse, because towards the end of his letter he says, "It is not likely that falsification of immunization records occurred to an extent sufficient to alter the results of the study."

Excuse number 13. "The vaccine was injected into the wrong part of the body."

The theory of vaccination is that it primes the whole body to resist infection.

EXCUSES FOR THE FAILURE OF MEASLES VACCINE

When there is no virulent wild measles virus in the environment, there is also no epidemic, and at these times the vaccine is said to be very successful. But when the measles virus becomes virulent in an area that has practiced vaccination, it becomes clear that measles vaccine causes individuals to get measles when they are older than the natural age for measles.

No matter in which part of the world the epidemic occurs, the statistics always show the same pattern. MMWR is a weekly publication produced by the Centers for Disease Control in Atlanta, USA. It publishes articles about diseases in all countries, not only in the USA. I read through all the data on measles epidemics in all the issues of MMWR published since the measles vaccine was invented. They all show the same thing; the bulk of vaccinated people with measles are in their teens or they are young adults, while the bulk of unvaccinated people with measles are children. It makes no difference what language the people speak, nor at what age the first jab is given, nor whether booster jabs are given to try and bolster waning immunity.

In 1991 there was a measles epidemic in New Zealand which clearly showed that the vaccine failed. The vaccinationists saw the epidemic as an opportunity to promote vaccination. They staged a brilliant campaign which succeeded in causing panic in many parents. Three months after the measles epidemic started, they conducted a five day blast in the media. On a Monday morning New Zealanders woke up to the "news" that a deadly virus had suddenly broken out and was sweeping through the population like a terrible reaper. Radio, TV and newspapers made it a prime news story. Civil defence vans with loud hailers built into their roofs cruised the streets of the poorer areas of Auckland, telling the population that a killer virus was on the rampage, and children needed an injection to be protected. The vans reminded me of the Casspirs that used to patrol the black townships in South Africa, except that instead of spewing out teargas, they were spewing out lies. And just like in Soweto, children were the targeted victims. The existence of these vehicles in New Zealand is justified by the threat from earthquakes and volcanoes, but they were being misused to promote a pharmaceutical product.

The propagandists said that even if children were already vaccinated, they should be done again, or they could die. People flocked in droves to vaccination clinics. Even little children who had been done only a year before, were done again. It did not seem to bother the parents that the first dose their children had been given, had been given with the promise of life-long immunity. Afterwards it was left to the committee of the Immunisation Awareness Society (IAS) to give emotional support to the parents of those who were severely brain damaged by the vaccine during the campaign.

The high intensity part of the campaign ended on the Friday of that week, with the announcement that the vaccination campaign had been successful, and the epidemic was now under control. In the following week, more new cases of measles broke out than had broken out during the propaganda week, but the media kept quiet about it.

If the Health Department had been honest they would have said;

* a measles epidemic started three months ago, and it has not yet reached its peak,
* vaccinated and unvaccinated children are getting measles,
* if children are not properly cared for while they have measles they can die,
* being vaccinated makes people get measles at an older age.

IAS tried to get these four points across to the public, but the brain dead media was not interested in allowing the public to have access to the facts. The media only repeated whatever came from the Health Department.

Sociologist Kevin Dew wrote his thesis about the Health Department's fear mongering campaign and about IAS's attempts to provide the public with factual information.[181] Kevin conducts his research without making the prior assumption that vaccination is safe and effective. He is in good company with writers like Herbert Spencer and Beatrix Potter. In his thesis he evaluated the validity of claims made by the Health Department against the findings of scientific studies. He showed how the Health Department created the "problem," and then presented themselves as having the "solution," due to their "superior knowledge." They then defined those who did not comply with the "solution" as deviants. He showed how the Health Department used the media as an agent of moral indignation, and how successful the campaign was as a means of achieving social control. He described how the Health Department tried to use him as part of their propaganda exercise as soon as they knew that he was writing about them. He remarked that studying the Health Department felt like being embroiled in politicking, whereas studying the IAS felt like doing research.

The epidemic lasted another eight months, and everybody knew someone who got measles. People were talking about the fact that vaccinated children were getting the measles "very badly." Some medicrats started to mutter excuses for the failure of the vaccine. The chosen excuses were;

*   The vaccine was given at the wrong age because in those days they did not know how to do things properly. (Half of the vaccinated children with measles had in fact been vaccinated at what was considered to be the "correct age" at the time of the epidemic.)
*   The vaccine had been "wrongly handled."
*   Unvaccinated children had caused the epidemic to break out and had made vaccinated children get it.
*   The vaccine had baked in the sun on the ships on the way from Europe.
*   and then finally they announced that one dose of vaccine was not enough, and a booster had to be given at age eleven, even to children who had already had measles as well as the vaccine.

A very promising young Auckland gymnast was prevented from participating in the Olympic games in Barcelona because she caught measles during this epidemic. New Zealanders had been very excited about her talent for gymnastics because she was said to be the best in the world and they were hoping she would win a gold medal. First she had to participate in trials in the USA in order to qualify for the Olympics. She had no symptoms when she departed for the USA, but she came out in spots and a fever once she got there, and was unable to participate. Her father said, "It's just one of those things. Her Plunket records show she was vaccinated at 11 months and the experts now say it should be 15 months."[182] What these self proclaimed "experts" were not telling the poor man is that thousands of children who had been vaccinated at the "correct age" of 15 months were also getting measles. They also did not tell him that if his daughter had never been vaccinated, she would most likely have had measles when she was much younger, and it would not have been able to interfere with her career later on. To all the wrongs which the measles vaccine has done, we can add that it robbed New Zealand of the chance to win a gold medal for gymnastics at the Barcelona Olympics.

The measles epidemic lasted 11 months, with 8000 cases, which is a significant number in a small country like New Zealand. At the beginning of the epidemic, New Zealand Health Department dogma still adhered to the belief that one dose of vaccine at the age of 15 months would give life-long immunity, because it is a live viral vaccine. But the statistics showed that half the children who got measles were teenagers who had been vaccinated, and half again had been vaccinated at the "correct age" of 15 months, while the others had been vaccinated at 12 months. The unvaccinated children who got measles were all younger than teenagers, as nature intended it.

The official report of the Communicable Disease Centre[183] did not publish the figures. The report stated that the epidemic had occurred because not enough children aged 12 - 15 months had been vaccinated, and because only 82% of children had been vaccinated by their second birthday. Towards the end of the report an evasive admission was made,

In addition to the failure to achieve high vaccination coverage levels, there is some evidence that primary and/or secondary vaccine failure also contributed to this epidemic, especially among older persons. To this end, the Department of Health recently announced a two-dose schedule for MMR vaccination, with the first dose to be administered at 12-15 months of age and the second to be given to *all* children at Form 1 [age 11].[183]

The term "primary vaccine failure" is used to describe a situation where a person does not make antibodies at the time of vaccination. "Secondary vaccine failure" is the terminology used when the person made antibodies at the time of vaccination, but the antibodies are presumed to have diminished in the blood before the disease was contracted. "Tertiary vaccine failure" is a term which is not used in medical jargon, but it should be used. It describes the situation where a person made lots of antibodies at the time of vaccination, and the antibodies were still there when the person got the disease. It is not generally acknowledged that people with a high level of antibodies can get measles, but it is documented.[184]

In New Zealand they publicly stated that the jab for 11-year-olds was being introduced because measles vaccine does not confer life-long immunity. Only a few months after it had been introduced, they started saying that it had been introduced purely as a catch up dose for the 40% of children who had missed out on the first dose. (Their own figures showed that only 18% had been missed.) From then on public health nurses and practice nurses were taught that the reason for giving the second dose is that 40% of children miss out on the first dose.

In Australia the second dose was introduced at the age of four years, with the promise that it would give life-long immunity, and children who have it will not need to be vaccinated again when they are young adults. We shall see.

Between 1975 and 1988, children in Finland were given two or three doses of measles vaccine before the age of seven.[176] No-one was vaccinated under the age of 14 months. In 1988 the measles virus became virulent in Finland, and thousands of children got measles. Some of the children who got it had had three doses of vaccine.[176]

In the 1999 measles epidemic in Melbourne, 84% of the reported cases were in people aged 18 to 30,[185] and in the 2001 epidemic in Melbourne, 88% were aged 18 to 34.[186] The official figures do not include cases of measles in vaccine free children whose parents kept their children well away from the medical establishment. The proportion of cases in young adults would have been lower if all children with measles had been included in the data. Nevertheless, the cases in young adults show that vaccine induced immunity wears off. After the 2001 outbreak, the health department put out a press release which urged young adults to roll up their sleeves for a second jab. The press release also said that people over the age of 34 did not need to worry because they had not been vaccinated, and therefore had lifelong immunity.

After a measles outbreak in Illinois, USA, the medical authorities investigated the circumstances of the outbreak to see if they could find out why the vaccine had failed.[136] They explored a number of possible excuses, but none could be applied. They could not use the excuse that the vaccination rate was too low. They investigated whether the vaccine had been injected at the wrong age, but found that all the high school students with measles had been vaccinated after the age of 15 months. They found they could not use the excuse that the vaccine had been "improperly stored," nor that globulin had been given at the same time as the vaccine, nor that the killed virus vaccine had been used.

They wondered if the people with measles had all been vaccinated with a "faulty vaccine lot," but the cases had all been vaccinated at different times from different batches. They use some rather contorted reasoning to discount the possibility that the failure could have been caused by waning immunity, and then they come up with a pathetic alternative; "chance clustering." "This outbreak may have resulted from chance clustering of otherwise randomly distributed vaccine failures in the community." They eagerly note that a lot of the high school students did not get measles, but they are forgetting that those teenagers who have not yet had measles still have many years of life ahead of them in which the artificially induced immunity will wear off.

Some American medical authorities use doublespeak terminology to conceal the failure of measles vaccine. They categorise cases of measles into "preventable" and "non-preventable." Their definition of preventable cases are those which occur in people who were not vaccinated, or who were vaccinated at an age that has since become known as the "wrong age." Their definition of "non-preventable" cases are those who got the disease despite being vaccinated at the "right age," or who were too young to have been vaccinated. So by dividing cases during an epidemic into "preventable" and "non-preventable," they avoid having to say what percentage of the cases occurred in vaccinated children. It makes it impossible for a reader to know how spectacularly the vaccine failed. If they say, for instance, that 70% of the cases were "non-preventable," the reader does not know what percentage were vaccinated, and what percentage were below the age for vaccination.

The Australian medicrats also use this terminology. When a vaccinated person gets measles they call it "non-preventable."[187] It is illogical to say that cases in the unvaccinated could have been prevented, when the vaccine has not worked in the "non-preventable" cases.

WHEN WHOOPING COUGH VACCINE FAILS

There is no need to make excuses for the failure of this vaccine when the condition is diagnosed as "viral whooping cough syndrome" or "croup." But when they can bring themselves to admit that it really is whooping cough, they often say that the child has caught a different strain to the one that was in the vaccine.

Sometimes the doctor changes the diagnosis as soon as she or he learns that the child is "fully immunised."

"He's got whooping cough! You should have had him immunised, you silly woman."
"But doctor, I did have him immunised."
"Oh well then it can't be whooping cough."

My friend Jeannette took her two children to the doctor when they had whooping cough because she wanted to get a certificate saying that they had had whooping cough. The elder child is vaccinated, while the younger child is not. This placed the doctor in a quandary because he wanted to say that the younger one had whooping cough but the older one had something else. By the end of the consultation he grudgingly agreed that both children had whooping cough. Where doctors are required to report cases of whooping cough to the authorities, they are more inclined to report cases in the unvaccinated than in the vaccinated.[188]

I was injected with one dose of DPT vaccine as a baby, and got whooping cough at the age of 33. It was called "viral whooping cough syndrome" because I was vaccinated, and because, although I whooped for over a month, I only threw up after each whoop for a few days. Chandra was four years old and she caught it from me, and she had the classic symptoms of whooping cough which lasted for months. So the germ I passed on to her suddenly reverted from being a virus to being a bacteria? I don't think so.

During the 1990-91 outbreak of whooping cough in New Zealand, I estimated that about half the cases in our area were occurring in vaccinated children. I tried to get the local medicrats to collect some figures, but they were not interested. Of course knowing what percentage of the people with whooping cough were previously vaccinated does not tell one the failure rate of the vaccine. To work that out, you need to know what percentage of the children and adults who live in the area are vaccinated, and how many of them have had whooping cough before. Another thing you need to know is how many of the children who do not get whooping cough during the current outbreak are going to get it when the disease comes back in about four years time. So it is actually not possible to know the failure rate of the vaccine without doing a large demographic study over 20 years.

While I was dreaming of collecting statistics in Auckland, two medicrats in Wellington were collecting data in their area, and they very obligingly published them in April 1991.[189] Near the beginning of the outbreak, whooping cough was made a notifiable disease in the Wellington area.

At that time the New Zealand schedule gave three doses of DPT before the age of five months, and considered someone who has had three doses to be "fully immunised." In this survey, only children who had proof of three doses of vaccine were classified as "immunised." Those who had had one or two doses, or were unsure of their vaccination history, were classified as "unimmunised." Of the 47 cases in individuals aged over 5 months, 30 were "immunised" and 17 were "unimmunised." Ten other cases were reported in babies under the age of 5 months. The number of doses of DPT vaccine each of these babies had had was not published.

So this means that 63% of the children with whooping cough, who were old enough to have had three doses, were "fully immunised." Now to some people these figures would imply that there is not much point in running the risk of a reaction to this vaccine, and it is a waste of time and taxpayers' money. But the medicrats said that the survey showed that it would be a good idea to accelerate the vaccination schedule so that babies are "fully immunised" by the age of three months, and to introduce a booster dose at the age of five years. One of the reasons they gave for this recommendation is that babies do not receive natural immunity from mothers who have been immunised.

In the USA they have a different definition of "fully immunised," with five doses of DPT being the required number for a preschooler. Sometimes the American authorities investigate and publish the details of whooping cough outbreaks. An outbreak which occurred in Oklahoma in 1983 was one that was investigated. Out of the cases with a known vaccination history, 36% were fully immunised according to the schedule, and another 46% had had some doses, with only 18% being unvaccinated.[190]

The chosen excuse for this Oklahoma epidemic was "low immunization levels in children appear to have been a major factor associated with this outbreak." But quite the opposite is true. The fact that there was a low background vaccination rate, and yet so many of the cases occurred in vaccinated children, is evidence that the low vaccination rate was not the cause of the outbreak. They did two surveys to find out what percentage of the background population was immunised. One came up with 65% and the other came up with 49%. If the latter figure is chosen (to be charitable to the vaccinationists), it can mathematically be said that this shows that the vaccine is 15% effective. That is without taking into account that those who were "protected" during this epidemic could still get it during a later epidemic.

The natural decline of whooping cough which has been happening since 1878 is a factor which the medicrats always choose to ignore when considering vaccine effectiveness. An outbreak of whooping cough in a community in Massachusetts in 1992 was another one that was investigated and published.[191] The report does not give the background vaccination rate, but it says that 96% of the school students with whooping cough had had "four or more" doses of the vaccine. Some vaccinationists want to introduce "routine booster immunization throughout life."[192] I will not be among their customers.

They could not use the "low vaccination rate" excuse in the 1991 epidemic in Cape Town, South Africa, because the vaccine failed against a high background vaccination rate. At that time someone who had had 3 doses was regarded as "fully immunised." 94.9% of the child population had had at least three doses of DPT. In this epidemic, 45% of those with whooping cough who were old enough to have had at least one dose, had had three or four doses.[164] At that time laboratory facilities for diagnosis of whooping cough were not available for black children, so the excuse was made that the cases of whooping cough in the vaccinated may have been caused by other germs. What people are forgetting when they come up with this excuse is that a natural dose of whooping cough causes lifelong immunity to all the germs that cause whooping cough, not only to the strain that caused the person to get the illness.

EXCUSES FOR THE FAILURE OF POLIO VACCINE

The polio vaccine is only put to the test when there is an outbreak of polio. Such an event happened in the summer of 1987-88, in the eastern half of Southern Africa. This is a lush, tropical region, (unlike the arid western half,) where millions of disenfranchised people lived in appalling slums. At that time South Africa was controlled by an illegitimate government which imposed a political system called apartheid. South Africa was theoretically partitioned off into "bantustans." "Bantustans" were invented by a psychopath named Verwoerd who wanted all the blacks in South Africa to be herded into small areas that would be granted "independence." Verwoerd deluded himself that this would make the international community start approving of apartheid, because with the blacks "gone" from South Africa, the whites would be seen as a majority, not a minority. The biggest bantustan was called KwaZulu, and it consisted of twenty-nine separate geographical areas, which were dotted around in the "white" province called Natal. Nowadays the whole region is called KwaZulu-Natal.

During the 1987-88 polio epidemic, every case of polio that was detected in South Africa or in the "bantustans" was typed into a computer in Cape Town. Flu symptoms and weakness of limbs without laboratory confirmation was classified as a suspected case of polio. If the symptom of flaccid paralysis was present, laboratory confirmation was not necessary for it to be recorded as a definite case of polio. This is a sensible approach to collecting polio statistics, but their common sense deserts them when it comes to explaining polio in the vaccinated.

The previous polio epidemic had occurred in 1982. The excuses for the failure of the vaccine during that one were that the vaccination rate was too low, and "the cold chain must have been broken." After the 1982 epidemic, a concerted effort was made to increase vaccination coverage, and to ensure that the cold chain was not broken. The latter had required a tremendous effort because of the warm climate and lack of electricity in far flung clinics. Their success meant they could not use the "cold chain must have been broken" excuse, nor the "lack of herd immunity" excuse, because they had themselves eliminated these excuses after 1982.

When the polio virus became naturally virulent again in 1987, the newspapers did some scaremongering about the extent of the epidemic, and the need for immunisation. There were the usual quotes from "medical experts" about the effectiveness of the vaccine. For example, "Dr. D….. said once a person had been immunised, he was protected against the disease for life," and "If a child is immunised and lives in even the very worst conditions, he or she will not get the virus, even if there is polio in the area," and so on.

Officialdom had realised, during the smaller epidemic of 1982, that three doses of vaccine did not cause immunity, so they had at that stage increased the number of doses which would purportedly create immunity to four. On paper the figure remained three, but parents were being told to have four doses "because three isn't enough to cause immunity." When the 1987-88 epidemic broke out, some individuals who had had four doses of oral polio vaccine got paralytic polio. At first the official line was that parents who said that their children had had four doses of vaccine must be mistaken because it is impossible to get polio after four doses of vaccine. Two weeks later the official line changed and they said that it was necessary to have five doses of polio vaccine to become immune. The epidemic came to its natural end before anyone who had had five doses of vaccine had an opportunity to get polio. As no children who had had five doses became paralysed by polio, they felt justified in saying that five doses create immunity.

In the official report they blamed the floods which occurred in KwaZulu-Natal for the failure of the vaccine.[193] Flash floods which sweep away everything in the valleys are a natural phenomenon which happen about every thirty years in this region. There had been a devastating flood two months before the epidemic broke out. Before the human population explosion, the area nearest to the sea was covered with thick jungle. The flash floods would carry away the jungle in the valleys about every thirty years, and despite the number of pythons and monkeys that drowned each time, life went on. By 1987 the jungle was gone and the area had become densely populated with slums, so lots of people drowned, and the makeshift dwellings and meagre possessions of thousands of disenfranchised people were swept away.

Seven hundred years ago the Chinese blamed an earthquake for starting the bubonic plague, but now we use science, not superstition, don't we? It is pathetic the way that the South African medicrats scraped the barrel for an excuse when none of the usual excuses could be used. The floods had covered less than 5% of the geographical area that was affected by the polio epidemic, and they had ended eight weeks before the first cases of polio appeared. It is ridiculous to claim that floods in KwaZulu made polio break out five hundred miles away in Qwa Qwa.

I emigrated from South Africa to New Zealand soon after this epidemic ended, and I met Hilary Butler a few weeks later. I mentioned the South African polio epidemic to her, and she wrote to the Centers for Disease Control (CDC) in Atlanta, USA, and asked for details. The CDC did not answer her letter, so she telephoned Dr. Anthony Morris, the FDA scientist who was fired for warning the public not to accept the swine flu vaccine of 1976. He telephoned the CDC, and they told him that the only epidemic of polio in Africa at that time had occurred in Senegal. Senegal is in West Africa, more than four thousand miles north west of KwaZulu-Natal. I thought that was an excellent way of denying the failure of the vaccine - just deny that the epidemic occurred.

I then wrote to the South African Department of Health, and they sent me a computer print out of the polio figures region by region, and month by month. The totals were 24 cases in 1987, and 172 cases in 1988. Hilary sent the CDC in Atlanta a photocopy for their records.

The CDC's attitude made me curious about the World Health Organisation's view of the epidemic. So I wrote to them and asked them how many cases of polio had occurred in South Africa during 1987 and 1988. I was amazed when they replied that there had been 27 cases in 1987 and 27 cases in 1988. On the 27th December 1990 I wrote to the doctor at the World Health Organisation who had supplied me with the figures, and told him that according to the official South African figures there were 24 cases in 1987 and 172 cases in 1988. I asked if he could explain to me why there is a discrepancy, and what source they use for their figures. I have still not had a reply to that letter, nor to a reminder.

Then I wrote to the South African Health Department and asked them how many doses of vaccine each case had had. In response they sent me a detailed report on the epidemic in the geographical region that was most affected. The thing that struck me most forcibly about the report was that there was absolutely no attempt at a cover up. There was the usual grappling for excuses at the end, but the investigators had tried, under difficult circumstances, to find out exactly what the correct statistics were.

The people who compiled the report had a major problem with reconciling the case reports that came from different sources. One patient could pass through as many as four different hospitals, and as there was a low level of literacy among hospital staff because of apartheid's educational system, the names were not always spelt correctly. Also, Zulu people use different names in different situations. In the final report, the compilers have included three suspected duplicates, because the information available to them was not sufficient to be completely certain that they were not duplicates.

When the polio virus becomes virulent there are far more cases of mild polio than of paralytic polio, but they do not get reported because they look like flu. These were of course not included in the data. Then there are the in between cases which are not classical polio, but are serious enough to make people go to hospital. The doctors know they are caused by the polio virus, but because the polio symptoms are too mild, they have to classify them as suspected cases, unless a lab test is available to confirm that they are polio.

The immunisation status of each case was given as none, incomplete, complete or unknown. One or two doses were regarded as incomplete, and three or more doses was regarded as complete. In the KwaZulu-Natal region, 49 confirmed cases occurred in people who had had no doses of vaccine. The World Health Organisation's grand total for all cases in South Africa is only five more than the number of cases that occurred in unvaccinated individuals in KwaZulu-Natal. The majority of all cases occurred in KwaZulu-Natal, so I wonder if the World Health Organisation was able to obtain the figures for immunisation status in the rest of South Africa, and it came to five. If I had not been living there at the time, and been very interested in the whole affair because I had a new baby, I would not have become aware that the World Health Organisation's figures differ from the official government figure.

While I was investigating the 1987 polio epidemic in South Africa, I discovered that the Minister of Health had revoked the law that made polio vaccine compulsory. The medicrats were dismayed by his action, and had asked all the newspapers not to report that polio vaccine was no longer compulsory. The newspapers had agreed to co-operate because they believed it was in the public interest. (Radio and TV were state controlled, whereas newspapers were politically censored but not state controlled.) One day the local state nurse and a doctor from Groote Schuur Hospital turned up on my doorstep to try and persuade me to vaccinate Kenneth. It was a fun encounter, and one of the most entertaining moments came when I mentioned that I knew that the law making the vaccine compulsory had been revoked.

In the country of Oman there was an outbreak of polio from January 1988 to March 1989.[155] As usual, vaccinated children caught polio. There were a variety of excuses, but because the situation had been studied, they could not just grasp at the usual excuses in the hopes that they applied. The studies showed that there had been no breaks in the cold chain, no sub-optimum vaccine potency, and no low antibody levels in the victims of polio who were vaccinated. They could also not use the excuse that herd immunity was lacking due to low vaccination rates, as they had just completed a vaccination campaign which had raised the percentage of children who were "fully immunised" to 87%.

One excuse they gave was that their vaccination campaigns had been so successful that children were no longer exposed to the wild virus. Another excuse was that babies were only "fully immunised" by the age of seven months, although that did not explain why more than half the victims of polio were "fully immunised." They did however admit that "sub-optimum efficacy" of the vaccine was a reason for the failure of the vaccine. That is a polite way of saying, "The vaccine did not work."

But having said all this, they then revert to the old "not enough doses" excuse in their conclusion, and they recommend four doses starting at birth and being completed at the age of 14 weeks. The next time a virulent virus comes along, the new schedule will fail, and they will be really short of excuses. In the conclusion they say that somebody had better invent a better vaccine. They actually say that twice. That gives lab workers around the world reason to bleat for more funds.

After an outbreak of polio in Israel in 1988, two groups of doctors were given the opportunity to make excuses for the failure of the vaccine.[194] Take a big breath before you read the next paragraph.

The one group said that the vaccine had failed because the oral vaccine that had been used 20 years previously wasn't potent enough against type 1 of the three strains of virus which you get in the vaccine, and because some children had been given only injected vaccine, which meant that they passed on the virus to susceptible people as they had no gut immunity. The other group said that the outbreak had been caused by long term exposure to contaminated sewage, and because the strain of wild virus which caused the epidemic was sufficiently different to the strains in the vaccine to overcome the immunity created by a vaccine strain that wasn't potent enough. Meanwhile the first group had said that the antibodies that the vaccine produced were wide spectrum enough to have covered the different strain of virus. What a lot of gobbledy-gook. Why don't they just admit that vaccination does not work?

As the long term exposure to contaminated sewage had been going on for some time, why had the victims not had polio before? And isn't being vaccinated supposed to protect one from germs no matter whether you catch them from the air, other people, or open sewage?

In the town of Vellore in India there was a polio outbreak in 1991-92.[154] The vaccination coverage for those years was 98% for three doses, and in 1992 it was 90% for four doses. All the children who got polio were "fully immunised."[154] In the surrounding rural communities the coverage rate for three doses was 80-85%, so they could not blame adjacent communities for causing the outbreak in Vellore. The three doctors who wrote to the *Lancet* about this outbreak say, "We believe it was due to sub-optimum vaccine efficacy and inadequate herd effect." Now I like those excuses. They are getting closer to the truth. It's a pity they cannot just come clean and say, "The vaccine did not work and herd immunity does not exist." They make the suggestion that seven doses of vaccine should be given, "with high coverage to achieve eradication." While they dream on, children around the world are being paralysed by this vaccine, and many more are suffering lesser side effects.

COVER UP OF THE FAILURE OF RABIES VACCINE

Louis Pasteur said that his rabies vaccine would work as long as it was given to the victim of a bite before any symptoms developed.[179] Once use of the vaccine became widespread, it was witnessed that vaccinated people often got rabies. These were excused by saying that anyone who got rabies within a month of starting the treatment was not protected by the vaccine, and could not be counted as a failure.[195]

This technique drastically reduced the number of failures that had to be acknowledged. So, for instance, the official failure rate of Pasteur's rabies vaccine at the Kasauli Institute in 1910, was given as only 0.19%. They arrived at this figure by excluding all deaths that occurred during the course of fourteen injections, and all those who died within fifteen days of completing the course. Out of 2073 people who were injected after being bitten or licked by suspected rabid animals, 26 died of rabies, but 14 died during the treatment, so they were not counted, and 8 died within 15 days of completion of the treatment, so they were not counted. Only four died after the 15-day cut off. Those four are the only ones counted for the statistic.[196]

Ardent vaccinationists like to view the 26 deaths as evidence that 2047 people were saved. What they overlook is that the cases that do not get rabies are not necessarily vaccine successes. We would only know how many of the vaccinated people were saved by the vaccine, if they were to collect statistics of rabies in people who were not injected with the vaccine after being licked or bitten by a suspected rabid animal. It was not in the interests of the newly founded vaccine industry to gather such information.

When a person gets rabies from the germ in the vaccine, the symptoms are usually not exactly the same as rabies. The old fashioned word for rabies is hydrophobia, so they called the rabies-like syndrome that occurred after vaccination "paralytic hydrophobia." A more recent word for the condition that is often caused by rabies vaccine is "neuroparalysis." Sir Graham Wilson has this to say about neuroparalysis,

> It was not long after the pasteurian method of protecting against rabies was taken into routine use that attention was drawn to cases of neuroparalysis occurring during or just after the course of treatment. Little was said about them in print. Among the directors of the Pasteur Institutes there was a conspiracy of silence, caused by a fear partly of bringing Pasteur's method into disrepute and partly of bringing blame upon themselves. Their position was not an easy one. Though little was acknowledged publicly, rumour was active and each fresh case furnished the occasion for local conversation and gossip. The poisonous atmosphere of covertly expressed criticism in which they moved reacted on the morale of the staff and made them miserable.[197]

He forgets that only people with a conscience feel miserable under these circumstances. Most people can stop themselves from being miserable by indulging in pathological denial. Denying reality is the way to stay happy if you are part of the vaccination machine. It is also the way to stay employed. However, a certain group of doctors decided not to indulge in pathological denial, nor to suffer the misery of guilty consciences. They gathered together data about side effects, and they testified against their colleagues who were dishonestly suppressing data about adverse reactions.[197] In April 1927, the director of the Pasteur Institute in Morocco, Dr. Remlinger, reported to the International Rabies Conference,

> We were impressed with the discrepancy between the number of observations published by directors of institutes and the number of cases orally acknowledged by them to have occurred ... We have come to the conclusion that certain institutes conceal their cases. On various occasions we have found in medical literature observations concerning paralysis of treatment, and we have afterwards failed to find in the report and statistics of the institutes concerned any mention of these unfortunate cases.[198]

When the people who stand to gain financially from favourable statistics are in complete control of the raw data, it is easy for them to omit to mention failures and side effects of their product. Although Dr. Remlinger came clean about rabies vaccine side effects and vaccine failures in 1927, the industry continued to foist Pasteur's vaccine onto the public until they had a new rabies vaccine that they could foist onto the public instead.

EXCUSES FOR THE FAILURE OF BCG VACCINE

The first vaccine for TB was invented by Robert Koch, and it was made with human TB germs. Its use was discontinued because it killed too many babies. The commercial void that this left was filled by two Frenchmen who thought of the idea of making a vaccine from the strain of germ which causes TB in cows. This vaccine is called BCG. It does kill a lot fewer people than Robert Koch's vaccine did, and it has been raking in money for the vaccine industry ever since 1921.

When I lived in Cape Town, I associated with a lot of medical people and medical students, and I often heard them muttering about the fact that BCG vaccine does not work. TB was rife in the black townships because of malnutrition and lack of proper housing. Most houses were made of pieces of corrugated iron that had been propped up next to one another in the mud, and Cape Town has a cold, damp climate.

The official stance of the South African Department of Health was that "BCG vaccine is 79% effective." This claim was based on a study which had been started in 1950 by the Medical Research Council in Britain, and had followed up the participants for ten years.[199] They said that out of the 12,699 unvaccinated participants, 213 got TB, and out of the 13,598 vaccinated participants, 48 got TB. "... this represents a reduction of 79% attributed to vaccination."[199] A doctor pointed out in the *British Medical Journal* that those who got TB from the vaccine were not included as cases of TB, and if they had been, there would have been no difference in the incidence of TB between the vaccinated and the unvaccinated.[200] This vaccine is not only useless, it is also harmful. It has some serious long term side effects, and it kills some babies and some teenagers outright. Homoeopathy cures TB very effectively and cheaply, so there is no excuse for using the vaccine, even in cold, damp slums. Despite the fraudulent finding that "the protective efficacy of this vaccine was thus substantial," the international muttering about the uselessness of BCG vaccine continued.

It was decided that the World Health Organisation should do a large study in a malnourished area to ascertain once and for all whether or not the vaccine was effective. The study involved two hundred and sixty thousand children, which made it large enough to ensure that there would be no quibbling afterwards about whether or not the study was representative. Well of course if the study had found that the vaccine decreased the incidence of TB, there would have been no quibbling afterwards, but the study found that BCG vaccine actually increases the risk of catching TB,[201,202] so the quibbling continues.

In 1980 the editor of the *Lancet* wrote,

> Thirteen years ago, D'Arcy Hart reviewed the conflicting evidence on BCG effectiveness and spoke of the need for a fresh field trial to clarify outstanding controversies, particularly in the face of increasing use of BCG in developing countries. There followed the latest Indian field trial with 260 000 participants, organised with the collaborative skills of the Indian Council of Medical Research, the World Health Organisation, and the United States Public Health Service. But it has not clarified - just the opposite. Though the 7 1/2 year follow up results reported in the Indian Journal of Medical Research are incomplete, they are negative - in fact, slightly more tuberculosis cases have appeared in vaccinated than in equal-sized placebo control groups. It looks like another zero effect.[203]

A negative effect is not a zero effect. And he says that the result has not clarified the situation, when it has clarified it very well. This editorial also lists eight excuses that have been put forward by others as reasons for the failure of the vaccine, then the editor says, "but there is no compelling evidence for any of them." Well, at least that is honest. The editorial ends off with a call for "clarity of judgment and courage to match the challenge." If the medicrats had any clarity of judgment and moral backbone they would have ceased using the vaccine as soon as the study result came out.

A year later there is another editorial in the *Lancet* which drags out eight excuses as reasons why BCG vaccination must be continued despite the result of the World Health Organisation's study in India.[204] A leading article in the medical journal called Tubercle has this to say,

> The widely publicised results of a large, controlled trial of BCG vaccination in South India showed, after 7 1/2 years of follow up, no evidence of a protective effect against pulmonary tuberculosis. This unexpected result, which has given rise to much discussion and speculation, has led to doubts about the value of BCG vaccination in general. Against this background a conference of experts was convened in Delhi … So far there has been no satisfactory explanation of the negative result of the Indian trial, despite an intensive search in every direction …[205]

It makes me chuckle to visualise teams of scientists with their heads down, conducting an intensive search in every direction - in every direction that is except the obvious one - which is facing up to the fact that the vaccine does not work. The Tubercle article goes on to suggest yet more possible excuses for the failure of the vaccine. Maybe these batches of vaccine were not potent enough. Maybe the wrong strains were used. Maybe the protective effect of the vaccine was masked by the fact that the whole population had been exposed to the wild germ before being vaccinated. Maybe the solution is to vaccinate "early in life" so that the recipients do not have a chance to meet the wild germ and become immune before they get vaccinated.

Sensible vaccinationists know that suppressing information about vaccine failures is the best way to avoid having to make excuses. On talkback radio in Auckland I heard a lady describe how she had been a teacher when teenagers were mass vaccinated with BCG in New Zealand schools. She said that 15 of the pupils at her school had contracted TB despite vaccination, and the Health Department had suppressed the information. "I believe in immunisation," she said, "but I don't think they should have done that."

We will have to wait until a new vaccine is introduced to replace BCG before they will admit that BCG does not work. The new vaccine will not work either, but it will make a lot of money.

BCG causes osteitis (bone inflammation) in 1 in 3000 well nourished babies,[206] and lots of other horrible side effects. TB is easily cured by homoeopathy, and TB germs do not become resistant to homoeopathic remedies like they do to drugs. There is no excuse for using BCG anywhere in the world.

HOW HOMOEOPATHY WORKS

Homoeopathic medicine is not a natural form of medicine. It is completely different to herbalism and naturopathy. All homoeopathic remedies are made by diluting a toxic substance and then shaking it, and then diluting it again and then shaking it again. The number that appears on the bottle after the name of the remedy tells you how many times the substance has been diluted and shaken. This simple procedure results in a range of remedies that can cure every type of disease without side effects. Naturally the pharmaceutical industry is not very enthusiastic about allowing the world's population to discover homoeopathy.

Being diluted, then shaken repeatedly, converts the substance from matter into energy. The energy which is trapped in the medicine has a unique natural frequency. When the medicine touches a mucous membrane in a person, the energy is released from the medicine and interacts with the electromagnetic field of the body. It does not work chemically, like a drug or herbal remedy does.

You can see how this works by tuning two strings of a guitar to the same note, and then plucking one of the two. The string tuned to the same note will vibrate, while the other four strings will remain still. To make a sick person better, a homoeopath has to choose a remedy that has a frequency that vibrates in sympathy with the sickness in the body. If a wrong remedy is chosen, it will not activate the required energy. It will have the same effect as the plucked guitar string has on the four strings that are not tuned to the same frequency.

Homoeopathic medicines do not cause side effects in the way that orthodox medicines and herbal medicines do. If an inquisitive child manages to get into the first aid cupboard and swallows a whole bottle of *Arnica 30*,

129

nothing will happen, whereas a child who swallows a whole bottle of paracetamol or a herbal medicine will be poisoned. However, homoeopathic remedies will cause side effects if they are taken many times a day for a few weeks by someone who does not have the corresponding symptoms. If a person repeatedly takes *arnica 30* when they have no need for it, they will start developing the symptoms of arnica poisoning. They will end up in the same condition as if they had drunk soup made from the arnica plant.

Homoeopathic medicine is very fragile. It loses its potency if moisture gets into it, or if a pungent aroma comes into contact with it. Eucalyptus oil, citronella oil, T-tree oil, mint and peppermint are some of the substances that make homoeopathic remedies lose potency. (Curry, chilli and spices like cinnamon do not have this effect.) If a homoeopathic remedy is stored in the same cupboard as a pungent substance, the smell will sneak in through the lid of the bottle and depotentise the remedy. X rays depotentise the remedies, as do the metal detectors used to scan luggage at airports. When a person has taken a homoeopathic remedy, it continues to work in the body for a period of time. If the person makes contact with a pungent aroma, the remedy "switches off" and stops working.

Dr. Samuel Hahnemann discovered homoeopathy in 1790.[207] He was determined to find a way of curing disease because he was unhappy about the fact that the drugs and methods he had been taught to use as a doctor always harmed, often killed and never cured his patients. As he was fluent in many languages, he chose to give up practicing medicine and earn an income by translating medical writings. In this way he became familiar with the views of ancient doctors like Hippocrates and Paracelsus, as well as with the beliefs that were current in his own time.

In 1790 one of his tasks was to translate a 1,170 page book about medicinal substances that had been written by Dr. William Cullen, who was a high profile pharmaceutical man in Edinburgh at the time. One of the things that Dr. Cullen said was that quinine cures malaria because of its tonic action on the stomach. However quinine does not cure malaria, but instead temporarily suppresses the symptoms of malaria. Therefore it looks, for a while, as if the patient is cured, but then the malaria starts up again.

Hahnemann felt sceptical of Cullen's claim. While working on the translation, he got up and took a dose of quinine. Thereafter he dosed himself twice daily for several days, and he developed the symptoms of malaria. The symptoms of malaria are the same as the symptoms of quinine poisoning. This convinced Hahnemann that Hippocrates and Paracelsus were correct in saying that "like cures like." The reason why quinine makes the symptoms of malaria disappear for a while is that quinine causes those very same symptoms in a healthy person.

But the most important part of the discovery was still to come. This was that repeated diluting and shaking makes the remedy able to bring about a permanent cure instead of just suppressing the symptoms. Hahnemann decided to dilute the quinine because it was so toxic, and as he was a trained chemist as well as a doctor, he banged the vial on the leather bound bible on his desk 100 times between each dilution, to ensure that there was an even distribution of the substance in the liquid. To his surprise he found that the diluted medicine was more powerful than the original substance. Later on he realised that the banging was a crucial part of making the medicine so powerful. When quinine in its crude state is given to someone suffering from a bout of malaria, it makes the symptoms of malaria retreat, only to come back later. But when quinine is homoeopathically potentised, it cures malaria once and for all without causing any side effects. The homoeopathic definition of the word cure is, "To restore health rapidly, gently, permanently; to remove and destroy the whole disease in the shortest, surest, least harmful way, according to clearly comprehensible principles."[208]

Hahnemann called his new discovery "homoeopathy," from the Greek words "homoios" (similar), and "pathos" (suffering). When a substance is potentised to make a remedy it is given a Latin sounding name so that people of every language will be able to refer to it without confusion.

Hahnemann soon realised that he could make remedies from toxic substances that were not recognised as drugs. For instance, people who worked in the copper mines exhibited symptoms of copper poisoning. He used potentised copper to cure these symptoms, whether or not they arose from exposure to copper. First he had to find a way of diluting non-soluble metals.

Modern homoeopaths use all the old remedies as well as new ones made from modern toxic substances like naphthalene and petroleum. Homoeopathy is not a placebo effect, and it works on animals as well as on humans.

Arsenicum is made by diluting and potentising arsenic. Arsenic is a very poisonous substance, but the remedy *arsenicum* is non-toxic. The remedy is not only used to treat arsenic poisoning. When a person eats rotten food they get what is called "food poisoning." The symptoms of food poisoning are usually the same as the symptoms of arsenic poisoning. Susceptible people can die from eating even a small amount of rancid food, but most people suffer horribly for a few days and then recover. This is one of the circumstances in which homoeopathy works astonishingly fast. *Arsenicum 30* cures the appropriate symptoms of food poisoning in less than an hour. If the All Blacks had known about *arsenicum 30*, they may have won the 1995 Rugby World Cup. Pharmaceutical medicine cannot cure food poisoning, nor malaria, nor copper poisoning, nor …

The big drawback of homoeopathy is that there is no single remedy for each disease, so we cannot say that A is the cure for cholera, and B is the cure for cancer. Each patient has to be individually assessed so that the right remedy can be given for their particular set of symptoms. Each person with cholera is different, and each person with cancer is different, although the people with cholera are a lot more alike than the people with cancer.

There are many remedies that can be used to cure tuberculosis (TB). The one which is right for a particular individual can only be chosen by carefully noting the symptoms of the patient. *Acalypha Indica* is one of the remedies for TB. A person who eats the plant in its natural form will start coughing up blood, will get progressively emaciated, and will be weaker in the mornings and gain strength during the day. The first two symptoms are typical of almost all cases of pulmonary TB, while the third symptom occurs only in some individuals. *Acalypha Indica* is the appropriate remedy for a person who has that idiosyncratic symptom, as well as the common symptoms.

Diseases that take a long time to develop need a few months of homoeopathic treatment to be fully cured, while diseases that take a short time to develop are cured very quickly by the right remedy. The range of remedies is huge, and extensive learning is needed to get to know them all. An amateur can practice homoeopathic first aid quite safely, as long as he or she does not give doses more frequently than necessary, and gets outside help if there is not a rapid improvement from the chosen remedy. Dr. Hahnemann used to give his patients first aid kits so that they could treat themselves for the regular ailments.

Ledum 30 is the first aid remedy for any puncture wound. It deals with the pain, and if given soon after the injury, it makes the body kill any tetanus germs that have entered through the wound. Bites and stings from small creatures that inject poison into the flesh are also puncture wounds, and *ledum* is the remedy to use for these. The remedy makes the pain fade rapidly, and it antidotes the poison which has entered, even when that poison has provoked an allergic reaction.

Spiders are a big hazard in Australia. In 1999 Chandra was bitten on the hand by a large spider that was hiding on the back of a towel. It took me ten minutes to find the *ledum 30*, and by then her hand was red, swollen and paralysed. This was 3 hours before she had to write an exam. The remedy halted the swelling, and then the swelling subsided and the redness disappeared. Mobility returned slowly. By the time she left for her exam, her hand was back to normal, except for two huge fang marks. This is what the pharmaceutical industry does not want you to know how to do. Under "orthodox" treatment she would have been given medications which do not work, some of which are harmful. Her exam would have had to be postponed. This example underlines an important aspect of homoeopathy. *Ledum 30* kills tetanus germs that have entered through a puncture wound, and it also antidotes poison from a bee sting or spider bite, but *ledum 30* does not cure tetanus if the tetanus germs have been allowed to spread in the body and have started causing paralysis. Another remedy is needed to cure a person who is suffering from symptoms of tetanus. That remedy is usually, but not always, *hypericum 30*.

When Chandra was eight she had an allergic reaction to a wasp sting at school. Her teacher telephoned me and said, "Chandra has been stung by a wasp on her hand and the swelling is going up her arm, and she says you have some medicine for it." I zoomed to school with *ledum 30*, and found that her whole hand was red and swollen, and the red swelling had engulfed her wrist and most of her forearm and was spreading upwards as I watched. As soon as the remedy made contact with the mucous membrane under her tongue, the redness and swelling stopped where it was and spread no further. After an hour the swelling had gone, but it took a few days for the redness to disappear completely. This is not welcome news for the makers of antihistamines.

When a child wakes in the night and screams from earache, the correct remedy can eliminate the pain and have the child sleeping again in a matter of minutes. The remedy also boosts the immune system to solve the ear problem in the long term. When homoeopathy is used, "orthodox" medicine loses customers for its antibiotics, pain killers and grommets.

In 2003 there was publicity of an experiment that was done to see whether some human immune system cells could still do what they naturally do after they had been homoeopathically diluted. A magician promised to pay a million pounds if they could. The magician's money was quite safe because once the cells were diluted, the experimenters did not try and make them do the opposite of what they normally do. They ignored the homoeopathic principle of "like cures like."

There is nothing magical about homoeopathy. Some Christians shun it because the electromagnetic force that alters the condition of the body cannot be seen under a microscope, and because many homoeopathic practitioners are occultists. Write to me if you are interested in this aspect.

The lower potencies are suitable for conditions that are largely physical, while higher potencies are suitable when there is a stronger psychological side to the condition. For instance, *arnica 6* is suitable for a bruise from bumping into a table, *arnica 30* is the potency for a sprained muscle, but you would go to the very high potency of *arnica 1m* for the deep shock of a car accident.

The amount taken each time is irrelevant. One pill has the same effect as three pills. However, the frequency with which it is given is important. If a second dose is given too soon, it stops the first dose from working. The length of time a remedy keeps on working depends on the potency used, the severity of the condition, and the vitality of the patient.

With some conditions it is easy to know when the remedy has stopped working and the next dose is required. When Kenneth broke one of the bones in his forearm, I could not get to *arnica 30* for ten minutes. He screamed terribly. The *arnica* switched off the pain instantly. As that is a severe kind of pain, the remedy wore off quickly. It was like a light being switched off; suddenly the pain was back. *Arnica* once again removed it instantly. The effect of the second dose lasted longer than the first, but suddenly the pain was back again. The effect of the third dose lasted even longer, and the fourth dose lasted over two hours. I decided I had made a mistake in thinking that a bone was broken, because he was playing happily with his train set on the floor. Then I noticed that when he leaned on his arm to reach a train, the broken bone stuck out sideways, so he did need to have it put in plaster. *Arnica* is a very effective pain killer, but only when the pain is caused by trauma.

If a person is undergoing drug treatment of any kind, homoeopathic remedies can be taken without them interacting with the drugs. However, homoeopathic remedies do interact with each other. Some remedies reinforce each other, while others counteract each other. You have to look up their clinical relationships to know the consequences of combining them.

One night at a restaurant my husband and I had the "seafood special" as an entree. The next morning Chandra had an accident and we needed *arnica* for shock. As the hours passed we began to suffer nausea, and we took more *arnica*, thinking the shock had caused the nausea. By midnight we were vomiting, and we realised we had food poisoning. The "seafood special" had been old fish with strong tasting mayonnaise piled on it. We took *arsenicum* and started to improve immediately. We were up all night with Chandra, who was full of beans after spending some of the day under general anaesthetic. We took more doses of *arsenicum* each time we began to slip back into feeling queasy again, and later I started taking *arnica* again for shock. By daybreak my husband was fully recovered from the food poisoning, but I was still sick, having ceased to progress when I restarted the *arnica*. Later I looked up the clinical relationship between the two remedies, and discovered that *arnica* prevents *arsenicum* from working.

Homoeopathic remedies continue working for a long time in the body, as long as they are not de-activated by a pungent aroma. Some homoeopaths are very slack about warning their patients to avoid strong smelling oils and mint toothpaste. Another homoeopathic story about Chandra arises from when she broke a metatarsal bone while on a teenage camp. Her foot swelled up like a balloon, but *arnica 30* made the swelling subside so rapidly that the camp director thought no bone was broken. The next day her foot was put in plaster, and over the next 6 weeks she took a dose of *arnica 30* whenever the break began to ache, which happened less and less frequently. At one point she accidentally brushed her teeth with mint flavoured toothpaste, instead of our usual mint free toothpaste. Within seconds the break became intensely painful again. The toothpaste had depotentised the *arnica 30* which had been silently working in her body.

Samuel Hahnemann wrote a lot about the principles and philosophy of homoeopathy. The book in which he summed it all up is called *Organon of Medicine*. He also documented the case histories of his own patients.

Books which give the symptoms that can be caused/cured by each substance are called "materia medica." The modern materia medicas contain some substances that were not available to the early homoeopaths, but the early materia medicas are just as useful now as they were when they were compiled. Medical textbooks become obsolete and have to be replaced, but homoeopathic books always remain valid. Knowledge about homoeopathy can increase, but homoeopathy does not change. The following materia medicas are useful in the home situation, but remember that access to one of these books does not make you into a homoeopath.

William Boericke MD, *Materia Medica with Repertory*, B Jain Publishers, New Delhi.

Dr. Sangeeta Chawla, *In Depth Materia Medica of the Human Mind*, Indian Books and Periodicals Syndicate, New Delhi, 1993.

John Henry Clarke MD, *A Dictionary of Practical Materia Medica*, Health Science Press, 1977 (originally published in 1900).

James Tyler Kent AM, MD, *Repertory of the Materia Medica*, B Jain Publishers Pvt Ltd., 1986 (originally published in 1905).

Roger Morrison MD, *Desk Top Guide to Keynotes and Confirmatory Symptoms*, Hahnemann Clinic Publishing, Albany, California, 1993.

Dr. F.R. Phatak, *Materia Medica of Homoeopathic Medicine*, Indian Books and Periodicals Syndicate, New Delhi, 1977.

Dr. M.L. Tyler, *Points to the Common Remedies*, B Jain Publishers, Pvt Ltd, New Delhi, 1991.

Frans Vermeulen, *Concordant Materia Medica*, Merlijn, Haarlem, 1994.

SOME POINTERS REGARDING THE PREVENTION AND TREATMENT OF MALEVOLENT INFECTIOUS DISEASES

There are a number of things that an individual can do to reduce the risk of catching the non-childhood diseases. Childhood diseases cannot be prevented, so knowing how to handle them is the answer to surviving them. However, steps can be taken to prevent malevolent infectious diseases, and they should be taken, because these diseases are harmful and have no long term benefits. A malevolent disease can only be caught when the germs are present in the person's environment. In some geographical regions the germs which cause typhoid and cholera are present in the water, and a traveller can get very sick or even die from drinking the water. The airborne malevolent diseases cannot be avoided through good hygiene, and it cannot be predicted when nor where they will put in an appearance. Avoiding junk food is the first step towards protecting oneself from airborne malevolent diseases.

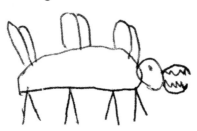

A fierce germ setting off to attack an innocent child

Sufficient rest is also essential for preventing some diseases, boring though it may sound.

Unfortunately it is not always possible to obtain wholesome food, because the food industry prefers to sell products with a long shelf life. Furthermore, our immune systems are under strain from all the pollutants in the air and water, the pesticides and additives in the food, and the poisonous metals in our teeth. On the other hand, we have many advantages which our ancestors lacked. Vitamin and mineral pills that are made of natural extracts go a long way towards compensating for modern food, and they can help one to survive if the germ does manage to cause symptoms of the disease.

Vitamin C has become such a cliché in the health field that it is easy to overlook how important it is to take extra doses of vitamin C when we are under attack from germs. The amount of vitamin C needed daily varies from person to person. The amount needed is affected by things like the genetic legacy, what damage has been done to the immune system in the past, and what poisons the bureaucrats add to the water. When germs come into the environment, the need increases dramatically. Vitamin C gets used up quickly in germ wars, so it needs to be replaced every few hours. Too much causes diarrhoea, so it is easy to know when the limit has been reached. Dr. Linus Pauling says,

> Vitamin C is not a wonder drug, a drug that cures a particular disease. It is instead a substance that participates in almost all of the chemical reactions that take place in our bodies, and is required for many of them. Our bodies can fight disease effectively only when we have in our organs and body fluids enough vitamin C to enable our natural protective mechanisms to operate effectively.[209]

The most enlightening part of the book from which that quote is taken is chapter 12, entitled *The Medical Establishment and Vitamin C*. Knowing the lengths to which the medical establishment goes in order to suppress information about vitamin C is sufficient to convince the health conscious reader that vitamin C supplementation is beneficial.

For those who want to know more about what vitamin C does once it gets inside the body, there is a book by Dr. Irwin Stone which explains how vitamin C has a direct effect on bacteria and viruses, how it breaks up the toxins which the germs produce, and how it helps the phagocytes in the immune system to eat germs faster.[210] Another good book[211] gives valuable information about vitamin C.

Each spring I receive phone calls from young people who are planning to spend their long student vacation travelling in impoverished countries. They want advice because they are scared of travel vaccines, and they are also scared of the infectious diseases that are prevalent in those countries. They have good reason to be scared of both. Only a fraction of deaths from travel vaccines make it into medical journals.[212,213] The fraction is so small that it is not even the tip of the iceberg, nor is it the penguin on the tip of the iceberg. It is the flea on the penguin on the tip of the iceberg. Vaccine mongers often tell prospective travellers that certain vaccines are "required" for visiting certain countries, when they are not. Some countries require visitors who are arriving from what they consider to be a yellow fever zone to either present a vaccination certificate or a letter from a doctor saying that vaccination is contra-indicated. Sometimes travel itineraries can be arranged to avoid the hassle of finding a co-operative doctor. For instance, Egypt considers Kenya to be a yellow fever zone, so if you go to Egypt first and then to Kenya, no paperwork is necessary. Yellow fever is the only vaccine required by any country.

Although there are no simple solutions to avoiding infectious diseases while travelling, there are many protective measures that are worth taking. It is particularly difficult to obtain nourishing food while travelling, so a good supply of non-acidic vitamin C pills is advisable, even for healthy youngsters. Vitamin C powder is impractical for travellers as it can easily be spoiled by moisture. It is better to use pills, but of course they must be good quality pills in a matrix which does not hinder absorption.

It is difficult to avoid waterborne germs when travelling in unhygienic countries. A good present to buy for a loved one who intends to travel to dubious areas is an electrical gadget which boils a small amount of water at a time, along with the relevant electrical connections for the countries they intend to visit. In remote areas where there is no electricity, the people use fire to cook their food, so a traveller can use the fire to boil water. Some hotels and restaurants do not boil the water when they make tea or coffee. Plush carpets and a grand reception hall are no guarantee that the water supply is not contaminated with typhoid or cholera. Even unpeeled fruit and bottled liquids can be contaminated. Those stories about fruit being injected with river water to make them heavier are not fairy tales. I bought a mandarin on the banks of a famous river which doubles as a sewer, and when I opened the skin, brown water came bursting out. When I looked at the skin carefully I could see where the water had been injected in. In another country that undervalues hygiene, I bought a bottled fizzy drink from a respectable looking shop, and there was a cockroach sealed inside it.

In theory homoeopathy can cure every disease, but homoeopaths are scarce in most countries except India. The pharmaceutical cartel has systematically worked on eliminating homoeopathy in every country, starting in the USA with the Flexner Report of 1911. So far their tentacles have failed to gain control of India. Homoeopathy can only save your life if the right remedy can be prescribed, and then obtained in time. Diseases like cholera, typhoid and typhus respond rapidly to the correct potentised similar, even when the patient is almost dead. But if you do not have the right remedy with you, and you cannot get it in time, you are in danger of dying. So doing your best to avoid the germs of these diseases is well worthwhile.

The only thing that modern medicine can do during acute stages of these malevolent diseases is to give life support. In regions where life support is available, it enables the patient to survive. Medical doctors are trained to think of each medicine as a cure for a particular disease. In homoeopathy there are many cures for each disease, but only one is suitable for a particular individual. Unless the right remedy is chosen for the specific symptoms of that particular person, the remedy will not work. This means that when an epidemic of a malevolent disease breaks out, each sick person has to be assessed by a homoeopath in order to achieve a high or 100% cure rate. Although most cases of cholera respond to potentised camphor (*camphora*) or potentised copper (*cuprum*), and most cases of polio respond to *gelsemium* or *lathyrus sativa*, you cannot call *camphora* and *cuprum* the remedies for cholera, nor can you call *gelsemium* and *lathyrus sativa* the remedies for polio, because they are not appropriate in every case. If a wrong remedy is chosen, it does not cure the disease.

Another disadvantage to homoeopathy is that the potentised energy in the medicine is very fragile. When travelling be sure to pack a type of toothpaste which does not contain mint. A number of manufacturers are now making toothpaste that is fluoride free and mint free. The fluoride is omitted for health reasons, and the mint is omitted because you never know when you might need a homoeopathic remedy. Don't use a deodorant which contains eucalyptus oil or tea tree oil.

Homoeopathic medicine can be depotentised by being packed in your luggage near something with a strong smell. Don't carry things like insect repellent in the same bag. Keep the remedies together in an airtight plastic tub. This protects them from moisture, odours and breakage, and also makes it easy to remove them from your cabin bag while going through the safety check before boarding an aircraft. The medicine becomes depotentised if it goes through the metal detectors, making it useless. When flying with homoeopathic remedies, keep the container in your hand luggage. Show the airport attendants who check for weapons what it is that you do not want to pass through the machine. A lot of airport attendants know that passengers do not want their homoeopathic medicine to be metal detected.

I once let my homoeopathic first aid kit get zapped by the metal detector rays because I was distracted. It was at a small airport in Africa, and the airport staff were struggling to help passengers embark as two jumbo jets were departing at the same time. My baby was in a carry papoose, and a steward grabbed it and almost put it though the machine. While I was extracting the baby from the papoose, the bag containing the first aid kit went through. The next time I used the *arnica*, the child who was hurt just kept on crying with pain. A few successive uses of the *arnica* showed that it was useless. Then I had occasion to use the *aconite* for a child who had caught a chill from being wet in the wind. It had no effect, and the child went on to get flu. I threw that whole kit away, and replaced it with fresh remedies from the local health shop. In some countries there is no local health shop, or laws pushed through by the drug companies mean that health shops cannot sell basic homoeopathic remedies. So guard your remedies well.

a) TB (Tuberculosis)

TB does not come and go in epidemics like measles and polio do. It is always there, and it is always looking for an opportunity to make people sick. It is caused by a bacterium that can attack any part of the body, but most commonly chooses the lungs. The bacteria are found living in the throats of a high percentage of the population, but only people who are run down become sick from it. Damp housing, malnutrition and chronic tiredness are risk factors that predispose a person to TB, and nowadays being infected with the HIV virus also makes people very vulnerable to TB. Overcrowding does not in itself cause TB. TB is associated with overcrowding, because poor people usually live in crowded conditions. Rich people who live in big houses are also at risk of coming down with TB if they do not eat sufficient nourishing food. A king of Sweden and a Hollywood star have died of TB.

A perfect diet of organically grown, unprocessed food is not necessary to prevent TB. If that were the case, most people in the world would be suffering from TB. Eating things like mincemeat, unpolished rice, pumpkin and apples prevents TB. Some people are too poor to buy enough of such simple fare, while others have been influenced by dysinformation which tells them to eat sugar and refined grains. In the old South Africa, radio and TV aggressively promoted sugar as the greatest benefit to health. Many people were illiterate because apartheid kept them out of school, and they believed that bright coloured synthetic drinks were better for them than milk. Whole wheat bread was cheaper than white bread, but people were told that white bread was better. So not only did they have very little money because their labour was exploited, but what little they had was wrongly spent. The results were things like high infant mortality and rampant TB. BCG vaccine was compulsory, and was given to newborn babies and to children without parental consent. It is possible that the vaccine increased the incidence of TB, as it does in India.[201,202] No record was kept of how many infants died from BCG, although sometimes deaths caused by the vaccine were reported.[214]

You do not need a first class diet to avoid TB. You need sufficient calories laced with some vitamins and minerals, and you need to be housed in an abode that is dry and warm. Affluent people who have sugar with every meal do not get TB, because they dilute the sugar with protein and minerals.

TB dwindles when a society becomes more affluent, and it resurges when the economy slumps. The USA and New Zealand both experienced great affluence after World War II. As a result, TB declined dramatically. BCG vaccine was used in New Zealand, but not in the USA. Medical mythology says that the vaccine caused the decline in New Zealand, and antibiotics caused the decline in the USA. When the New Zealand economy collapsed in 1987, the incidence of TB began to rise dramatically. An economic downturn in the USA also caused an increase in TB there, and this was aggravated by the spread of the HIV virus, which lowers resistance to TB.

Some of the symptoms of TB include; continuous cough that lasts more than four weeks, loss of appetite, night sweats, pains in the chest, breathlessness, tiredness, weakness and loss of weight. Coughing up blood is a sign that the disease is well advanced. Not all of these symptoms are present in each case, and there are other symptoms as well.

There are drugs that are effective against the old strains of TB, and the new and old strains can be vanquished by homoeopathy. To a homoeopath, the strain of TB bacteria that is causing the disease is irrelevant. Only the symptoms matter. Most cases of TB respond to *Koch Tuberculinum 30*, which is made by homoeopathically potentising a vaccine that was invented by Robert Koch. This vaccine was made from human TB germs, and it killed so many babies that it was withdrawn. Once it is homoeopathically potentised, this deadly vaccine saves lives. It has the potential to save millions more lives because enough medicine to cure one person costs less than a dollar. If governments were to introduce homoeopathy to treat TB, the most expensive part for them would be maintaining clinic buildings in poor areas, and paying the salaries of the people who administer the remedy.

An old fashioned way of curing TB was by the patients having a lengthy stay in a sanatorium, where they ate wholesome foods, got lots of rest, and breathed fresh air. TB that is not treated by one means or another is usually fatal. You may have heard stories about TB curing itself spontaneously without treatment. This never happens unless there is a fundamental change in the person's living conditions and diet. For instance it has happened in situations where prisoners of war with TB have been released, and gone home to warm housing and plentiful food.

b) POLIO

There are three main strains of polio virus, with over 250 subtypes, and the Coxsackie virus also causes polio. Epidemics are more frequent in warm weather, but they also occur in winter. The pandemic of polio about which we hear so much began in the 1880s, reached a peak in the 1920s, and abated during the 1960s. In the 1920s it was overshadowed by the "Spanish" flu epidemic, which might be why it is not well remembered from that time. The long term history of polio is not known, but the disease is occasionally mentioned in historical documents. Some mummified bodies from Ancient Egypt show evidence of polio, and there is no reason to believe that the virus will not become virulent again in the future.

Polio is a very bad disease that can lead to death or permanent physical disability. If an epidemic of polio breaks out in the region where you live, there are three lifestyle factors that need careful attention. These are the types of food that are being consumed, whether sufficient rest is being taken, and the avoidance of chills.

When the polio virus becomes virulent, it floats through the air and is breathed in by everybody. Some of the people who breathe it in will suffer no symptoms, while others will suffer mild or severe symptoms of polio. Polio can easily be mistaken for flu during the early stages, as the symptoms are a sore throat, fever, tiredness, and a headache. When it is known that there is a polio virus in the environment, it is safer to regard every case of flu as suspected polio, and to treat it homoeopathically and chiropractically so that it is cured before it does damage. A feature of polio is that the early symptoms sometimes clear up, and the patient seems better, but then the symptoms come back again a few days later and quickly progress to full blown polio.

If polio progresses beyond what looks like flu symptoms, there will be nausea or vomiting, the headache will be severe, and there will be stiffness in the neck and back. Once these symptoms appear there is great danger that part of the body could become paralysed. The paralysis can cause death, especially if it affects the lungs. Nerves get damaged by the polio virus, and some get destroyed. When this happens the victim suffers a degree of disability for the rest of his or her life. If the victim is not fully grown when the nerves are damaged, the affected limbs will not grow properly afterwards, so that the person ends up with one or more limb that is small and withered.

Survivors of polio are also afflicted with the onset of new symptoms 30 or 40 years after they have had the disease. This is because the nerves that were not damaged by the polio get worn out over the decades, by having to do the work of the damaged nerves as well as their own work. This problem is called post polio syndrome.

A health conscious family can protect themselves against this nasty virus - but it requires time, effort and hassle. Take a careful look at what you eat over the next 48 hours. If the wild polio virus suddenly became virulent, would your family's diet be good enough for them to breathe in the virus and suffer no ill effects? You do not add sugar to your food, but are you eating packaged foods that have had sugar added by the manufacturers? Flour is added to many products, which of course is refined flour because it does not go rancid as fast as whole flour. You need to be sure that children are properly nourished when there is a polio virus in the environment, and the first step is cutting out all refined foods. The second step is to eat animal protein, or soya protein or almonds.

Of course you do not eat white bread, except for now and then - more often than you think. And then there's pasta and pizza and pies. Well of course you only eat the whole wheat kind, except when you're in a hurry - which is most of the time. We kid ourselves that we eat a wholesome diet, but we do not, because it is just so doggone difficult to organise a wholesome diet. Most of the time we get away with it, but during a polio epidemic the risk is too high to be negligent about children's food. Children do not crave sugary things if they eat enough wholesome food. Organising solid food for them is difficult, expensive, and time consuming, but polio is a worse option. Most children like melted cheese on whole wheat bread, and sausages made of pure meat, and unpolished rice, and stir fried vegetables. (Most hate boiled vegetables.)

If you run a sugar free home you will still have the problem that people in the outside world will try and pressurise your children into consuming sugar. Some children are good at resisting this pressure, while others succumb. Both adults and children who are addicted to sugar feel emotionally threatened when they encounter someone who does not partake of the habit, and their retaliation against the sugar free offender can be quite unkind.

The immune system cannot work properly if there is a deficiency of protein or vitamin B.[215] When grains are refined, the vitamin B in their outer layer is thrown away. Eating white bread, white rice, white pasta and white pastry severely compromises the immune system. Refined starch is also the biggest cause of heart attacks.[216,217,218] The anti-cholesterol brigade tells people to eat cereals, without mentioning that the cereals must be unrefined. They also scare people off eating meat, while encouraging them to eat sugar. A lack of vitamin B is what makes cholesterol cling to artery walls. This irresponsible behaviour on the part of the "experts" not only fails to protect people from heart attacks, it also makes people more vulnerable to infectious diseases.

Children can be chronically tired if they have difficulty sleeping, or if they have bad bedtime habits. Tiredness makes them vulnerable to polio. Most cases of insomnia can be cured by calcium supplements, or by homoeopathic treatment for inability to absorb calcium. Bad bedtime habits are much harder to cure, especially when the parents are overworked and tired.

In childhood diseases, getting chilled can bring on complications, but with polio, a chill can be the factor which makes the person catch the disease in the first place. A classic example of how polio can be caught is the way that Franklin D. Roosevelt caught it in 1921. He was an adult with 5 children. His biographer, Allen Churchill, writes,

> Although Franklin seemed outwardly healthy, he had suffered an unusual number of serious illnesses as a man. Following his five week attack of typhoid in 1912 he had had acute appendicitis, lumbago, tonsillitis, pneumonia, double pneumonia, and influenza, together with frequent sinus attacks and head colds which may have been caused by the overdose of chloroform at birth. In December, 1919, his tonsils had been removed, and after that he seemed less prone to sickness.[219]

This sets the scene. Taking the tonsils out made him "better," because it pushed the illness inward.

> On the afternoon of August 9, roughhousing with his boys on the deck of the Black Yacht, he toppled off into the freezing Bay of Fundy. He laughed this off as a great joke, but the icy waters dealt his body a severe shock.

> The next afternoon he took Anna, James, and Elliot out in his small sailboat Vireo. On an island close to Campobello they spied a forest fire. The four landed, cut evergreen boughs, and spent several hours vigorously fighting it. Back on Campobello, a hot weary Franklin suggested a refreshing dip in Lake Glen Severn, a mile and a half away. With the children after him, he ran at dogtrot to the lake. The swim failed to invigorate him - the only time in his life this has happened, he told Eleanor on his return to the cottage. So he suggested another dip into the colder waters of the bay. In wet bathing suits, the four finally jogged back to the house.

> Here Franklin found his daily mail and newspapers. Out of doors, still wearing the damp bathing suit in air turning chill, he sat and read for thirty minutes. All at once a shattering chill and sharp pains shot through him. He went to bed. Next morning he was feverish and still in pain. He also complained that his right leg was weak. When he tried to get up, the right knee buckled. Next, both legs became affected. By the third day the paralysis had spread to nearly every muscle from the chest down.[219]

Remember that this happened at a time when the polio virus was virulent in the environment. Sitting around in a cold wind after a swim will not make you get polio if there is no polio virus in the air. This tragedy and many others made it obvious to health authorities that chills are a major risk factor in catching polio. In 1948 the New Zealand Health Department warned parents of the danger with this poster.

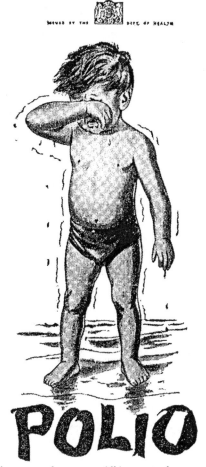

This summer, keep your children out of very cold water. See that they do not stay too long in swimming, and that they get dried and reclothed quickly. Chills and fatigue are allies of the poliomyelitis virus.

Why did they know that then when they do not know it now? It reminds me of the way that the Ancient Greeks knew so much about mathematics and astronomy, yet their knowledge was forgotten and had to be rediscovered all over again during the Renaissance.

At kindergarten I chatted to a granny who had had polio in 1956. At the time she was mother to a toddler and a baby, so she was generally tired. One morning she woke up with "flu" and she was feeling really rotten. Her mother offered to come around and help with the daily chores, but she refused the offer because she did not want to burden her mother. She felt that she must hang the nappies on the line before she had a rest. Her mother had a feeling that something was wrong, and came to the house without telephoning again. She found her daughter collapsed on the ground under the washing line, and called an ambulance. The woman, who is now a granny herself, spent a long time in hospital with polio, and when she was discharged she could only walk very slowly. She still cannot walk at a normal pace. She told me that all the other polio victims that were in the hospital at the same time as she was had also been very tired at the time that they contracted the disease. She now regrets that she tried to do too much on that morning, because it was by overexerting herself that she made the "flu" reach the paralytic stage of polio.

Having had one's tonsils removed increases the risk of catching polio.[220,221] Studies from 1910 to 1953 found that when tonsils had recently been removed, the risk was very high, but there was still an increased risk after ten years.[221] Some health departments instructed doctors to refrain from removing tonsils while the polio virus was virulent.

The tonsils are the first line of defence. They are made of lymphoid tissue, and this tissue is swarming with immune system cells. If the tonsils become sore and inflamed, it is because they are being overloaded with toxins and underfed with nutrients. Massive doses of vitamin C will fix them, as I learned in 1977. I was living in Africa near a hospital called Settler's Hospital, and there were lots of severely poverty stricken, disenfranchised people living in the same town. I was approached by a woman who asked me to give her five rand so that she could have her tonsils out at the hospital. Five rand was two weeks wages for a Black person who was employed, and this woman, like the majority of Blacks in the town, was unemployed. I did not feel like parting with five rand, so I shone a light on her tonsils. The sight was revolting. The flesh had split into canyons that were filled with green and yellow pus. This condition is called quinsy. I looked it up in Adelle Davis, and vitamin C was recommended. I had an unopened bottle of vitamin C on the shelf which had cost two rand. The bottle had been sitting there ever since I had bought it with the intention of doing the right thing and taking a pill every day. So I gave her the bottle and told her how much to take and how often. I was really trying to save myself three rand. A few days later the woman came round and I looked at her throat again. The flesh of her tonsils was smooth and healthy. And it stayed healthy. I had not only saved myself some money, I had also inadvertently saved her from losing an important part of her immune system.

Weleda's *Zinnober D6* taken alternately with *Erysidoron 1* on the hour, rapidly converts struggling, overloaded tonsils into healthy, hardworking tonsils. The barbaric act of removing the tonsils lowers a person's immunity for the rest of his or her life.

When the polio virus is naturally virulent in the environment, injecting vaccine material into a person increases the risk of him or her contracting polio. After a vaccine has been administered, there is a period in which a person has lower resistance to infections. Usually this is not a problem because there seldom are the germs of an infectious disease in the environment, but when the germs are present, the likelihood of succumbing to them is greatly increased by being vaccinated against another disease. The first person to publicise the phenomenon of suppressed immunity after vaccination was Almroth Wright, the inventor of the typhoid vaccine. In 1901 he called the period of suppressed immunity which follows vaccination the "negative phase of diminished bactericidal power."[222] In 1967 Sir Graham Wilson labelled disease which occurs as a result of this suppressed immunity "provocation disease."[223]

The polio virus was still virulent in the 1940s and 1950s. It was an empirically observable fact that children were more likely to come down with polio if they had recently been vaccinated against diphtheria, whooping cough, or with the combined diphtheria and whooping cough vaccine. An official investigation into the 1949 epidemic in Britain found that the risk of contracting polio was greatly increased for 28 days after vaccination, and that the period of greatest risk was from 8 to 17 days after.[224] The chief medical officer in Britain then told the regional medical officers to use their own discretion, and vaccination was suspended in many areas until the natural virulence of the polio virus abated.[225,226] In 1951 the Health Department of New York City suspended vaccination against whooping cough and diphtheria from June 15 to October 1 in order to avoid cases of provocation polio.[227]

Sir Graham Wilson says,

Working on the London County Council figures, Benjamin and Gore (1952) calculated that during 1949 the risk of contracting poliomyelitis [polio] was nearly four times as high in children of 9 - 24 months who had received an injection of combined diphtheria and pertussis [whooping cough] vaccine within the previous six weeks as in a control uninoculated group.[228]

The injected polio vaccine also increases the risk of contracting polio shortly after vaccination. An interesting point that emerges from Graham Wilson's collection of data is that the injected polio vaccine causes provocation polio when used during an epidemic, while the oral polio vaccine does not. Also of interest is the fact that those brands of vaccine which had had aluminium added to them, had a worse provocation effect than the brands without aluminium.

The polio virus was not globally virulent during the later part of the 20th century, but it has become virulent in limited areas from time to time. When this happens, recent vaccination increases the risk of catching polio. For instance, the polio virus put in an appearance in the country of Oman in 1988. A study found that 35% of the cases of polio in babies aged from five to eleven months had been provoked by injection of DPT vaccine.[229] Of course a vaccine can only provoke polio when there is a polio virus in the environment, but it is clear that one way of protecting yourself if the polio virus becomes virulent in your area is to avoid all vaccines.

Paralytic polio has been cured in a number of different ways. If someone in my family came down with polio, I would have them treated by a homoeopath right away, and by a chiropractor or osteopath as soon as possible. Polio is a fast acting disease and there is no time to waste. The appropriate potentised remedy, selected by a properly trained homoeopath, will hit right at the core of the polio, and you will see an improvement in the patient in a matter of minutes.

Don't be tempted to try and choose the remedy yourself. A good homoeopath has the materia medica inside his or her brain, and can select a remedy that corresponds to all the prevailing symptoms, not just to some of the symptoms. You can afford to experiment with treating flu yourself, because if you do not succeed in choosing a remedy that makes the patient's body kill the virus, then the patient is only left with flu or post viral fatigue syndrome. But polio is a much more serious disease. Failure to kill the virus can result in death or life-long paralysis.

Modern medicine calls polio an incurable disease because they cannot cure it, but intensive care in hospital can prevent victims from dying during the acute phase. The iron lung prevents death from lung paralysis, and intravenous fluids help to sustain life, but medical treatment cannot prevent nerve damage.

I was a child during the era when the polio virus was still virulent, and I remember the unlucky ones with their callipers hobbling around at school. For them the effect was going to be life-long. One classmate was in a wheelchair as a result of polio when we were only six. At playtime he sat in his wheelchair and did French knitting with a wooden cotton reel that had four tacks nailed into it. He made a brightly coloured rope that seemed miles long. He coiled it and made it into a big carpet. He had time on his hands because he could not run around the playground with us. It was all quite unnecessary because there were a lot of properly qualified homoeopaths in

Johannesburg. One of them, Dr. Archie Taylor Smith, is mentioned by Dr. Dorothy Shepherd in her book on how to treat infectious diseases homoeopathically.[230] She quotes the remedies he recommends for the different types of onset "to break up the disease in its early stages." Treatment in the next stage prevents paralysis, while treatment during paralysis prevents death and nerve damage.

I remember my mother telling her friends that homoeopathy was the way to treat polio, and I remember her mentioning the name of Dr. Archie Taylor Smith among others. My mother also spoke about Archie's success at treating a girl from Bulawayo in Rhodesia for brain damage from DPT vaccine. The girl's parents drove the 550 miles from Bulawayo to Johannesburg on very underdeveloped roads once a month to see Archie. The child never became normal, but Archie's choice of remedies accomplished a remarkable improvement. In another suburb in Johannesburg there lived a batch of little boys who were destined to become my brothers-in-law two decades later. They were treated successfully by Archie for a number of ailments, and he cured their father of a life threatening condition. The things which homoeopathy can do seem amazing to people who have no first hand experience of it.

The polio virus does damage when it moves from the gastro-intestinal tract into the cells and attacks the nervous system, so it is a good idea to keep the skeleton free of subluxations. Subluxations are partial dislocations of the bones. When the vertebrae of the spine are out of position, they impede the flow of information along the nerves. An adjustment to correct the position of the bones in the neck is particularly helpful to stop giving flu or polio germs an advantage.

It surprised me to learn that chiropractic and osteopathic care can help to alleviate residual paralysis after the acute stage of polio has passed. The first time I heard about this was in 1972, when my mother and I went on a bird club camp in the Magaliesburg mountains. A woman who walked with a peculiar gait started putting up a tent next to ours. Her body was crooked, and her movements were rather awkward. My mother, with her usual tact, said, "Let me help you. You look as though you have a crick in your neck." The lady was not phased by that, and she told us that she had had polio at seventeen, and the specialist had told her she would never walk again. At twenty-one she had started chiropractic treatment, and was up and about in a matter of weeks. Some years later she was walking up Adderley Street in Cape Town when the specialist came walking down the street. He was astounded to see her walking, and when she told him that a chiropractor had done it, he was furious, and reprimanded her for going to a "quack."

When the polio vaccine was being developed there was a fund raising effort called the *March of Dimes* which used posters to advertise their cause.

One of the posters showed a photograph of a little girl called Winifred Gardella who had lost the ability to walk because of polio. In the photo she was standing supported by crutches with her legs in callipers. Medical treatment was unable to improve her condition, but later a chiropractor named Lewis Robertson got her walking again.[231]

Good old vitamin C comes to the rescue again when the polio virus is wreaking havoc in the body, but it has to be injected. A person with polio is too sick to swallow megadoses of vitamin C. Dr. Linus Pauling says,

> Dr. Fred R Klenner, a physician in Reidsville, North Carolina, was the first person to report the successful treatment on polio patients by injecting large amounts of ascorbic acid.[232]

Adelle Davis says,

> Some years ago it was my good fortune to visit with Dr. Klenner and hear him lecture ... Dr. Klenner told of an eighteen-month-old girl suffering from polio. The mother reported that the child had become paralysed following a convulsion, after which she soon lost consciousness. When Dr. Klenner first saw the child, her little body was blue, stiff and cold to the touch; he could neither hear her heart sound nor feel her pulse, her rectal temperature was 100 degrees F. The only sign of life he could detect was a suggestion of moisture condensed on a mirror held to her mouth. The mother was convinced that the child was already dead. Dr. Klenner injected 6,000 milligrams of vitamin C into her blood; four hours later the child was cheerful and alert, holding a bottle with her right hand, though her left side was paralysed. A second injection was given; soon the child was laughing and holding her bottle with both hands, all signs of paralysis gone. Dr. Klenner quite understandably speaks of vitamin C as "the antibiotic par excellence." A physician who later obtained striking results at the Los Angeles County Hospital by treating severe infections with vitamin C matched Dr. Klenner's enthusiasm with the remark, "if anything should be called a miracle drug, it is vitamin C."
> With his extremely ill patients, Dr. Klenner found that no vitamin C whatsoever could be detected in the blood only a few minutes after massive doses were injected; nor was any vitamin C found in the urine. It is his belief that this vitamin combines immediately with toxins and/or virus, thus causing the fever to drop.[233]

You can see why the makers of paracetamol, who happen to control the curricula at medical schools, do not want doctors to know about vitamin C. Drugs which reduce fever do so by crippling the immune system, not by helping the immune system fight the invader. I wonder how many millions of children have died when a shot of vitamin C could have saved them. Few doctors have the savvy to use injections of vitamin C in a crisis, and in some countries doctors know that they would face persecution by the medical establishment if they did use it. Dr. Archie Kalokerinos, who works in the Australian outback, is one of the modern doctors who uses vitamin C injections to save lives.

In Australia and New Zealand the Kenny treatment[234] was used to treat polio while it was still around. Sister Kenny was an Australian nurse who devised a method of reducing paralysis by using heat and massage. The treatment aims to relax the muscles that have gone into spasm, and to stimulate the muscles that have gone limp. The patient is wrapped in thick woollen blankets that have been warmed, and the blankets are replaced with warmer ones as soon as they cool down. The modern medical tenet of chilling a seriously ill patient is in direct contrast to this.

Because Sister Kenny's treatment was drug free, certain elements tried to suppress it, and Sister Kenny herself was persecuted. Nowadays it is acknowledged that the treatment was helpful. Although the treatment meant that polio victims did not lose the ability to walk, it unfortunately did not save polio victims from suffering post polio syndrome in their old age. The only way to prevent the nerve damage which inevitably leads to post polio syndrome is to stop the virus from doing the damage by intervening early in the acute phase with a potentised homoeopathic remedy, or with megadoses of vitamin C.

c) TETANUS

Tetanus germs can only cause disease if they enter the bloodstream. They do not create disease when they are breathed in or swallowed. When the germs get into human blood they thrive if the blood lacks oxygen. This is why tetanus seldom occurs in fit, healthy adults. The very old and the very young are most at risk from tetanus. Flesh that has been injured lacks oxygen, which is why men with war wounds are so susceptible to the disease. The germs gain entry to the blood through a wound or a prick or a splinter. Tetanus germs can exist on anything in the environment, but there are always lots of germs in soil on which cattle walk, and in cattle dung.

Even though the blood of most healthy individuals is an unfavourable environment for tetanus germs, everyone should take steps to avert tetanus after a wound. This is because it is a fast acting and potentially fatal disease. Ideally every wound should be washed with a mixture of *hypericum* tincture and *calendula* tincture. In some countries this is sold ready mixed under the name *hypercal tincture*. No pharmaceutical product is as effective as these plant extracts. If they are not available, wash the wound with soap or disinfectant.

It is not possible to wash a puncture wound that has been made by something like a pin, a thorn, or an animal's tooth. These are problematic wounds because tetanus germs can be delivered deep into the flesh, out of the reach of disinfectants. The homoeopathic remedy *ledum 30* should be taken after all puncture wounds. If an innocent looking little splinter gets under the skin, it is worth taking a dose of *ledum 30* because there are often tetanus germs on wood. After a bite from an animal the patient should take *ledum 30*, even if it looks as if the flesh was torn open enough for effective washing.

When redness appears around the mouth of a puncture wound, it is a sign that germs are causing a problem, but lack of redness does not mean that the person is safe from tetanus. Pharmaceutical medicine treats redness around a wound with a drug that makes the redness go away. When there is redness around a wound it means that the capillaries have become wider to allow macrophages to travel to the scene. Macrophages are big immune system cells that can swallow up invading germs, toxins and damaged cells. A capillary is the smallest kind of blood vessel, and each cell of the body has a capillary running past it. Macrophages are too big to fit down the pipe of a normal capillary, so the capillaries get wider when macrophages are needed in a particular area. The response of modern medicine to this little miracle of nature is to say that the red area is "inflamed," and a drug must be given to stop the "inflammation." "Anti-inflammatories" are very effective drugs. The redness disappears, so the doctors congratulate themselves for "curing" the problem, when what they have actually done is to stop macrophages from getting to a place where they are badly needed.

Most deaths from tetanus occur in babies in impoverished countries. When a baby is born in a community which lives in close proximity with animals, the umbilical cord is often cut with an implement that is contaminated with cow dung. In these communities the floors and walls of huts are often plastered with a mixture of cow dung and clay. This mixture forms a practical building material, but unfortunately the cow dung component is usually contaminated with tetanus germs. Before the umbilical cord dries and drops off, it is like an open wound. When a cutting implement has been lying on a floor that looks clean, but has tetanus germs incorporated into it, the germs go from the implement into the umbilical cord and then into the baby's blood stream. Hygiene is 100% effective at preventing tetanus in newborns. In one part of Nigeria infant mortality from tetanus dropped to nil after traditional midwives were issued with stainless steel scissors for cutting the cord, and were shown how to keep the scissors sterile.

Elderly people are a high risk group for tetanus because of their slowed down circulation. A high proportion of tetanus victims in Australia and New Zealand are elderly. Their vaccination status is not given in the statistics. Statistics about the people who are paralysed by tetanus vaccine are also not provided.

Tetanus bacteria and tetanus toxoid can be inactivated by vitamin C,[235] so it is a good idea to take megadoses of vitamin C after any kind of wound. The money spent on the vitamin C will not have been wasted if there were no tetanus germs in the wound, because vitamin C helps wounds to heal and helps the immune system kill other germs that might have entered the wound.

An experiment was done in a hospital in Dhaka, Bangladesh, to see if vitamin C helped in the treatment of tetanus.[236] The subjects consisted of one hundred and seventeen people who were hospitalised with tetanus. They were divided into two age groups; those up to 12 years, and those over 12 years. Each group was then divided into those who received the conventional treatment plus vitamin C, and those who received only the conventional treatment. Unfortunately they did not create a group which was given vitamin C but no conventional treatment. The amount of vitamin C that was given was only 1000 mg of ascorbic acid, and yet it made a tremendous difference to survival rates. No deaths occurred in the children who were given this small amount of vitamin C, while 74.2% of the children who were not given vitamin C died. The amount of vitamin C being so small meant that it did not have such a great impact on the age group with the bigger body weight. 37% of the adults who were given 1000 mg of vitamin C died, while 67% of those not given vitamin C died. This experiment was published in a medical journal in 1984. It clearly shows that injections of vitamin C save the lives of people with tetanus, yet no public hospital in the world has started using vitamin C injections as a treatment for tetanus. Tax payer funded hospitals do not exist to make people well - they exist to make the pharmaceutical industry rich.

Homoeopathy can also cure tetanus after symptoms appear. To work quickly, the correct remedy needs to be given in the right potency and with the right frequency. If it is repeated too soon it will stop the first dose from working, and the patient could die. If the symptoms of lockjaw develop a few days after infection occurs, it means that the disease is going to proceed fast, and quick action must be taken. If symptoms appear two weeks after the wound, there is less danger of death, but the sooner homoeopathic treatment commences, the less residual nerve damage there will be. The presence of fever is also a bad sign, but of course the treatment should not focus on making the fever go away, it should focus on ridding the body of the cause of the fever.

Medical treatment uses things like muscle relaxants and antibiotics, and of course someone else's blood with antibodies in it (immune serum globulin). The modern drugs they use to deal with the symptoms of muscle tightening are much safer than the old fashioned ones they used to use. Old statistics on tetanus are meaningless, because many of the patients actually died from curare poisoning, not from tetanus. Medics are still quite happy to inject tetanus toxoid at the same time as immune serum globulin into a person who is already suffering from tetanus.

In World War I the British soldiers were vaccinated against tetanus. According to figures tabled by Winston Churchill in the House of Commons in July 1920, the rate of tetanus on the western front was 4.3 times higher than during the Boer War, where no vaccine was used.[237]

One day in a dark shed I stood on a rusty nail that was pointing directly upwards. It went through my shoe and deep into my foot. It did not hurt because it went into a fleshy spot, but I was emotionally upset because of the fear of tetanus. Most rusty nails in farmland Australia do have tetanus germs on them. I have no reason to assume that my blood is aerobic enough to kill those germs, and it is not possible to kill the germs from the outside because of the shape of the wound. I took a dose of *ledum 30*, but I had no confidence in it because Kenneth had taken the bottle on a camp, and it had been confiscated and stored with other medicines for a while, so it may have been depotentised. If I started going rigid, there was no-one to drive me to a homoeopath. Then Chandra reminded me of the Bangladesh study with vitamin C. Of course! I had a bottle of non-acidic calcium ascorbate with bioflavinoids in the cupboard. I stopped worrying. The perfectly round mark on the sole of my foot lasted three months, but I suffered no systemic effect. Perhaps I did not need the vitamin C and I would not have developed tetanus anyway, but the vitamin C certainly cured my emotional problem. I knew that a small amount of vitamin C can cure people with the full blown disease, so a large amount would definitely protect me from developing the disease.

d) DIPHTHERIA

When diphtheria was still prevalent, the homoeopaths successfully cured people by choosing the correct potentised similar for each individual case. One of the worst features of diphtheria is that a membrane forms at the back of the throat. If the membrane grows right across the opening of the throat it can cause suffocation. There are other conditions that can also bring on this membrane, most notably glandular fever (infectious mononucleosis). The exact appearance of this membrane helps the homoeopath choose a remedy for the individual with diphtheria.

Antibiotics can kill the germs that cause diphtheria, but they make no impact on the course of the disease, and do not reduce the death rate. In the past medical treatment of diphtheria involved injecting patients with horse blood containing a high level of antibodies.

Diphtheria has not disappeared, although it has undergone a considerable natural decline during this century (see graphs in myth number four). No-one can predict what it is going to do in the future. If it were to return in a big way, the homoeopaths would once again treat it successfully, but not necessarily using the same set of remedies as they used before. Each case would have to be individually assessed before a remedy is chosen.

f) CHOLERA

Cholera is a waterborne disease, so unboiled water is to be avoided when travelling in countries where cholera is endemic. Even if you are young and fit and healthy, don't make the mistake of thinking that you would be immune if you swallowed some cholera germs. It is a good idea to try and oversee the cooking of all food that you are going to eat. Don't assume that an expensive hotel has an hygienic kitchen, just because there are plush carpets on the floor of the dining room. Salad may have been washed with contaminated water. Also, don't assume that tea and coffee are made with boiled water. It is safer to make your own hot drinks with a gadget that you immerse in a cup of water. Some travellers carry with them an assortment of homoeopathic remedies for diarrhoeal type diseases, just in case.

In vaccine myth number five I have described how cholera started in India 1300 years ago, and how in 1817 it suddenly started spreading across the earth. A second wave started in 1826, and it spread steadily towards Western Europe. The homoeopaths were the only people who were successful at treating this disease as it crossed Europe.

Dr. Frederick Hervey Foster Quin was an English doctor who met Dr. Samuel Hahnemann in 1826.[238] The meeting resulted in his conversion to homoeopathy. In 1831 Dr. Quin travelled from Western Europe to what was then called Moravia, in Eastern Europe, to study the approaching cholera epidemic. Soon after his arrival in Moravia he was suddenly struck down with the violent form of cholera while eating dinner. (Cholera often strikes suddenly. During one of the waves that crossed Europe, scores of people at a grand ball in France suddenly fell down with the sickness.) Dr. Quin was carried to a bed, and when he came out of the coma he treated himself with a remedy. He began to recover, and then he started treating others while still sick and weak. "I was overworking from morning to night treating cases of cholera, all the other doctors being bedridden."[239]

Cholera is one of those diseases which strikes very fast and can kill within a day. In response to these fast acting diseases, homoeopathy works very quickly to effect a cure. Onlookers are stunned by the rapidity with which a patient reverts from being at death's door to being well. Diseases that take a long time to develop, like arthritis, take much longer to be cured by homoeopathy.

After Dr. Quin left Moravia, the mayor of the town where he had worked sent him a letter of gratitude for starting to work before he was fully recovered. In the letter he mentions that from the time that Dr. Quin started treating the victims of cholera, no patient died.[240]

Dr. Quin founded the British Homoeopathic Society in 1844.[241,242] At one time Dr. Quin was personal physician to the bloke who later became the King of Belgium. Homoeopathy still remains available to the privileged few, while the inhabitants of Belgium's former colonies die in droves from cholera. The World Health Organisation (WHO) should arrange for homoeopaths to enter refugee camps during cholera epidemics and treat each affected individual with the correct remedy. A trained homoeopath would only take a few minutes to assess and prescribe for each patient. The medicine to save the patient's life would only cost a few cents, which is the main reason why the pharmaceutical industry does not allow WHO to use it. Malaria and bilharzia (schistosoma) are the biggest killers in Africa. Both diseases can be cured with homoeopathic medicine costing less than a dollar for each individual.

In recent years modern medicine has developed techniques for replacing the water lost by the person with cholera. This often keeps the patient alive until the cholera bacillus works its way out, but the instruments needed for this treatment are expensive and not available in areas where cholera prevails. The homoeopaths do not need to do rehydration, because the right remedy works so fast.

g) TYPHOID

The germs that cause typhoid are good survivors. When they enter a human body, they can live there for years, and they shed billions of offspring which go into the sewage. They do this whether or not the human they have entered gets clinical symptoms of the disease. This means that typhoid can be caught by drinking water that is contaminated with sewage, or from food prepared by someone with faeces on their hands. The typhoid germ belongs to the salmonella family. All types of salmonella are good survivors, and many of them cause serious symptoms that can lead to death. They thrive in hot weather, but they also survive in cold weather. Typhoid is caused by Salmonella Typhi, which is the worst member of the salmonella family. It does not always strike fast. Sometimes it starts by looking like a bad case of flu, and sometimes it starts with mental symptoms or nausea and vomiting. The wide variety of symptoms the typhoid germ can cause means there is an even bigger range of possible homoeopathic remedies for it than for a disease like cholera. All kinds of salmonella contaminate water in countries where sewage is not properly disposed of, so always boil the water in dubious places.

Gastro-enteritis from salmonella is sometimes called "food poisoning," but it is not caused by the food being rancid. Perfectly fresh food can carry salmonella, and there is no warning smell or taste. Flies can carry salmonella on their feet. Always cover food so that flies cannot land on it. Salmonella germs go through phases of increased virulence, but it is safer to practice hygiene as if they are always virulent. Outbreaks of salmonella poisoning occur in modern cities when the germ becomes virulent, because a few people do not practice hygiene.

A vaccine for typhoid was invented early in the history of the vaccine industry. The "success" of this vaccine is often quoted as justification for the practice of vaccination in general. It is claimed by vaccine promoters that typhoid was rampant during the Boer War because vaccination was not used, while it hardly occurred during World War I because vaccination was used. The historical evidence is fragmentary, but the information available certainly does not support such a view. Lets look at the data which does exist regarding typhoid in the Boer War (1899 to 1902), the Russo-Japanese War (1904 to 1905), and World War I (1914 to 1918).

In the Boer War, 400,000 doses of typhoid vaccine were dispatched for the protection of the British soldiers. It is not known how many doses were actually administered. The soldiers did not live in hygienic conditions, and they drank contaminated water. Typhoid took a heavy toll on the soldiers, even though a common geranium, *pelargonium reniforme*, which grew at their feet, could have saved them. The natives taught some of the British to use it. Horses were dosed by wrapping the root in a cloth and tying it to the bit, so that a small amount mingled with the saliva.[243]

Only two years after the Boer War ended the Russo-Japanese war broke out. It was the first of the high tech wars. Both Russia and Japan wanted control of Korea and Manchuria, and in this particular squabble, machine guns, howitzers, mines, and battleships with torpedoes were used. It was a practice run for the arms industry which made such a fortune out of World War I. Professor Kitasato, the co-inventor of the tetanus and diphtheria vaccine, tried to persuade the Japanese army to buy the typhoid vaccine which the English had used in the Boer War.[244] The Japanese army declined. Hygiene had been traditional in Japan for a long time, and they attempted to keep food and water clean for the soldiers. They were not entirely successful. The rate of typhoid was one sixth that of the British troops during the Boer War.

Chlorine had been used to sterilise water for the first time in 1897 in Maidstone, England, during an epidemic of typhoid.[244] That epidemic came to an abrupt halt because the chlorine killed the typhoid germs in the water. In World War I, most of the water on the western front was chlorinated, but it was difficult to take the bulky chlorinating apparatus to the troops at Gallipoli. The unfortunate soldiers at Gallipoli sometimes drank from muddy pools of water while hoping to avoid being shot by the unseen enemy. Most of the Allied soldiers at Gallipoli, including all of the ANZACS (Australian and New Zealand soldiers), had been vaccinated against typhoid. Australian soldiers who refused vaccination were taken off the ships before they left Australia. Typhoid hardly affected the men in the trenches on the Western front, whereas there were 96,684 victims of typhoid at Gallipoli.[245]

The water at Gallipoli contained paratyphoid as well as typhoid bacteria. Some of the soldiers who were admitted to hospital at Lemnos because of typhoid symptoms had their blood tested to see whether they had antibodies to typhoid or to paratyphoid.[246] The type of antibodies which were found were interpreted as indicating which type of germ had caused the illness. Some soldiers were found to have antibodies to both typhoid and paratyphoid, so their vaccination status was checked, and if they were vaccinated, they were regarded as a case of paratyphoid. Despite the shenanigans, the survey still found that 96% of the individuals who had typhoid antibodies and no paratyphoid antibodies, had been vaccinated against typhoid.

So we see that vaccination *was* used, to an unknown extent, during the Boer War. We also see that chlorination protected the Allied soldiers on the western front during World War I, while on the eastern front, ninety six thousand soldiers who had been vaccinated against typhoid got typhoid because they were exposed to typhoid in the water they drank. Yet vaccinationists still claim that it was the use of typhoid vaccine during World War I that established vaccination as an effective medical procedure.

When a homoeopath is confronted with a patient with any kind of salmonella poisoning, he or she does not need to know the name of the germ that caused the problem. The homoeopath must take note of the symptoms which are showing themselves in that particular patient, and after deciding on the right remedy, must move on to the next patient and start all over again.

Penicillin was able to kill salmonella typhi until the germs mutated. New antibiotics are effective until the strain mutates again. The medics tend not to use antibiotics any more, because they acknowledge that by killing the good bacteria in the intestine, they do the patient more harm than good. They prefer to take the better course of supporting the patient through the infection, rather than trying to kill the infective agent. Life support greatly reduces the death rate, but of course is not available in far flung poverty stricken areas.

h) TYPHUS

The symptoms of typhus are very different to the symptoms of typhoid, and the organism that causes typhus is completely different to the organism that causes typhoid. Typhus is caused by a tiny germ called rickettsia prowazekii. It is neither a bacterium nor a virus. Typhus is carried by lice, but there is a mild relative of typhus that is carried by fleas as well as lice.

Typhus breaks out when malnourished people are crowded together, so you are not likely to encounter the disease in a suburb in a democratic country. But it is difficult to avoid typhus if a political force is causing you to live in a crowded place, and is depriving you of washing facilities and food. Thousands of people die every year from typhus in poor areas of the world. These deaths do not make headlines, even when there is media interest in a political crisis in the area.

Typhus thrives on wars and other social upheavals. When twelve million people were kidnapped from Africa and shipped to America to be sold as slaves, about 10% of them died of typhus on the way over, and their bodies were thrown into the sea. In 1899 the Boers were in possession of the gold and diamonds of central southern Africa. The British wanted it for themselves, and as they could not beat the Boers militarily, they burned down their homes and herded the Boer women and children into concentration camps. Twenty thousand women and children died of typhus and typhoid. In 1948 the Boers regained possession of the gold and diamonds, and they herded the Blacks into concentration camps called bantustans, and hundreds of thousands of Blacks died of typhus and typhoid. No-one counted how many died.

A rumour has arisen in "health" publications that the ancient Greek doctor Hippocrates cured typhus during the siege of Athens in 440 BC. The doctor Hippocrates was not even there, and the symptoms, which are described in detail, are not those of typhus.[247]

The first recorded instance of typhus being cured was when Dr. Samuel Hahnemann, the person who discovered homoeopathy, cured 178 people during an outbreak in 1813. The opportunity for him to do this was created by Napoleon Bonaparte. After Napoleon was forced to retreat from Russia in 1812, he gathered up a new army and marched against Prussia and Austria. He won a battle at Dresden, and then marched on to Leipzig. For three days a battle raged in and around Leipzig, and then Napoleon retreated back to France. Eighty thousand corpses were left in the city of Leipzig, and there were another eighty thousand wounded soldiers. A handful of doctors from the university did their best to tend the wounded. To make matters worse, an epidemic of typhus broke out.[248]

Dr. Hahnemann happened to be in Leipzig at the time. He treated 180 people who had typhus, and only two died, one of whom was a very old man. He chose the appropriate remedy by observing the symptoms of each patient who had typhus, and giving them the homoeopathic similar. He needed only two remedies, because there was not a great variation in symptoms. This seemingly amazing feat of curing typhus made the fame of Dr. Hahnemann spread throughout Europe.[248] All the people who get typhus today could be cured cheaply and quickly.

In World War II many Allied soldiers were sprayed with DDT insecticide to protect them from getting typhus.[249] It is an effective measure because no lice means no typhus. Pity about the side effects, but being poisoned is better than getting typhus. The American allies used DDT in the Pacific during World War II, and some of it floated down to Antarctica. The penguins there still harbour DDT in their body tissue because DDT is a persistent chemical.

> DDT was used against lice in a dusting powder applied to fully clothed people, and had the most important property of persistent action after one application, thus preventing reinfestation.[249]

Photos were taken of Allied soldiers being powdered with clouds of DDT during a typhus epidemic in Naples. There were only two cases of typhus among the Allied soldiers in Naples, one of whom died. Both soldiers had been vaccinated.[249] It would be great to see an end to prisoner of war camps, refugee camps, chemical farming, vaccination, and the suppression of homoeopathy. That would put an end to typhus.

i) HEPATITIS B

Hepat is the Greek word for liver, and hepatitis refers to inflammation of the liver. Hepatitis can be caused by toxins or by germs. Hepatitis A, hepatitis B and hepatitis C are all caused by viruses that attack the liver. Hepatitis A can be caught from cutlery and crockery that has not been properly washed, from food that has been prepared by someone who does not wash their hands, or from shellfish that is harvested from a part of the sea that is contaminated with sewage. Hepatitis B and hepatitis C are different in that they need to enter a person's blood in order to cause infection. As with the virus that causes AIDS, the risk factors for catching hepatitis B and C are promiscuous sex, contaminated blood products, and contaminated needles. The hepatitis B virus can also be transmitted from a mother to her baby during pregnancy or birth, but only if the mother has the virus living in her body.

The symptoms of hepatitis B include nausea, yellowness, tiredness, loss of appetite, pain in the liver, sore joints, sore muscles, a skin rash and dark coloured urine. However, when a person is infected with hepatitis B it does not always cause symptoms to appear. Some people become infected with the virus and do not show any symptoms at all. Furthermore, not all symptoms are present in all cases where symptoms do occur.

Sometimes the virus continues to live in the body of a person it has infected for a long time. This can happen whether or not the virus caused any symptoms when it first infected the person. So a person who has been exposed to one of the risk factors for catching hepatitis B may be carrying the virus in his or her body, even though he or she has never experienced the acute symptoms of hepatitis B. In some carriers the virus causes liver damage, and in rare cases, liver cancer. Certain racial groups are more prone to chronic infection, but no group is immune.

Hepatitis B can be a difficult disease to diagnose because the symptoms vary between individuals. If hepatitis B were suspected in a member of my family, I would want a blood test for confirmation even though homoeopaths do not need to know the cause of liver troubles in order to be able to cure them. Drugs that are used to treat people who are carriers of the hepatitis B virus have the problem that they do not work very well, and they have unpleasant side effects.[250]

With any kind of hepatitis, the liver struggles to process fat. Adelle Davis describes how supplementing with large enough doses of vitamins B, C and E and eating protein foods supports the liver through any kind of hepatitis.[251] From my own experience of liver damage from yellow fever vaccine, I recommend desiccated or freeze dried liver pills, rather than vegetarian forms of vitamin B. Supplements should continue for months after hepatitis, because the liver remains fragile. Livers have to work hard in these days of environmental toxins, and they need all the help they can get.

The Australian pamphlet that promotes hepatitis B vaccination on the day of birth is possibly the most despicable health department pamphlet I have ever seen. The first trick is that the pamphlet is given to mothers when they are already in labour, instead of being given out during pregnancy. A woman who is in labour is usually not able to think clearly, be assertive, think of the right questions to ask, nor go to the library to do some research. This is precisely why the pamphlet is given to mothers at this time. The pamphlet contains 4 blatant lies, 6 clever half truths, lots of omissions and 2 serious omissions. The first serious omission is that it does not mention that the vaccine is made from genetically engineered yeast. There is a public outcry in Australia about the fact that the government subsidises genetically engineered crops while not supporting sustainable agriculture. Yet no-one is talking about the fact that the government injects genetically engineered yeast into babies on the day that they are born.

The other serious omission on the pamphlet is that it does not mention that if the mother's blood has not been exposed to hepatitis B infection, the baby cannot catch hepatitis B from her. A baby is not old enough to be promiscuous or to share needles with other drug addicts, so the only way that he or she can become infected with hepatitis B is through contaminated medical products or instruments. That is not likely to happen in a country that screens blood products and cleans medical instruments. In any case, catching an acute infection of hepatitis B is not nearly as dangerous as being injected with genetically engineered yeast on the day you are born.

One of the clever half-truths on the pamphlet is the statement that the risk of becoming a hepatitis B carrier is highest during infancy and early childhood. This is half true, because if the baby's blood is exposed to the hepatitis B virus during infancy or early childhood, the risk of him or her becoming a carrier is higher than it is from exposure to the virus when he or she is older. However, what the pamphlet does not say is that the risk of the baby's blood being exposed to hepatitis B during infancy and early childhood is much lower than it is during adolescence or adulthood.

In the blatant lie category the pamphlet says, "Serious side effects of hepatitis immunisation are rare." When medical people are presented with a case of severe side effects, they usually just deny that the vaccine is the cause. A baby born at Box Hill hospital in Melbourne in September 2002 was doing well. It was contented while awake, and feeding and sleeping well. When it was two days old it was injected with hepatitis B vaccine at 4 pm. It immediately stopped feeding, and it cried constantly. The mother was very concerned, but the nurses were not. It continued crying until it died at 7 am. The newspaper published the death notices, but not the cause of death.

In 1988 the hepatitis B vaccine made with human blood was introduced into New Zealand. The policy was that newborns were vaccinated a few days after birth, and a nurse had to stand and watch the babies for 20 minutes so that if one had a bad reaction to the vaccine, she could inject it with adrenaline. After a few months a nurse telephoned Hilary Butler and told her that the policy had been changed. Nurses had now been instructed to carry adrenaline and a syringe at all times, because some babies were going into shock more than 20 minutes after the vaccination, and some were dying in the time that it took for the nurse to gallop to the store and fetch adrenaline after she noticed the reaction. A normal brain would think that the policy should have been changed to suspend vaccination, but bureaucratic brains are not normal.

The vaccine was introduced in both Australia and New Zealand with the claim that a child could catch hepatitis B in the playground from the scabs or open wounds of carrier children. The New Zealand government employed Saatchi and Saatchi to make a terrifying TV advertisement that promoted fear of the disease, and confidence in the vaccine. The advertisement featured empty playground equipment and a doll that fell to the ground. Saatchi and Saatchi have great talent. The advertisement was so chilling, bordering on spooky, it sent a shudder down one's spine. After the vaccine was introduced, the theory that children could catch hepatitis B from other children was put to the test by a study in Sydney, and it was found that hepatitis B is not passed on from child to child.[19,20]

Some institutions that employ nurses make hepatitis B vaccine compulsory for their staff. I know nurses who have chosen to make a career change rather than have the stuff injected into their bodies.

j) RABIES

After a bite from an animal that is carrying rabies, the germ can live in the body for up to two years, although once six months has gone by without any sign of rabies, the chance of the disease developing is very much reduced. The fact that an animal bites does not automatically mean that it has rabies. Rabies is a very rare disease, and always has been. A bite from an animal seldom results in rabies, but when it does, the consequences are dire, unless homoeopathic treatment is used. Rabies can enter a human without a bite. A young girl in South Africa got rabies from the saliva of a cow which splashed into her eye. The poor girl suffered terribly and then died, quite unnecessarily, as there are so many good homoeopaths in South Africa.

An old medical book says, "If the symptoms of rabies have begun to appear, all treatment is useless to save life ..."[252] It is typical of pharmaceutical medicine to call a disease incurable because it cannot cure it. There are modern and old fashioned drugs which relieve spasms, and they can save a victim of rabies who would otherwise have died from the throat closing up. However, drugs cannot stop the virus from attacking and destroying the brain, whereas homoeopathy can.

The primary homoeopathic cure for rabies is lachesis. This is made from the venom of a deadly snake that lives in the Amazon jungle. This is how John Henry Clarke describes the discovery,

> To the genius and heroism of Hering the world owes this remedy and many another of which this has been the forerunner. When Hering's first experiments were made he was botanising and zoologising on the Upper Amazon for the German Government. Except his wife, all those about him were natives, who told him so much about the dreaded Surukuku that he offered a good reward for a live specimen. At last one was brought in a bamboo box, and those who brought it immediately fled, and all his native servants with them. Hering stunned the snake with a blow on the head as the box opened, then, holding its head in a forked stick, he pressed its venom out of the poison bag upon sugar of milk.[253]

Hering made low potency dilutions with the poison, and handling the poison made him suffer from the fumes. He went into an altered state, which included fever, tossing, delerium and mania. The next day his wife described his symptoms and how he had behaved, and Hering wrote down what she said. That was the first proving of lachesis.[253]

Another remedy for rabies is lyssin, which is made by homoeopathically potentising the saliva of a rabid dog. This remedy was thought of by Dr. Hering, made by Dr. Swann, and introduced in 1833,[254] fifty two years before Louis Pasteur injected Joseph Meister with rabbit spinal cords. Once potentised, the saliva loses all toxicity, unlike what happens in a crude vaccine. The manufacture of lyssin does not involve the infliction of pain on animals, and the use of it does not cause pain to humans.

"SMALLPOX WAS ERADICATED BY VACCINATION"

Vaccine Myth number Nine: Edward Jenner discovered that by inoculating people with cowpox he could make them immune to smallpox. He took cowpox pus from the teat of a cow and scratched it into a human. This meant that it was no longer necessary to inoculate people with pus from a human smallpox pustule. After the introduction of cowpox vaccination, smallpox disappeared from England. In the 20th century the World Health Organization vaccinated everyone, and the disease has now been eliminated from every country in the world.

I was taught at school that Edward Jenner observed that dairymaids who caught cowpox from cows never got smallpox afterwards. I was told that this observation led him to carry out scientific experiments, which proved that by inoculating people with cowpox, one could prevent them from getting smallpox. I was also taught that smallpox had been a terrible disease that had killed someone from every family, until Edward Jenner saved us by discovering how to prevent it. For three decades that misinformation sat in my head as part of my general knowledge. Then I was stunned to learn that the only part that was true, was that smallpox had been a deadly disease in Jenner's time.

All infectious diseases come and go on a natural cycle, which human beings cannot predict, nor can they alter. Smallpox entered Europe from the

Middle East in the 6th century AD, and while it became more common in the 11th century, it remained a mild disease until the 17th century. Smallpox suddenly became a virulent disease in the 17th century.[255] The reason why smallpox became so virulent in the 17th century is not known. For that matter, the reason why any disease becomes virulent for a time, and then fades away, is unknown. Between the time that smallpox entered Europe, and the time that it became the most feared disease in Europe, a number of other diseases came and went, like bubonic plague, sweating sickness and leprosy.

Sweating sickness was the greatest cause of death in England at one time, and yet it has completely disappeared without any action being taken against it by human beings. Its disappearance was so absolute that the germs which caused the disease were no longer available to be studied when microscopes were invented. Leprosy and bubonic plague are still present on the planet, but they have become quite rare. They waned in Europe without any help from human beings.

The history of smallpox indicates that, like other diseases, smallpox came and went of its own accord, and struck various countries at different times, with different levels of severity. The introduction of hygiene to some parts of the world has had absolutely nothing to do with the disappearance of smallpox. It is not possible to know whether the vaccine made smallpox wane faster than it would have waned without vaccination, because scientific studies were never done to see whether or not the vaccine worked. Edward Jenner's research was ridiculously unscientific, and once the vaccinators had succeeded in getting the medical establishment to accept the vaccine, there was no need to do scientific experiments to justify it. All that was needed was politicians who were prepared to pass laws making vaccination compulsory.

In 1853 vaccination was made compulsory in England, and each of the epidemics which followed were progressively larger and more lethal. Nearly 100% of the cases and the deaths were in vaccinated people. Some anti-vaccinationists accused the practice of vaccination of causing the epidemics and of causing their severity, but the vaccine cannot do that. What was happening was that the disease was naturally increasing in virulence, and the vaccine made no difference. After smallpox reached its peak, it dwindled, and then ceased to occur, just like English sweating sickness.

From the start the vaccine industry said that it was going to eradicate smallpox. In 1877 an anti-vaccinationist wrote,

> ... if it were possible to 'stamp out' smallpox by vaccination, that desirable result would long ago have been accomplished. The doctors have had it all their own way for seventy-six years.[256]

After 180 years they eventually "succeeded," coincidentally with the natural demise of smallpox. While researching the history of smallpox vaccination I became so fascinated by the topic that I have started another book about it. So all I am going to do here is to point to some of the evidence which shows that vaccination did not bring an end to smallpox, and that it caused devastating illness for millions of people.

With modern vaccines they use a hypodermic syringe to neatly inject all the poisons deep into the flesh, but smallpox vaccination was not so tidy. They did it by scratching lacerations into the skin, and then pushing pus into the wound that they had made. When this resulted in a flare-up, it was said that the vaccination had "taken." If there was no flare-up, it was said that the vaccination "had not taken," and needed to be done again.

Sometimes the flare-up involved the whole limb, causing a great deal of pain and suffering. Sometimes it involved the whole body, and the person died. Sometimes the vaccination caused cancer at the site of vaccination,[257,258,259] and in other cases it caused systemic cancer. The start of the vaccination era was the start of the cancer era. Encephalitis and urticaria were common side effects of vaccination. Some people were permanently disabled, while others were hampered by poor health for the rest of their lives, unless they consulted with a homoeopath who knew how to treat vaccine damage. Orthodox medicine treated the side effects of vaccination with mercury. In those days orthodox medicine treated just about everything with mercury. Mercury was the paracetamol of the 18th century. Before vaccination with cowpox was introduced, variolation had been practiced. Variolation was different to vaccination in that some pus was taken from a human smallpox pustule instead of from a cow, and the pus was scratched into the skin of anyone who was willing to undergo the procedure. Mercury had been used to treat the side effects of variolation. The Empress of Russia took mercury in an attempt to counteract the side effects of variolation in 1768.[260]

The medical establishment dismissed discussion of side effects with the claim that severe side effects were just "one in a million." However, shortly before smallpox vaccination ceased, some countries attempted to find out what the incidence of side effects really was. The American authorities conducted a survey of side effects in 1968.[259] The method they used meant that they missed a lot, and they also did some pruning to make the results look better. Despite this they were left with the figure that more than one person per thousand suffered a severe reaction to his or her first smallpox vaccination. Instead of "one in a million," they found it was over a thousand in a million.

Reports of serious reactions were collected in Bavaria between 1956 and 1965.[261] The method of gathering reports failed to detect all the cases,[261] but it was a sincere attempt to assess the side effects. The finding was that 1 out of every 8000 children died from vaccination, and that the younger a child is when vaccinated, the higher the risk of death is.[261]

The mythical history of smallpox vaccination is lovingly nurtured by the modern vaccine industry. Children's books are a major source of brainwashing. The myths are continually repeated in the media, so that people incorporate the false history into their world view. It does not stop. In August 2002 the *British Medical Journal* published an article[262] on the "history" of the anti-vaccination movement. The article portrays non-believers as silly people who need to be treated gently, and it portrays smallpox vaccination as safe and effective. A favourite myth of the vaccinationists is that people objected to compulsory vaccination for intellectual reasons, rather than for health reasons, and this article reinforces that idea. It also gets its facts about Edward Jenner wrong. The article states,

Widespread vaccination began in the early 1800s following Edward Jenner's presentation of an article to the Royal Society of London in 1796 detailing his success in preventing smallpox in 13 people by inoculation with live infectious material from the pustules or scabs of people infected with cowpox. The process induced cowpox, a mild viral disease that conferred immunity to smallpox.

Well, it is true that Jenner presented an article to the Royal Society in 1796, but the latter were very wise and would not publish it.[263] Two years later Jenner had a slightly different version of his article published by a vanity publisher.[264] The writers of the *British Medical Journal* article are not correct in saying that Jenner presented 13 cases which detailed his success in preventing smallpox. Jenner presented 23 cases, and only one case comes anywhere near to inoculating someone with cowpox to try and prevent smallpox. Most of the cases he presented were descriptions of people who had had cowpox naturally at some time in the past, and then did not catch smallpox when exposed to people with smallpox, or did not get full blown smallpox when inoculated with pus from a person with smallpox. Presumably he presented these cases because he believed that they demonstrated that the subjects were made immune by having had cowpox. Of course they demonstrated nothing of the kind. Lots of people can be exposed to smallpox without getting it. Without a control group of people who have not previously had cowpox being included in the investigation, it is not possible to know whether or not the cowpox made any difference to the subjects' chances of catching smallpox.

Some of Jenner's cases were people who had previously had smallpox, and then did not catch cowpox when exposed, or else they only got a mild dose of cowpox. He does not explain what this is supposed to prove, but presumably it is supposed to indicate that smallpox can create immunity to cowpox. The fact that some people who had had smallpox still got cowpox does not seem to bother him. One of the cases had had natural cowpox three times, with no decrease in severity. Jenner stated that cowpox could not prevent itself but it could prevent smallpox. In the real world smallpox did not prevent itself either. A Swiss doctor showed mathematically that a person who had had smallpox once was 63% more likely to get it again in the next epidemic than a person who had never had it.[265]

Three of the cases had had natural horsepox, not cowpox. Two of these were challenged by having pus from a smallpox pustule scratched into their skin, and they did not get very sick from it. One of the two was later exposed to smallpox and did not catch it. The third case was exposed to smallpox 20 years after having horsepox, and did get smallpox. From this Edward Jenner deduces that horsepox has to be cultivated on the nipple of a cow before it can create immunity to smallpox in a human being. I am afraid the logic of this escapes me.

In all, 16 of the 23 cases were not inoculated with anything, and 6 of the cases were not challenged with anything. Some of the "cases" involve a group of people, and it is difficult to know which individual out of that group Jenner intends to be the one that proves his point.

Case number 17 was an eight year old boy named James Phipps. Jenner inoculated him with "matter" which was taken from the hand of a dairymaid with cowpox. James became quite sick, but he recovered. Six weeks later Jenner inoculated him with smallpox pus, and he did not react. Children's story books tell us that Jenner proved that his vaccine worked by experimenting on a boy named James Phipps. They do not mention that James was not exposed to real smallpox. The vaccine industry has latched onto this case as "proof" that vaccination works. One case, who was not exposed to wild smallpox, with no control cases, is the backbone of the propaganda machine which makes people grow up believing in vaccination.

Case number 18 was a five year old boy named John Baker, whom Jenner inoculated with pus from the hand of a man who had caught horsepox from a horse. Jenner reports that the boy had a reaction to the inoculation, then got better, and then he came down with a "contagious fever ... soon after this experiment was made."[266] As Jenner believed that horsepox could not prevent smallpox unless it had first been grown on a cow, he wanted to see if horsepox worked when it had been grown on a human. But, says Jenner in his *Inquiry*, he could not administer the challenge dose because "the boy had been rendered unfit for inoculation."[267]

169

The reason why the boy had become unfit for inoculation was because he had died. Jenner does not mention the fact that the boy had died in his *Inquiry*, but in other writings he mentions that this boy died after a bad reaction to the cowpox vaccination.[268,269] The name of John Baker is not mentioned in children's story books. In the long term, the name John Baker will go down in history as the first person to die from Jennerian vaccination.

So out of 23 cases which were supposed to prove that inoculation with cowpox makes a person immune to the wild smallpox virus, none were inoculated with cowpox and then exposed to the wild smallpox virus, one was vaccinated with cowpox and then challenged with smallpox pus, one was vaccinated with attenuated horsepox and died before he could be challenged, and there were no controls at all.

I wrote to the authors of the article in the *British Medical Journal* twice and asked them which 13 of Jenner's 23 cases are the ones to which they were referring when they said that he succeeded in preventing smallpox in 13 people by inoculation with live infectious material from the pustules or scabs of people infected with cowpox. They did not reply. So I sent a referenced letter to the editor of the *British Medical Journal*. It said,

> Dear Editor,
> Wolfe and Sharp's inaccurate and patronising "history" of the anti-vaccination movement uses omission and implication to perpetuate the myths of smallpox vaccination. They mention an epidemic in Sweden which subsided after the vaccination rate was increased, but they do not mention any of the epidemics which broke out after mass vaccination. One of the epidemics that is never mentioned by vaccinationists broke out in Italy from 1887-89 against a background vaccination rate of 98.5%. Attack rates and death rates were higher in the re-vaccinated than in the vaccinated, and also higher in those whose vaccinations had "taken."
> Wolf and Sharp mention widespread protests and riots against vaccination, including one of 100 000 people in Leicester. But they imply that people objected to compulsory vaccination because it infringed their liberty. One hundred thousand illiterate, disenfranchised people did not demonstrate in the streets of Leicester because of an intellectual concept about civil rights. They protested because vaccination maimed and killed their babies.
> The authors of the article state that Edward Jenner demonstrated his success at preventing smallpox in 13 people by inoculating them with cowpox. Jenner presented 23 cases in his Inquiry. I have twice asked the authors to inform me which 13 were the cases to which they were referring, but they do not reply. I contend that they have

never read Jenner's Inquiry, and as with the rest of their article, they are just repeating popular myths which promote the concept of vaccination. If they had taken the time to read Jenner's Inquiry, they would have known that out of 23 cases which were supposed to prove that inoculation with cowpox makes a person immune to the wild smallpox virus, none were inoculated with cowpox and then exposed to the wild smallpox virus, one was vaccinated with cowpox and then challenged with smallpox pus, and there were no controls at all.

Apologists for Jenner claim that his method is not important as the cowpox and vaccinia vaccines were effective. But a huge amount of data, including that presented by WHO, shows that it was not. In 1899 the president of the AMA said that doctors who do not believe in vaccination are "mad" and "misguided." Modern doctors suffer more than name-calling when they don't believe in the faith.

The *British Medical Journal* acknowledged receipt of my letter, but as expected, they did not publish it. They have allowed a minority group to be disparaged on their pages, and have given the group no right of reply. It is typical of the behaviour of most media outlets in regards to vaccination. In the "debate" about vaccination, the playing field is so unlevel, that the debate cannot proceed.

During the 1887-89 smallpox epidemic in Italy over forty seven thousand people died of smallpox.[174] At that time Italy had a 98.5% vaccination rate. A 95% vaccination rate is supposed to provide "herd immunity," and therefore is supposed to prevent smallpox in the unvaccinated as well as in the vaccinated. The Italian epidemic is one of many that showed that neither the vaccinated nor the unvaccinated were protected.

On the 8th May 1980 the World Health Organisation declared that they had eliminated smallpox from the planet. They published a 1400 page book about how they had done it.[270] This book gives details about the coming and going of smallpox epidemics in some European countries, but it does not mention Italy at all. This is a deliberate omission. Despite many omissions of this nature, a careful reading of this book reveals that the demise of smallpox was coincidental to the world wide vaccination campaign.

At first it was claimed that one vaccination would give life long immunity. When vaccinated people got smallpox, more doses were introduced, and it was called "re-vaccination." There were many epidemics which showed that re-vaccination did not work. The Italian epidemic mentioned above is one of them.

In his first article Jenner says, "what renders the Cow-pox virus so extremely singular, is, that the person who has been thus affected is for ever after secure from the infection of the Small Pox."[271] But 10 years later, when it was obvious that vaccination did not prevent smallpox, he did a complete about-face, and claimed that re-vaccination was necessary. He published an article in support of re-vaccination, in which he described cases of people who had smallpox more than once as part of his argument.[272] The authors of the World Health Organisation's 1400 page book say that Jenner never abandoned the stance that one vaccination is sufficient to create lifelong immunity.[273] As with many things, they are wrong.

During the 1887-89 epidemic in Italy, the incidence of deaths from smallpox in people under the age of 20 was exactly the same in males as in females. Men were re-vaccinated at the age of 20 for military purposes, while women were not. Yet in people older than 20, the death rate from smallpox was much higher in men than in women.[174] In the town of Vittoria in Sicily, there was official proof that all the people had been vaccinated during their six monthly vaccination campaigns. When the epidemic of 1887-89 broke out, the number of deaths from smallpox was 2,100.[174] As the total population of the village was only 2,600, this meant that less than 20% of the population was left alive. It is no wonder that this example, and examples from other villages in Sicily, Sardinia and Calabria are not mentioned by anyone trying to promote the myths of vaccination. The spectacular failure of vaccination in intensively vaccinated areas like Japan and the Philippines is also not a popular topic with vaccinationists.

When re-vaccination was introduced, the length of time that immunity created by vaccination was supposed to last was arbitrarily set at seven years. It then continually decreased until two years became the official length of immunity. When people caught smallpox soon after vaccination, that was said to be because the vaccination "had not taken." So here we have a situation where the vaccinators win no matter what happens. If the vaccinated person does not catch smallpox, then they say that he or she was protected by vaccination. If the person catches smallpox more than two years after vaccination, they say it is because he or she was remiss about being re-vaccinated. If the person catches smallpox within two years of vaccination, they say it is because the vaccination "did not take."

The World Health Organisation claims that re-vaccination was what conquered smallpox. On page 273 of their book there is a table which compares the number of smallpox deaths in Germany and Austria from 1866 to 1897. Re-vaccination was made compulsory in Germany in 1874. In the text they say,

The results, when compared with the prevailing situation in Austria, in which general conditions were similar but re-vaccination had not been introduced, were dramatic (Table 6.4) and hardly require comment.[274]

But a look at Table 6.4 shows that the results very much require comment. The figures show that there was the same drop in Austria between 1874 and 1875 as there was in Germany. And between 1873 and 1874 the drop in Austria was more than double the drop in Germany. And they show that smallpox continued to rise and fall in Germany with the same disregard for re-vaccination as it had shown for vaccination. And they show that there was an overall decline in Austria as well as in Germany, despite the fact that Austria was doing the "wrong thing" by not re-vaccinating. Their own "proof" shows that they are talking nonsense.

If a terrorist were to release smallpox from a laboratory, a few people would get smallpox, but the virus would not spread into the community because it lacks the natural virulence which it had 200 years ago. The vaccine industry would vaccinate as many people as they could, and they would claim that their actions were the reason why it did not spread.

"LOUIS PASTEUR DEFEATED RABIES"

Vaccine Myth number Ten: Louis Pasteur discovered germs, which are tiny creatures that pounce on people and cause disease. He saved the French wine industry and silk industry from ruin, and made milk safe to drink by inventing pasteurisation. He conducted public experiments with sheep, which showed that when they had been vaccinated, they were safe from anthrax. He invented a vaccine which cured and prevented rabies, thereby saving the world from mad dogs.

Louis Pasteur was a pioneer of scientific fraud. It is significant that he is the darling of the vaccine industry. The true story of Louis Pasteur's life is far more interesting than the one they teach in schools.

Popular mythology holds that Pasteur was the first person to think of the germ theory, but the theory was already written down nearly 300 years before Pasteur was born. In 1546 a bloke called Fracastoro published a treatise on contagious disease in which he said that these diseases are caused by particles which are too small to be seen. He said that the particles move from person to person by contact, or they travel on items that an infected person has touched, or they travel through the air. He also said that the particles can reproduce themselves within the human body.[275,276] Germs were first seen through a microscope by Antonius van Leenwenhoek in 1675.[277] He called them "little animals," but he did not associate them with disease. The theory that germs cause disease was causing heated debate long before Pasteur came on the scene, and there are still people today who deny that infectious diseases are caused by germs.

The extent of Louis Pasteur's fraud is quite amazing. He plagiarised the research of other scientists, and he made pronouncements that he had experimentally proven certain "facts" when he had not done the experiments. He deliberately lied about what he had done in his experiments with the anthrax vaccine for sheep, and with the rabies vaccine for humans. He put far more effort into cultivating favour with the aristocracy than he put into cultivating things in his laboratory, and his greatest affectation was that of pretending to be a humble person. He made himself into a celebrity during his life time, and the cult of hero worship which was built up during his life time still exists after more than a century. None of the adulation is justified. The products he invented have harmed millions of people, and the commercial success of his endeavours has hindered scientific inquiry into how to make people healthy.

Louis Pasteur "laid the foundations of his own legend,"[278] both through his behaviour and through his writing.[279] The myths about him are perpetuated in books, cartoons, a Hollywood movie, websites, school curricula, and by journalists who think they are referring to historical fact when they mention Louis Pasteur in the media. For almost a century nearly every child in French and English speaking countries was taught that Louis Pasteur saved the world from germs. Nowadays fewer children are exposed to the myth, because school curricula are filled with other things.

Right from the start there were vociferous critics of Louis Pasteur. Some of them published articles or pamphlets saying that his work was unscientific, and that his vaccines were killing people and animals, while not preventing disease. In 1923 Ethel Douglas Hume published a lengthy book in which she showed that Pasteur was dishonest, and that his vaccines were harmful and ineffective.[280] In 1937 and 1938 Pasteur's nephew, Adrien Loir, published some essays about his famous uncle which exposed more of the deception.[281]

Before he died, Louis Pasteur instructed his family never to allow anyone access to his notebooks.[282,283] His grandson donated them to a library in 1964,[283,284] and in 1971 some historians were permitted to have access to them.[282] Gerald Geison of Princeton University studied them, and at the 1993 meeting of the American Association for the Advancement of Science, he spoke about the dishonesty which he had unearthed.[282,283] Later he published a book detailing what he had discovered.[281]

One of Pasteur's co-workers was a scientist named Antoine Béchamp. Béchamp held some strange views, but he did discover that fermentation is caused by yeast, and that the disease that was killing French silkworms was caused by little parasites. Béchamp and Pasteur both published a lot of articles, and Ethel Douglas Hume took on the task of reading these articles. She documented the sequence in which Béchamp made his discoveries, and Louis Pasteur first denounced them, and then stole them.[280]

Pasteur believed in spontaneous generation.[285] This is the theory that small things appear out of nothing, spontaneously. Pasteur was in line with the thinking of the times. For instance, it was believed that maggots appeared spontaneously out of rotting meat. In Pasteur's day it had already been scientifically proven by an Italian scientist that maggots cannot appear in meat unless flies first land on the meat and lay eggs, but this finding had not yet been accepted by the scientific establishment. One of Pasteur's experiments aimed to "prove" the popular theory of spontaneous generation. He lied that he had managed to make yeast appear by spontaneous generation in a medium formed only of sugar, a salt of ammonia and of mineral elements, when he had actually added yeast to the mixture.[286]

The misconception that Pasteur saved the French silk industry from ruin has been entrenched in medical mythology. This is not only due to the personality of Louis Pasteur, it is also because bureaucracies suffer from corporate paralysis when a wrong needs to be put right. Silkworms had started dying en masse in 1850. The silk farmers were desperate because production dropped from 30 million kilograms per year to 8 million kilograms per year. After Pasteur had allegedly "saved" the industry, silk production dropped to 2 million kilograms per year.[287]

Béchamp investigated silkworm disease and found that a parasite which came from the air was making the silkworms sick. He experimented, and found that the parasite could be killed by the vapour of creosote, without harming the silkworms. However, Louis Pasteur had been appointed by the Minister of Health to solve the problem, so the bureaucrats ignored Béchamp.

No one who understands anything of departmental red tape will wonder that, instead of at once accepting Béchamp's verdict, agricultural societies waited to hear the pronouncement of the official representative. Plenty of patience had to be exercised.[288]

Louis Pasteur flitted around, ingratiating himself with the Empress Eugenie and Napoleon III, and occasionally making pronouncements about silkworms. He also found time to launch attacks against Béchamp for saying that the disease was caused by a parasite.

On June 18, 1866, Béchamp sent a report to the Academy of Science on how the silkworms could be saved by making them hatch in the presence of creosote, so that the fumes of the creosote would kill the parasites.[289] His advice was ignored, and the silk industry suffered more and more from the ravages of the disease. What made matters worse for the silk farmers was that Pasteur said that healthy eggs from healthy moths would be disease-free, so some entrepreneurs jumped on the band wagon, and the farmers paid high prices for these eggs, only to see the caterpillars sicken and die because of the parasite.

After a year of waiting for some words of wisdom from the celebrity Pasteur, the scientific world was treated to,

> I am very much inclined to believe that there is not actual disease of silk-worms. I cannot better make clear my opinion of silk-worm disease than by comparing it to the effects of pulmonary phthisis. My observations of this year have fortified me in the opinion that these little organisms are neither animalcules nor cryptogamic plants. It appears to me that it is chiefly the cellular tissue of all the organs that is transformed into corpuscles or produces them.[290]

When Pasteur finally realised that Béchamp was right about silkworm disease, he had no qualms about publicly claiming that he himself had discovered what Béchamp had discovered. It was, however, too late for the silk industry. The Academy of Science and some government officials knew the truth about what had happened, but the mythological version became regarded as historical fact.

Popular mythology says, "Pasteur proved the value of vaccination by vaccinating sheep against a disease called anthrax."[291] Fifty sheep were used in this experiment, and by the time the public came to see the results, half the sheep lay dead or were dying. The vaccine appeared to be 100% effective. Yet it did not produce those results for farmers who bought it to protect their stocks from anthrax. By reading Pasteur's personal notebooks, Gerald Geison discovered that Pasteur had lied to the officials and the public about the type of vaccine he had used.[282,283,292] Geison suggests that this lie was told for the purposes of personal advancement.[292] The track record of the vaccine suggests that the problem went deeper than the method of manufacture.

In March 1882, a commission that had been established by the Italian authorities to investigate whether or not Pasteur's anthrax vaccine worked, tested Pasteur's vaccine at Turin University. They injected half of a group of sheep with it, and then challenged all the sheep with an injection of blood from a sheep that had died of anthrax the day before. Every single one of the vaccinated and unvaccinated sheep died.[293] Angry letters passed backwards and forwards between Pasteur and the professors at Turin. On the 10th June, 1883, the professors of Turin published a document detailing the way Pasteur had contradicted himself in his correspondence with them. The document highlighted Pasteur's ignorance about anthrax and septicaemia, and it was published in French two months later. But the adoring public adored on.

A factory for manufacturing vaccines had been opened at Odessa in Russia. They trialled Pasteur's anthrax vaccine on a farm near Kachowka by vaccinating 4564 sheep, and 81% of the sheep died from the vaccine.[294] Pasteur ended up paying financial compensation to some of the farmers whose stock had been killed by the vaccine,[295] which is more than can be said for the British, American and Australian governments. They will not pay compensation to the families of the soldiers who have been killed by anthrax vaccine, nor to the soldiers whose lives have been ruined by the health problems caused by the vaccine. Because of the nature of the anthrax germ, anthrax vaccines made by any method will always be the most deadly of vaccines. These vaccines kill and cause terrible infirmity in the fittest and healthiest of our young men. It is not likely that an anthrax vaccine will ever be developed which is able to protect a person in the case of a biological warfare attack.[296]

A commission set up in Hungary recommended that Pasteur's anthrax vaccine should be prohibited,[295] and in 1881 the Hungarian government said,

> The worst diseases, pneumonia, catarrhal fever, etc., have exclusively struck down the animals subjected to injection. It follows from this that the Pasteur inoculation tends to accelerate the action of certain latent diseases and to hasten the mortal issue of other grave affections.[297]

This is the same phenomenon that Sir Graham Wilson called "provocation disease" eighty five years later, in his book *The Hazards of Immunization*.[223] The sickness is not a direct reaction to the vaccine, it is a reaction to the fact that the vaccine has compromised the immune system. The phenomenon has been well documented with regards to polio,[224,226,228,229] but it is not generally acknowledged by the medical establishment. The phenomenon is seldom mentioned in the medical literature. One exception is in a study of 3801 Swedish children who had been injected with DPT vaccine.[298] Three of the children died of a bacterial infection in the weeks following vaccination, and the study authors believed that their deaths were caused by provocation. Without doing really big studies, it is not possible to know how often vaccination causes unrelated diseases.

The story of Joseph Meister still features on many a school curriculum. This boy was bitten by a rabid dog, and his mother brought him to Pasteur because she had heard that he had a treatment for rabies. Joseph was injected each day for 11 days with stuff made in Pasteur's laboratory, and he did not develop rabies. Schoolchildren are taught that this proved that the vaccine Pasteur had invented for rabies was effective, and that since then, thousands of people have been saved from rabies by the vaccine.

Schoolchildren are not taught that for 52 years homoeopaths all over the world had already been successfully curing cases of rabies in humans.[254] Dying of rabies is a prolonged and painful experience. The victim suffers severe pain and terrible mental anguish. The pharmaceutical industry prevents people from having access to homoeopathic cures, simply because it would damage their profits.

Pasteur claimed that before he injected the vaccine into Joseph Meister, he had already tested it on a large number of dogs which had suffered bites from rabid animals. But Gerald Geison found in the notebooks that he had experimented on only a few dogs, and not in the same way as with Joseph Meister.[282,299] Pasteur had given the vaccine to 26 dogs which had been bitten by rabid animals, and 10 of them had died.[300] There were also 7 dogs which Pasteur had used as controls. They had been given no treatment after being bitten by a rabid animal, and 4 of them never developed rabies.[301] This means that out of the dogs that were vaccinated, 62% survived, while out of the ones that had no treatment, 57% survived.[302] It was a good indication of what the vaccine would do in the real world. Geison also found that some of the dogs had not been injected with the same potion as that which had been injected into Joseph Meister.[303] Some had been injected with rabbit brain, some with guinea pig brain, and the rest with rabbit spinal cords. The latter is what had been injected into Joseph Meister. When he had used rabbit spinal cords on the dogs, he had injected dried out ones first, and then moved on to fresher cords. But with Joseph he had used the fresh cords first, and then moved on to drier ones. These gruesome details are not important in the big picture, because rabies vaccine is a disgusting, harmful substance no matter how it is made. However, the details are relevant in that Louis Pasteur lied about what he had done. The vaccine industry was founded on lies, and the lies have just kept on coming.

Three months later Pasteur treated a shepherd boy who had been bitten by a rabid dog, and this boy also survived. The vaccine was greeted with enthusiastic approval by most of the medical establishment, and by most of the public. No studies were ever done to see whether it worked, nor what side effects it caused.

The vaccine to be injected into people who had not yet been bitten was made in different ways at different times. At first it was made by taking bits of brain from a rabid dog and "inoculating it directly onto the surface of the brain of a healthy dog through a hole drilled into its skull."[304] Later it was made by placing brain from a dog into a monkey, and through a series of monkeys.[305] Then later it was made by inoculating the spinal marrow of a rabid dog onto the brain of a rabbit through a hole bored in its skull, and then from rabbit to rabbit through holes in their skulls.[306] With the latter method, he took the spinal cord of each rabbit that had died, cut it into strips several centimetres long, suspended it in a flask for about two weeks, made a broth with it, and then injected it into dogs.[307] According to Ethel Douglas

Hume, the broth contained cow matter as well.[308] The World Health Organisation defined Pasteur's vaccine as,

> ...a suspension of infected tissue from the central nervous system of an animal.[309]

Lionel Dole's comment is,

> The manner in which Pasteur made rabbits "rabid" by boring holes in their skulls and inserting filth into their brains was not science but simply brutal quackery.[310]

One of Pasteur's co-workers thought that injecting the saliva of humans who were healthy, and the saliva of humans who had died of rabies, into rabbits, was a worthwhile pastime. He found that the two types of saliva were equally harmful to the rabbit.[311]

There are numerous written records of the failure of the rabies vaccine, and of it causing death. In 1890 a doctor published a list of people who had died after being vaccinated with Pasteur's rabies vaccine, while the dogs that had bitten them remained healthy.[179] The National Anti-Vivisection Society collected the names of 1,220 people who died from the vaccine between 1885 and 1901.[312] Just like all the people whom the vaccine industry has killed, these people do not count in the eyes of "science." They are "anecdotal evidence." Louis Pasteur's cousin-by-marriage, Dr. Michel Peter, spoke out about deaths that were happening after the treatment, and questioned the secretiveness of Pasteur's research. He was hissed and booed when he tried to speak at the Academy of Medicine.[313]

Manufacturing vaccines became a booming commercial enterprise, with Pasteur Institutes opening up in many countries. At the International Rabies Conference held in Paris in 1927, the Director of the Pasteur Institute in Morocco reported that certain of the other institutes were concealing cases of rabies vaccine failure.[198]

The vaccine not only failed to prevent rabies in many people, it also caused rabies in recipients. A postman named Pierre Rascol, and another man, were attacked by a dog. The postman's clothing was sufficient to protect him from having his skin penetrated, but the other man was badly bitten. The postal authorities required Rascol to undergo a course of rabies injections, but the other man was not treated. A month after the course of injections was started, Rascol developed symptoms of rabies, and two days later he died. The other man remained well.[179]

Eleanor McBean tells the funny albeit tragic story of what happened to a young English girl in staid Victorian times. She went to the "baths" with her friends, and came home with a bite. Her parents rushed her off for Pasteur treatments, and she then got ill and died. On the way home from her funeral, her friends told her parents that she had not been bitten by a dog, but by her boyfriend.[314] Would the wrath of a Victorian father have been worse than the jab of a Pasteurian needle?

In October 1920, King Alexander of Greece was bitten by a monkey. An "expert" from Paris was summoned to give him the course of vaccinations, and the king died.[196] We do not know if he died from the monkey bite or from the injections, but can you imagine the fanfare there would have been if he had survived? Schoolchildren all over the world would enthusiastically be taught that Louis Pasteur saved the life of the King of Greece.

By 1982 it was admitted that Louis Pasteur's vaccine does not work. A host of new rabies vaccines are available instead. They are made with flesh from aborted babies,[315,316,317,318] goats' brains,[319] hamsters' kidneys,[320] fertilised eggs,[321] and dogs' kidneys.[322]

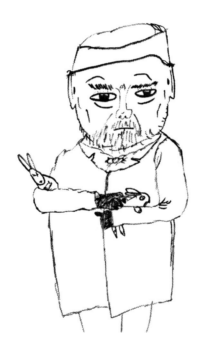

Louis Pasteur loved
rabbits so much that he bored holes
in their skulls and inserted rabid
dogs' brains onto their brains.

"VACCINES ARE SCIENTIFICALLY TESTED FOR SAFETY AND EFFECTIVENESS"

Vaccine Myth number Eleven: Before a vaccine is licensed for use, it is tested for safety and effectiveness. The vaccine is first tested on animals, and if it proves to be safe and effective, it is then tested on a small group of humans, then on a larger group of humans. If the vaccine does not prevent the disease it is supposed to prevent, it is discarded. The exact dosage needed to produce immunity is worked out according to the weight of the person. If the vaccine causes bad side effects during the trials, it is not released for mass immunisation. If, despite all these precautions, the vaccine causes bad side effects once it is used on the general population, it is immediately recalled.

Vaccines are not properly trialled before release, nor are they properly monitored after release. Commerce is the driving force behind vaccines, not science. Since its historical beginnings, the testing of vaccines has been left to the people who manufacture and sell the vaccine, when it should be done by people who are financially independent of the manufacturer. The way that the vaccine industry pretends to research vaccines has become more sophisticated since the days of Jenner and Pasteur, but it has not become more scientific. Vaccines which are licensed cause a high incidence of serious side effects, and they fail to prevent the target disease when the germ becomes virulent in the environment. This shows that they are not being properly tested before they are released.

The USA is the heart of the vaccine industry, even though there are independent manufacturers in other countries. Just as stock exchanges around the world react to happenings on Wall Street, so too does the vaccine industry regard the USA as its point of reference.

Originally there was no pretence at testing drugs before they were marketed, but things changed in 1937 when a "wonder drug" called Elixer Sulfanilamide killed 73 people in the USA. This was in the good old days when Franklin D. Roosevelt was president. He was an unusual politician, because he believed that people are more important than profits. In response to the 73 deaths, he created a government body that is supposed to check the safety and effectiveness of substances that are destined for consumption by the public.

In 1938 the Federal Food, Drug and Cosmetics Act was passed. It prohibited the sale of foods that were dangerous to health, and prohibited the sale of foods, drugs and cosmetics that were packaged in unsanitary or contaminated containers. The Food and Drug Administration (FDA) was established to enforce the new law. It was a noble concept. Independent government monitors were going to check that all newly invented medicines and food additives were effective and safe for consumption. But of course it has not worked out that way.

The situation at present is that the manufacturer collects raw data on the product by doing a series of studies. They then compile a report which they submit to the FDA. People at the FDA read the report, and if it sounds good, they license the substance for sale to the public. The FDA does not look at the manufacturer's raw data to see if the report is an honest representation of the information collected. "Unlike almost every other federal agency, the FDA lacks the legal clout to subpoena a company's internal records."[323]

A further problem is that the law regarding vaccines is different to the law regarding drugs. Manufacturers have to present data to the FDA that their drugs are safe, and pure, and effective, but the manufacturers of vaccines do not have to supply evidence that their product is pure nor effective. They only have to produce evidence that the vaccine is "safe."[324] So the FDA is not required to take an interest in how rancid the rotten monkey kidney in the vaccine has become, nor what other viruses and bacteria are in the vaccine, nor whether or not the vaccine is capable of preventing the disease.

Most health conscious people are aware that there is corruption within the drug industry, but few realise the extent of the corruption. Criminologist John Braithwaite has written a book about fraud, bribery, and unethical marketing practices within the pharmaceutical industry.[325] The chapter on safety testing reveals that researchers deliberately withhold information about harmful effects that they observe. They even go to the extent of replacing animals that die from the substance with healthy animals, and of forging the signatures of human participants, after the humans have died from the substance.

The media seldom reports on the behaviour of the drug companies, but an exception was a BBC Panorama documentary[326] on a drug called Halcion. They showed how the information presented to the FDA by the makers of Halcion was fraudulent as it omitted to mention frequent side effects like insanity and violent aggression. One person within the FDA was dissatisfied with the reports about the drug, but the FDA suppressed her concerns. When some doctors spoke out about side effects they had seen, the drug company bribed other doctors to say that the product was safe.

The FDA is supposed to protect the public, but historically it has been more inclined to protect money interests. When 225 reports of death caused by Hib vaccine came in between 1 November 1990 and 31 July 1992, they set about trying to discredit the reports, instead of trying to determine whether or not the vaccine is safe. The situation will not improve until the voting public demands that clinical trials be done by people other than those hoping to market the product.

In 2000 there was a Congressional committee investigation into the fact that the individuals who make US policy on vaccination are on the payroll of drug companies that manufacture vaccines. The committee found that, "US government officials are failing to enforce conflict of interest regulations and are allowing experts with industry ties to sit on vaccine approval panels."[327] During the hearing a congressman whose grandchild is autistic as a result of vaccination pointed out that there are 700,000 doctors in the USA, so it should be possible to find 15 doctors who do not have financial ties with the drug companies.[328] I have noticed that the names of these government officials/drug company representatives appear quite often as authors of pro-vaccination articles in medical journals. Professor Gordon Stewart says that the international vaccination scene is controlled by a "closed circle" of about 100 people.[329]

Some countries simply accept a drug or vaccine once it has been approved by the American FDA, but Australia and New Zealand have their own panels of bureaucrats to approve medicines. All that these bureaucrats do is to read the material handed to them by the manufacturer, and approve the product if the promotional material makes it look good.

Britain has the Committee on the Safety of Medicines and the National Institute for Biological Standards and Control, which are supposed to ensure vaccine safety. In 1989 I started correspondence with these two groups regarding how they had tested the measles vaccine. Their answers were evasive. Now 445 families are suing the British government for severe damage done to their children by measles, mumps and rubella vaccine, and they still refuse to provide information about their testing procedures to the lawyers. Before I even wrote the first letter in 1989 I held the suspicion that they did not test vaccines properly, because I had personal contact with so many cases of serious vaccine damage. Now even the newspapers in Britain are beginning to express their suspicion that MMR vaccine was not properly tested.

THE TESTING OF DPT VACCINE.

DPT vaccine is supposed to prevent whooping cough, tetanus and diphtheria. Most cases of whooping cough are caused by a bacterium called bordatella pertussis, and for more than sixty years the vaccine was made with billions of these bacteria in each dose. The number of bacteria that cause a natural infection is not known, but what is known is that when the bacteria are breathed in naturally, they meet the immune system in the mucous membranes, whereas when they are injected directly into the blood they elude this part of the immune system. The ineffectiveness of the vaccine combined with the serious side effects it caused made Sweden and Germany stop using it.[330] Hundreds of articles were published in medical journals describing serious side effects of the vaccine. One such article says of other reports,

> … convulsive seizures and lethargy dominate the clinical manifestations in the affected child. These are often coupled with other features indicative of grave damage to the brain.[331]

Articles like this one and all the others are no longer published in the English language medical journals. The drug companies have orchestrated a successful cover-up of side effects. Their methods have included denying individual cases, paying doctors to do fraudulent studies, and vilifying journalists who expose the truth.

The new genetically engineered acellular whooping cough vaccine causes less of the non-serious side effects of the type that the medical establishment are willing to acknowledge, but it causes the same incidence of serious side effects as the whole cell whooping cough vaccine.[332]

In 1954 it was pointed out that whooping cough vaccine only causes central nervous system damage, unlike other vaccines which cause neuritis and myelitis.[333]

This peculiarity, taken together with the very short incubation period, the frequent occurrence of convulsions after the first dose of vaccine in a young infant, and the high proportion of patients having persistent cerebral damage, does suggest that the mechanism of production is different from that of the demyelinating type of encephalitis.[334]

Demyelination is when the myelin sheath, which is the insulation around each nerve, gets stripped off. When this happens the nerve that has lost its protective sheath cannot transfer messages from the brain to the body. Time will tell whether the genetically engineered acellular whooping cough vaccine restricts itself to attacking the central nervous system, or does general demyelination like the other vaccines. The vaccine industry will not collect data, but ever since vaccination has been invented, individuals or groups have collected anecdotal data. That is how we will know.

DPT vaccine was invented in the 1920s, and was used in various countries before mass vaccination began. A number of doctors reported that the vaccine caused convulsions, collapse and death.[335] The Medical Research Council in Britain ran three clinical trials from 1946 to 1957 to see if the vaccine was effective at reducing the incidence of whooping cough.[336] The babies in the trials were aged 6 to 18 months.[336] Children who had contra-indications to vaccination were excluded from the British trials, which decreased the number of serious reactions. Yet the rate of reported convulsions was more than one per thousand.[336] It was found that vaccinated children have a lower rate of whooping cough than unvaccinated children during the three years following vaccination.[336]

Mass vaccination of babies in the USA was already underway before the results of the British trials came out. The British trials on babies aged 6 to 18 months were cited by the US Health Authorities as proof that the vaccine is safe for babies aged only six weeks,[337] but the British trials were not properly designed to test safety, and were done on much older children. There was no suggestion that the dosage should be decreased in the USA, even though the recipients had a much smaller body weight.[338] Six week old babies manufacture only a few antibodies, so a second dose of vaccine was introduced in the USA to increase the density of antibodies. Later on a third dose was introduced. Some countries now use four, and some use five doses.

The establishment tried to trivialise concerns about brain damage from the vaccine by saying, "The few have to suffer for the general good." In 1976 the media in Britain allowed parents of vaccine damaged children to speak out, and this caused the vaccination rate to drop from 76% to 42%. Whooping cough comes and goes according to a natural cycle, and when the next peak in whooping cough cases came, there were fewer deaths than there had been in the previous epidemic.[158] This pattern of fewer deaths with each peak, which had started a hundred years earlier, has continued to the present time.

Each batch of whooping cough vaccine is tested on mice for safety and effectiveness before it is released. This is done to make it appear that the vaccine is being scientifically produced. To test each batch for effectiveness, the mice are vaccinated, then three weeks later they have a challenge dose of pertussis bacteria injected into their brains. If more than a certain number of mice survive, that is taken to mean that the vaccine will prevent whooping cough in humans.[339] To test each batch for safety, the vaccine is injected into the abdomens of young mice, and if the mice continue to gain weight, that is taken to mean that the vaccine will not cause brain damage in a human baby.[339] The breed of mouse that is used determines whether 4% or 43% die from the same batch of vaccine.[340]

These methods of testing the vaccine obviously do not work because the vaccine does cause death and severe as well as mild brain damage in human babies. The researchers do not ask the mice if they have a headache after vaccination, and they do not test the mice for dyslexia when they start school.

Neurological damage does not prevent growth in mammals. The fact that the mice continue to grow bigger does not mean that they have not suffered neurological damage. Human babies who are neurologically damaged by the vaccine continue to grow bigger. They grow to adult size, but their brain remains damaged. If the motor section of the human brain is damaged, they grow bigger, but they cannot look after themselves. If the intellectual segment is damaged, their body keeps growing, but their mind does not mature. I speak with parents of children in their 20s and 30s who have the mentality and behaviour of toddlers. The vaccine industry and government agencies that coercively promote vaccination are not interested in hearing about the problems associated with controlling and caring for adult sized toddlers. When doing the mouse toxicity test, some laboratories are careful to use a breed of mouse which has a low susceptibility to the toxic effects of the vaccine,[341] but when doing mass vaccination of humans, the industry is not careful to exclude vulnerable children.

The original DPT vaccine is still batch tested on mice.[342] The new genetically engineered vaccines are batch tested by counting antigens and measuring levels of toxin.[342] This new method still does not address the issue of whether or not the substance which has been manufactured is harmful to humans. That is supposed to be gauged by post marketing surveillance.[342] As post marketing surveillance is not done, the validity of this type of batch testing cannot be assessed.

In 1981 an article which claimed to relate the findings of an FDA study on DPT vaccine was published in a medical journal.[343] This was the first study on DPT side effects in humans conducted by the American medical establishment. It should of course have been done *before* the vaccine was introduced and made compulsory in some states, not decades after it was introduced. But even at this late stage, it was not a sincere exercise. One of the researchers admitted that the study was being done to produce data which would convince American parents to accept DPT. They were concerned about the way British parents were refusing the vaccine, and they were scared that "public panic might spread to the United States."[344]

Early on in the study the researchers found that the frequency of adverse reactions was 50 times higher than they had anticipated.[344] They curtailed the study, but they deny that the unfavourable findings were the reason for the curtailment.[345] The article concludes with the statement,

> Convulsions and hypotonic hyporesponsive episodes each occurred in 1:1,750 immunizations. No evidence of encephalopathy or permanent brain damage was seen in any vaccine recipients. In view of lack of neurologic sequelae and death associated with DTP immunization in the study, it seems prudent to continue the routine utilization of pertussis immunization in infancy and childhood. This study supports the conclusion of others: that the benefits of pertussis immunization far outweigh the risks.[343]

This article is used by vaccinationists around the world to support the view that DPT vaccine is an acceptable risk. Doctors are presented with this statement as evidence that they should continue to inject DPT vaccine into their infant patients. It is reasonable for doctors to believe that articles in medical journals represent scientific studies done by reputable authorities. They have no way of knowing that the statement is fraudulent because it is not a true reflection of the findings of the study. Doctors also do not have time to read and analyse the article, which would in itself throw some doubt on the conclusion of the article.

Harris Coulter and Barbara Loe Fisher read the unpublished report, which had been handed to the FDA on March 18, 1980, and they found discrepancies between the data in it and the version published in the medical journal.[346]

To keep the figures low, the study doctors had only recorded symptoms which occurred within 48 hours of the injections, they had excluded the symptom of unusual high pitched screaming, and they did not allow children who had reacted badly to a previous dose to enrol in the study, even though in the real world those children's parents are bullied into having subsequent doses. Another trick was to record the number of reactions per jab, not per child, when each child is expected to have 5 jabs.

The children whose serious reactions were acknowledged were not followed up to see if they suffered long term damage. This is one of the most seriously dishonest aspects of the article. The abstract at the beginning says, "No sequelae were detected following these reactions." (Sequelae are morbid conditions occurring as a consequence of another condition or event.) The reader has no way of knowing that the reason sequelae were not detected, was because they were not looked for.

After the study was completed, voices within the system, and activists outside of the system, tried to pressurise the study doctors to follow up the children who had exhibited neurological symptoms during the first 48 hours after vaccination, to see if they were suffering any long term consequences. The FDA devoted their energy and some taxpayers' money to making excuses to resist doing a follow up.[347] The refusal to follow up is bad enough, but it is scandalous that despite having refused to follow up, they have the audacity to imply that they know that the children who demonstrated neurological reactions soon after vaccination, did not suffer any long term damage. In the body of the article they imply it once again.

No evidence of encephalopathy or permanent brain damage was seen in any vaccine recipients.

No mention of the fact that they refused, under pressure, to look for any evidence. Six years earlier a French study had found that 16 out of 20 children who had exhibited neurological symptoms soon after vaccination had neurological or epileptic sequelae.[348]

The American article also makes the statement, "No deaths occurred within 48 hours of immunization." This is true. But two of the babies in the trial did die soon after vaccination. One child developed a runny nose 72 hours after vaccination, and was found dead in his cot 84 hours after the injection. The other child exhibited typical symptoms of DPT reaction; excessive sleeping, decreased appetite, lethargy and diarrhoea, and was found dead by her father on the fourth day.[349] The latter death was labelled SIDS, although it does not fit the criteria for SIDS. The death rate among the trial babies was four times higher than the national average for SIDS.[349]

It is outrageous that this article is still presented as proof that DPT vaccine is safe. The American parents group called National Vaccination Information Center (NVIC) has publicly named one of the doctors involved in this study as being on the payroll of drug companies, and has called for his dismissal.[350] The interests of children will never be served while those who are supposed to be responsible for their welfare have financial interests in the pharmaceutical industry. Governments are not going to change the system - it is going to be parents who have to do it.

The drug companies also use fraudulent trials to prevent vaccine damaged children from obtaining compensation. This behaviour had long been suspected by anti-vaccinationists, but it was confirmed in 1993 during a court case which revealed drug company tactics.[351] Despite the efforts of the drug companies, a number of families in Britain had succeeded in winning compensation for vaccine damage. Then in 1988, in the case of Loveday versus Crown, the judge made the finding that the plaintiff had not provided sufficient evidence that DPT vaccine causes brain damage.[352,353] The vaccine bureaucracy took it and ran with it, presenting it around the world as if the court case had finally and conclusively proven that DPT does not cause brain damage.

Soon after the Loveday case came the case of Kenneth Best. Kenneth suffered the same life ruination as all the other victims of DPT, but the way that his mother persevered in fighting the system for over 20 years was so unusual that the BBC made a documentary[354] which told the story. Kenneth's mother, Margaret Best, lived on a low income, and received no state assistance in coping with her vaccine damaged child. He is incontinent as well as having no intellect. Usually coping with a brain damaged child uses up all of a family's time and resources, but Margaret somehow also found the energy to fight the giant. The measures she took to obtain compensation were extreme, but extreme hindrance requires extreme measures. One of the things that she did was to stage a sit-in with a group of her friends at a government office in order to get hold of her son's medical records. Medical records are actually the patient's property. She should have been given them as soon as she asked for them. After 15 years of battling she won a court ruling that the drug company that made the vaccine, Wellcome, had to allow her to see their documents relating to DPT. Of course drug companies do not want the public to see their internal paperwork, and for three years they succeeded in disobeying the court order. Eventually Wellcome shipped a roomful of files to Dublin, perhaps thinking that she would be daunted by the volume of reading. Margaret and five friends took two weeks to photocopy every page. Then the files were returned to Wellcome. Margaret and a friend took 18 months to read the photocopies. Among the things they discovered is that Wellcome pays doctors to write fraudulent articles for medical journals about the safety of DPT, and that they release batches of vaccine which have failed mouse toxicity tests. The drug company had even paid a British doctor to try and discredit a German doctor who had provided part of the evidence about DPT vaccine that had made the German government take whooping cough vaccine off the schedule in Germany.[351]

After 20 years Kenneth was finally awarded a large amount of financial compensation for what the vaccine had done to him. The money will help his mother care for her adult sized toddler, and it also means that he will be cared for after she dies. In talking to parents of vaccine damaged children, I find that the parents' biggest worry is about what will happen to their child after they die.

At one of the lectures I gave to Public Health nurses, they started barking that a big court case had "proved conclusively" that DPT vaccine never causes brain damage. I told them about Margaret Best's great effort and her great victory, and the corruption that she had unearthed, and I showed them photos of the family. But some of those very same Public Health nurses went on telling parents that a big court case had proved conclusively that DPT vaccine never causes brain damage.

So from this court case we know the names of some doctors whose articles in medical journals are not telling the truth. But how many of the other articles are also fraudulent? At least we know that the articles that make a finding against vaccination are unlikely to be fraudulent, because researchers cannot gain financially from making vaccination look worse than it is. In fact, they open themselves to vengeance from the industry, the bureaucracy, and their colleagues by publishing unfavourable data. Even the most unprejudiced of editors has no way of knowing when a study is fraudulent. Some medical journals have psychological ties to the pharmaceutical industry but no financial ties (like *Lancet* and *BMJ*), some are censored by and financially biased towards drug company interests (like *JAMA*), and then there are magazines for doctors that are funded by the drug companies. Some of these magazines masquerade as medical journals, and they sit there on the shelves in medical libraries along with the genuine medical journals.

Barbara Loe Fisher and Harris Coulter used the empirical method to document the wide range of side effects that DPT vaccine causes.[355] They reveal the varied ways in which severe brain damage first manifests itself, and they show that mild forms of brain damage like dyslexia and dysgraphia are also caused by DPT. They unearthed the fact that DPT also causes a host of other maladies, including the immune system damage which leads to repeated ear infections and tonsilitis.

Ear, throat and nose problems are nowadays regarded as "normal" in children, because they are so common. But they were not common before DPT was introduced. DPT has created a boom in Ear Throat and Nose specialisation. In the Northern suburbs of Johannesburg, most children go through the antibiotics-grommits-tonsils-out routine. I thought that the reason why my little girl Chandra was the odd one out was because of her good diet, and the fact that her ears were always protected from cold by a bonnet I had knitted with cute little ear flaps. When I read the book *DPT: A Shot in the Dark*,[355] I realised that the fact that she had never been injected with DPT was the main reason why she has never had ear infections, tonsilitis or swollen adenoids. I had rejected DPT because I was scared of brain damage and cot death, and unwittingly I had saved her from a whole lot of other troubles too.

The medical establishment scorns empirical findings because they are based on anecdotal evidence, and are not the result of a field trial that compares the rate of chronic diseases in the vaccinated and the unvaccinated. If anyone in the medical establishment had ever done a comparative field trial they would have the right to criticise. As I mentioned earlier, Dr. Michel Odent conducted two comparative field trials which showed that DPT vaccine causes asthma.[5,6,7,8] Dr. Odent is not a member of the medical establishment. He is a true doctor, as his life's work with babies shows.

A VACCINE TRIAL IN NEW ZEALAND

Modern vaccines are tried out on human beings to see whether they produce antibodies. If they do, the vaccine is declared able to produce immunity. There is no requirement to prove that antibodies reflect immunity. The manufacturers of the vaccine have total control over which side effects are going to be acknowledged during the trials, and which are going to be ignored.

In September 1990, while I was living in New Zealand, I received a phone call from someone whose sister had been asked by her doctor to allow her baby to take part in an experiment with a new vaccine. The caller wanted IAS to get the trial halted. We knew that that would be impossible, but we decided to investigate the details of the experiment, and then to ask the Minister of Health to appoint an independent, unbiased individual to monitor the results of the experiment.

The vaccine was intended to prevent a disease called haemophilus influenza type b, which is called Hib for short. It is a rare disease, but it does cause death or serious damage in some babies. Babies are unable to make antibodies to the germ that causes Hib, even when they have the full blown disease. This poses a problem for the vaccine industry because they can only justify the use of a vaccine if it makes antibodies. To add to their commercial troubles, adults of European extraction had been shown to produce antibodies in response to the vaccine, but adults of other races did not.

The aim of the New Zealand experiment was to find out whether attaching the outer shell of the Hib germ to diphtheria toxoid could cause babies under 18 months of age to produce antibodies to Hib. The drug company was particularly interested in finding out what the antibody response would be in Maori and Polynesian babies.

Two doctors who were in full time employment with the New Zealand Health Department were being paid by a multinational drug company to do the trial. We asked two people who worked for the Health Department to go and interview them on our behalf. The trial doctors fell into the trap of assuming that the interviewers were devotees of vaccination, and they enthusiastically answered the questions. The only question they would not answer was how much they were being paid by the drug company.

The study was not designed to assess side effects, but passive reporting by parents was permitted. It was then up to the two doctors to decide which of the parents' reports to include in the data. Our two moles who interviewed the two doctors asked about side effects, and the response was most enlightening. The doctors said that the side effects would be a local reaction at the injection site, like redness, swelling or heat, and where it did occur, it would go away pretty quickly. They said that some children might experience a mild fever as in DPT, but the fever would be much lower with Hib. They said that there are no serious long term effects of the vaccine, because it had already been safely administered to thousands and thousands of children. They said they would encourage the mothers to monitor temperatures, and they would be providing a follow up service. One of them could be paged at all times. They did not give a cut off point for the follow up, but they were quite adamant that anything relating to the vaccine would be happening close to the time of the shot.

This confirmed all our fears about the likelihood of getting a true report on any side effects which may occur. The doctors had made up their minds, before they had even started, which symptoms they were going to acknowledge as side effects. They had also made up their minds that all side effects would show up soon after vaccination, and there would be no permanent damage done. We know that when a mother rushes to get medical help during the acute stage of a baby's vaccine reaction, the doctors and nurses prescribe a painkiller, and deny that the baby is having a vaccine reaction. We had no reason to believe that if a mother in a panic paged one of these doctors, she would be treated any differently.

As the researchers already "knew" before they started the study that all side effects would show up soon after vaccination, any side effects which took two or three weeks to emerge would be discounted. As the germ itself is capable of causing permanent brain damage, it is absurd to suggest that the surface antigen of the germ that has been attached to a foreign protein cannot do the same. If any babies suffered severe reactions to the vaccine, the study doctors could simply choose to believe that it was a coincidence, and then fail to mention it in the report. It is especially easy to ignore subtle symptoms that are a precursor to a long term handicap.

My greatest concern was that if a baby died from the vaccine, it could be replaced by another baby in the final report, because the two doctors who were being paid by the drug company were the only people who knew the names of all the babies who started into the experiment. So we asked the Minister of Health to appoint an independent ombudsman to monitor all the babies who started in to the experiment, and we recommended that the ombudsman should be a person who has credibility with both the medical establishment and with consumer groups.

We expected to be fobbed off, and we were fobbed off. Perhaps this was partly because the Ministry of Health was very busy at the time fobbing off all the people who were trying to warn them that the Factor 9 blood product being used in New Zealand at that time was contaminated with hepatitis C. So the study went ahead without an independent observer being able to note any cases of encephalitis, seizure or death that might have occurred.

When our moles had interviewed the study doctors during the recruitment for the trial, they had queried whether the number of babies in the study was big enough to be valid. Our moles wrote in their report, "The intention is to have 2 groups with 50 in each. However they may go for 60 in each group to allow for dropouts along the way. They have had approval from the Ethics Committee & the FDA that the numbers in their study will be statistically significant."

As the Maori cot death rate at that time was 8 per 1000, there was a strong possibility of a death occurring within the trial group. That would of course not necessarily have meant that the vaccine was responsible for the death, but it would have been good if an unbiased observer had had viewing rights. It is common practice in medical trials to treat deaths as "dropouts along the way," instead of investigating the cause of death. Statistically they are treated as if they had moved to another city.

We tried to find out from the Ethics Committee what protocols had been accepted before they gave permission for the trial to go ahead, but the committee lost the file for a few years, and then when they found it again, they said that the contents were none of our business. In any case, even if they did give approval for a good method of recording side effects, that does not mean that the side effects would have been honestly recorded.

The only indication we had that the study was over, was a newspaper report in September 1992, which said that the vaccine had not proven effective in Maoris and Pacific Islanders.[356] A spokesperson for the Health Department was quoted as saying that a Hib vaccine for babies of six months would not be introduced unless it were "proven effective" in Maoris and Pacific Islanders, because that would be "poor public health practice." Shortly afterwards, a different brand of Hib vaccine, made in exactly the same way as the one in the trial (conjugated polysaccharide), was included in the New Zealand schedule. The vaccine was started at six weeks, not at six months. I wrote to the Ministry of Health and asked if this brand of vaccine had been tested to see whether it made antibodies in Maoris and Pacific Islanders, and the reply I received said that it had not.

During the first 18 months that Hib vaccine was in use in the USA, the FDA received 182 reports of death caused by the vaccine. The FDA conducted a complicated whitewash, and proclaimed the vaccine to be free of responsibility. One of the contortions they used for the whitewash was to say that the rate of adverse events was not known, because none of the trials had been big enough to detect them.

THE EFFECTIVENESS AND SIDE EFFECTS OF VACCINES ARE MONITORED AFTER THEY ARE INTRODUCED

Vaccine Myth number Twelve: Once a vaccine has been introduced, the medical authorities keep a record of the side effects. They also keep a record of the vaccination status of people who catch the disease, so that they can assess how effective the vaccine is. They compile data about side effects by getting doctors and nurses to report any side effects which occur. Every vaccine reaction is then recorded in a central data collecting system.

The biggest factor which prevents an accurate appraisal of side effects is the pathological denial into which most doctors and nurses retreat when they see a case of vaccine damage. Pathological denial is a term used to describe the reaction of a person who does not want to face up to the reality of the consequences of his or her actions. Medical people even resort to pathological denial when a large group of children have the same violent reaction to a vaccine in the same place at the same time.

A friend of mine's cousin had a violent reaction to BCG vaccine at the age of 13, and died after 3 days. The doctors and nurses who were involved with the case went to absurd lengths to deny that the vaccine was the cause. One of them even said that her death was more likely to have been caused by some seagull poo landing on her sandwich at playtime, than by the vaccine. The girl's mother managed to establish that other children in New

Zealand had died from that vaccination campaign, but she never got official acknowledgment.

Families who are victims of vaccine damage are seldom aware of other families who are also victims. They tend to think that their child is just a rare unlucky exception. It is impossible for them to get an overview of the situation in a vacuum of information.

Hilary Butler has been contacted by a lot of parents with vaccine damaged children who have received no help from the authorities whose job it is to help them. One day she noticed that two of these families lived in the same suburb in Wellington. She put them in touch with each other, and they discovered that they lived in the same block, around the corner from one another, yet they had never met. Both families had boys who had had violent reactions within hours of the measles vaccine, and have ongoing behavioural problems as well as recurrent immune system disease. They are both intellectually damaged in specific areas, and in both of them the immune system damage flares up periodically with the same dramatic symptoms. They were both being seen by the same paediatrician, who was telling both the mothers that the fact that the brain damage occurred at the time of vaccination was just a coincidence. One of the mothers had said to the doctor, "You say that my child can't have been affected by the vaccine because it only happens to one in a million. Well how do you know that he's not that one in a million. Someone has to be the one in a million. How do you know that its not my child?" But the doctor still would not admit it. One day the two mothers confronted him together, and he almost admitted that the vaccine was the cause. Afterwards they talked to his receptionist, and she told them that four other mothers who brought their children to him regularly had told her that their child's condition was caused by vaccination.

My phone number is made available at Citizens Advice Bureaus and on the internet for people who want information and support, so I get a steady stream of phone calls from people who are having to endure the consequences of a vaccine reaction. Because of the media blackout on the topic, people who are not personally affected by a vaccine reaction are blissfully unaware that vaccination is causing so much death, disease and distress.

Each vial of vaccine comes with a piece of paper with information about how the vaccine is to be administered, and any other information the manufacturer feels like including. There is a section about side effects, but they are not obliged to list all reactions that they know to occur from their particular product. Yet sometimes they do mention symptoms that have serious long term implications. I sometimes wonder whether doctors read package inserts. I know of cases where mothers have pointed out to their doctors that the very symptoms that their children have suffered are mentioned on the package insert, but the doctors still insisted that it must have been "something else" that caused the symptoms, because it definitely could not have been the vaccine.

When there is a convulsion after vaccination they say it is a coincidence. When there is another convulsion after the next vaccination, they say that too is a coincidence. Convulsions are not uncommon in the first year of life, so it is possible for a convulsion to occur after vaccination without it being caused by the vaccination. However, when it happens a second time, the likelihood of it being a coincidence is greatly diminished. The chance of a convulsion which is not caused by vaccination happening in the three days after vaccination is one in four thousand, and the chance of it happening a second time after a subsequent vaccination without being caused by the vaccination is one in five million.[357] Yet many parents are told that the second one is also a coincidence.

Ultimately the responsibility for monitoring the effect of a vaccine does not lie with the drug company nor with the doctor. It lies with the government agents who bought the vaccine from the manufacturers and foisted it on the population. They are the ones who should be on the lookout for an upsurge of any kind of disease or disorder after a new vaccine is introduced, and they should withdraw the vaccine as soon as there is doubt about its safety. Unfortunately bureaucracies do not work like that in English speaking countries. Not only do they fail to monitor side effects, but they refuse to listen when other people point out side effects. When consumer groups like the Association for Vaccine Damaged Children offer them a golden opportunity to study side effects, they run away and hide.[358] A culture of denial prevails, and doctors who do not partake of the denial are viewed as traitors.

Professor Gordon Stewart hit the nail on the head when he said in 1984,

> The crux of the matter is the risk benefit equation. Assumption that this favours vaccination creates the danger, not only of accepting a hypothesis which is untested but also, because the assumption is already adopted as policy, of creating conditions whereby it can never be tested.[159]

Vaccines are introduced on the assumption that they will be safe, and once they are part of the schedule, any evidence that they are not safe is ignored because they are already a part of the schedule.

A CASE OF MASS PATHOLOGICAL DENIAL

A startling example of mass pathological denial occurred during a meningitis vaccination campaign held in New Zealand schools in 1987. A polysaccharide vaccine was used, and it was designed to give immunity to one strain of bacterial meningitis for two or three years. The way that the information was presented to parents led many to believe that it would make their child immune to all types of meningitis for life.

When this vaccine was used at a primary school in a town called Drury, which is just 10 miles south of Auckland, two mothers who had brought their preschoolers to school to be vaccinated saw children reacting violently to the injection. They decided to stay at school to see what was going to happen. Some of the children vomited or collapsed within minutes of being injected with the vaccine, while others took a few hours to become ill. These mothers saw scores of children seriously affected by the vaccine. One of the two mothers described it to me later as, "It was like one of those old Florence Nightingale movies. The war wounded were lying all around."

The children did not all have the same reaction. Interestingly the trend was for the older children to react immediately, while the younger ones took longer to become affected. Some of the children got severe headaches, some got dizzy, some got fevers, some fainted, some got tingling sensations in their arms and hands, some vomited, some lost control over their legs, some got numb feet, some could not concentrate on the person who was speaking to them, some got sore necks, some got glassy eyes, some lost eye/hand co-ordination, some slowly became floppy and slowly fell off their chairs while trying to do schoolwork. Some children were only beginning to react when it was time to go home. Some of them went home by bus and had to be carried off the busses. Some of the children slept abnormally that afternoon.

Most of the children suffered more than one of these symptoms, and they had all been perfectly fit and healthy before being injected with the vaccine. All of these symptoms, including the vomiting, can be caused by neurological disturbance.

The two mothers who witnessed these reactions went to the press, and two newspapers decided not to withhold the information from the public. A journalist contacted the medical officer of health for comment, and was told that only 14 children had shown any symptoms, and the symptoms had no physical cause, they were just caused by mass hysteria. The reason he gave for the hysteria was that the vaccine had been delayed for an hour, and "all sorts of nasty rumours developed, and the youngsters got themselves worked up into quite a state." It is true that the vaccine had been delayed for an hour, but the children were not aware that it had been delayed. They were just working in their classrooms until they were called out to be jabbed.

Another person in the Health Department said that the neurological effects were not caused by the vaccine, they were caused by an unrelated meningitis virus which was "rippling through the community" at the time. It is of course absurd to suggest that a large group of children suddenly got very sick from a virus in the air, just minutes after they are injected with a bacteria that causes the same symptoms, and that the injection of the bacteria had absolutely nothing to do with the symptoms. But it worked as a public relations exercise.

The Health Department did not have it all their own way. After ten days the medical officer of health admitted that the reactions were not psychological, and said that they were now treating all complaints with concern. Despite this quiet admission, much of the New Zealand public is still left with the impression that there was an incident of mass hysteria after vaccination at a school. The medical officer also said that side effects like this had not been heard of before, and were apparently not known to the makers of the vaccine. "It is potentially of world-wide importance."[359]

Eventually it emerged that the same thing had happened at another school at the start of the campaign, but the director-general of health had decided to suppress the information, so as not to jeopardise the rest of the campaign. It had then happened at other schools as well, and they had managed to keep it out of the press, until the incident at Drury Primary School. The thing that I find most shocking about all this is that so many teachers kept quiet about what they saw. One expects the doctors and nurses who are promoting the campaign to be callous and dishonest, and only concerned with preserving the status of modern medicine. But teachers are supposed to care about the welfare of children, and in New Zealand they will not lose their jobs if they speak out about a pharmaceutical product.

Once the cat was out of the bag, the Health Department decided to improve its image. When the publicity first started, various medicrats made statements which contradicted one another, so to avoid further embarrassment the chief bigwig issued a decree that only he and one other bigwig were allowed to make statements to the press. They also advertised a phone number for parents to call if they were concerned about their child's reaction. The phone number was only available for a short time, and some parents who tried to use it received no answer. I was not living in New Zealand when all this happened, but I have since spoken to a number of parents whose children were affected by the vaccine. Two of them told me that they contacted the phone company to see if there was something wrong with the phone line because they could not get through.

Two paediatric neurologists were appointed to examine the 546 victims who had managed to make contact. One of the neurologists is an individual who has been appointed to assess other cases with which IAS has been involved in compensation claims. His behaviour towards the parents of these cases suggests that he has made up his mind that there is no such thing as vaccine damage. I believe that this prejudice very strongly clouds his judgment.

Six weeks after the reactions had first reached the media, the official report came out saying that there was no evidence to suggest that the reactions were associated with permanent harm, but that children under the age of two who had reacted badly should not have the booster shot. Two weeks later a group of medicrats declared that there was no evidence of long term damage in any of the children, and there was no clear link between neurological problems experienced by some children and the vaccine. This was going beyond the findings of the official report. They had no new data on which to base this declaration, they just made it up.

They said that the same vaccine was used in a major campaign in Finland in the 1970s, and no neurological reactions were reported there. I can think of a number of possible reasons why no neurological reactions were reported in Finland. Perhaps it is because the medicrats in Finland are also pathological liars, and were more successful at keeping the truth under wraps. Perhaps there were much fewer reactions in Finland, and it was easier to keep it out of the press. Or perhaps Finnish children are made of stronger stuff, and none of them experienced bad reactions to the vaccine. But even if all the children in Finland were strong enough to cope with this injection, that still does not alter the fact that thousands of New Zealand children were not strong enough to cope with it.

This episode in history was not a case of mass hysteria by "youngsters" who got themselves worked up about a needle. It was a case of adults in a position of responsibility and power resorting to mass pathological denial in order to protect their own status. When children lose the use of their legs for three hours after an injection, what has actually happened to them? What did the vaccine do that made that possible? What are the long term implications of such a symptom? The Health Department should be researching the biological reality of this symptom, instead of pretending that they know the symptoms are not important. No attempt was ever made to find out what the immediate reactions indicated about the long term side effects of the vaccine.

Hilary Butler documented the story of one girl who was damaged by the vaccine and was still in pain and could not play sport five years after the injection.[360] I have received phone calls from many people whose children were damaged by that campaign, and were still suffering effects of the vaccine years later. Most of them were suffering from mild unco-ordination, which affected their movements, and made them unsuccessful at sports which they had previously enjoyed. All of these people telephoned me because they were being pressurised to accept yet another vaccine for the damaged child or for one of its siblings, and they wanted IAS to help them avoid it. Some have told me that they did not know about the hotline at the time that it was available, while others made contact with the Health

Department, but were successfully told to get lost. Two have told me that their children were examined by the paediatric neurologists and given a clean bill of health when they were still affected by the vaccine.

Two doctors reviewed the official report that was presented by the paediatric neurologists, and published an article in the *New Zealand Medical Journal*.[361] This article keeps on harping about the possibility that other things may have caused the severe symptoms, and they will not let go of that psychological bit. "The initial explanation seemed to be related to a delay in the arrival of the vaccine, and therefore an anxious waiting period for the children at the school." They make this claim despite the fact that it had been admitted in the press that there had not been an anxious waiting period.

Although it is regrettable that the true figures were well pruned and trimmed, at least there is something in a medical journal to say that something happened. They said that there were 63 reports of headache, stiff neck and myalgia within 48 hours of vaccination, although, "other causes, particularly viral illness, cannot be excluded." They also mentioned 152 cases of fever, and 85 of fever, rash and local reaction.

There were 92 reports suggesting peripheral nerve involvement. Motor symptoms consisted of 80 reports of unexplained weakness and subjective "heaviness" unrelated to injection site, and there were 57 reports of sensory symptoms suggesting paraesthesia or dysaesthesia. Both categories occurred in some children, and in younger children, reluctance to use a limb may have been due to either. The majority of cases, both sensory and motor, were transient and had gone within 48 hours of immunisation although symptoms persisted for up to three weeks in some cases. These symptoms could have been vaccine related as they are less likely to be related to intercurrent illness, and many episodes occurred within a plausible time interval. On the other hand it is clear that absolute causality cannot be ascribed on the basis of the data.

So they are not quite admitting that the vaccine was responsible, and they are certainly not admitting that some children were permanently damaged.

All reported cases of fainting, nausea and dizziness occurred within 24 hours and can probably be ascribed to psychological effects of the procedure.

No, probably not.

Other symptoms which were reported only occasionally were considered too subject to confounding to warrant further consideration.

In other words, "Some children suffered unusual symptoms from the vaccine, but as there were not a large group of each of these symptoms, we will choose to ignore them."

Although this report is mildly infuriating, it at least makes it official that there were some neurological side effects. This is important because one of the features of medical denial is that it is often claimed that something cannot be happening here if it has not been reported as having happened somewhere else. So although the incidence of reactions is greatly reduced in this report, and although the children who are still suffering bad effects years afterwards are not acknowledged, the fact that the report was published in a medical journal means that medicrats in other countries will not be justified in brushing aside similar events in their own country on the grounds that "there has never before been a report of serious reactions to this vaccine anywhere in the world."

It would be interesting to know what percentage of medicrats actually take cognisance of things that are printed in medical journals. Two and a half years after this report was published, a journalist interviewed a highly placed New Zealand medicrat about vaccination. When discussing the Drury incident, the medicrat told her that a specialist had been called in to check the reactions, and had concluded that it was a case of mass hysteria, and there were no problems with the vaccine.

Five years after the event IAS had discussions with a number of school principles about an MMR vaccination campaign that was planned in schools. Many of these principals were still under the impression that the Drury incident had been a case of mass hysteria. A lie once told is very powerful.

The person who was the Medical Assessor for New Zealand at the time reported to the World Health Assembly in Geneva that there had been problems with the vaccine. The World Health Organisation had two excuses for not acting on his report. The first was that he had no controls.[362] According to them, he should have selected some children who were not injected with the vaccine, and investigated whether they were vomiting and collapsing at 11 am on vaccination day. Their second excuse was that no other country had reported any side effects.[363] The first excuse is almost valid because all data should have controls. Even though it is quite obvious to anyone with common sense that those children were vomiting and collapsing because of the vaccine, to be scientifically correct, the Medical Assessor should have sent evidence that children of the same age who had not been vaccinated, were not vomiting and collapsing at the same time on the same day. If the World Health Organisation actually cared about the welfare of children, they would have investigated the matter for themselves. They could easily do it, seeing as they have billions of dollars to work with. Their second excuse for ignoring his report has no validity, because most countries that bought the vaccine make no effort to record the side effects of any vaccine.

Later the Medical Assessor spoke on radio about side effects of vaccination, and was verbally rebuked for doing this. When his contract with the Health Department was due for renewal, which normally happens automatically, it was not renewed. Basically he got fired for talking about vaccine reactions.

In 1987 Hilary Butler published a paper which documented the events of this mass vaccination campaign.[364] In it she discusses the immunological reasons why those particular reactions occurred. She mentions that some doctors recognised the syndrome and diagnosed correctly, while

> ... the hospitals, paediatric neurologists and Health Department chose to ignore such blatantly obvious facts. As one doctor put it: "Well, we'll never really know, until in maybe five years time in some other country, the same syndrome is reported in the literature." Such statements are somewhat of an oxymoron, since in the hypothetical five years time, said doctors would probably look at the literature and say "Can't be - never happened before!" and it wouldn't get within an arm's length of a medical journal. This is the way that information which should be classified as *fact* and reported, is continually ridiculed and put-down as *anecdotal*.[365]

These were prophetic words. In 1991 there was a minor controversy in South Africa about the death of a child after a meningitis vaccination campaign in schools. My friend Arlene in Cape Town wrote to a member of parliament who was in parliament on an anti-apartheid ticket and expressed her concern about the child's death. The child who had died had a black skin, so there would have been no point in contacting a pro-apartheid parliamentarian about the death. The member of parliament replied that he knew that the death was not caused by the vaccine, because no other country had reported side effects.

I wrote to the World Health Organisation and asked how they monitor the side effects of vaccines in South Africa. They replied that they do not, and they gave me the address of the Medicines Control Council in Cape Town, and suggested I should ask them how the South Africans monitor side effects.

I knew very well that the South African medical authorities did not monitor side effects of vaccines, but I wanted them to put it in writing. So I wrote to the Medicines Control Council and asked them how they monitor side effects. They replied that they have a system for the voluntary reporting of adverse drug reactions by medical doctors, dentists and pharmacists and the pharmaceutical industry, but they do not have a system that specifically solicits adverse reactions to vaccines. Their letter ended, "Because the system is a voluntary reporting system it does not allow for monitoring the incidence of adverse reports."

It was a very tidy arrangement for the drug companies. The World Health Organisation promoted vaccination around the world but made no effort to find out what side effects occur. The governments which accepted the vaccines did not monitor side effects. Yet the World Health Organisation could reject a report from an official in New Zealand because there were no similar reports from other countries. Things are done differently now, as you will see below.

Consumer groups that are run by volunteers are now documenting the side effects of the new genetically engineered meningococcal meningitis vaccine. They can only document the cases which are reported to them, and of course most cases do not get reported to them because media censorship prevents most victims of vaccine damage from knowing that consumer groups exist, let alone that there is the option of reporting the reaction to a consumer group when their doctor refuses to report it to the official body.

RELIANCE ON PASSIVE REPORTING

In the USA they now have the Vaccine Adverse Event Reporting System (VAERS). This only came into existence because of the efforts of a group of parents.[366] The group called itself *DPT - Dissatisfied Parents Together*, and they were comprised mainly of people whose children had been killed or severely damaged by DPT vaccine. After a tremendous struggle the group managed to bring the National Childhood Vaccine Injury Compensation Act into existence.

> Like David against Goliath, DPT represented essentially powerless vaccine injured victims pitted against three of the most powerful and wealthy segments of our society: the pharmaceutical industry, organised medicine, and the federal government.[366]

The group worked very hard for four and a half years to compile and submit legislation to create VAERS. When the prospects of success were looking very bleak, the drug companies said that they would allow the law to be passed, as long as it went through at the same time as a law that they wanted introduced. Their legislation makes it possible for them to sell new drugs to countries outside the USA without having to wait for the drug to be passed by the FDA.[366] This is not as bad as it sounds for those of us who live outside of the USA, because the FDA is a corrupt organisation that passes unsafe drugs anyway. So the law creating VAERS and the drug companies' law were passed at the same time.

VAERS is a branch of the FDA. The Act states that a doctor must report a side effect of a vaccine to the FDA if they "judge the event warrants reporting."[367] If a doctor decides to retreat into pathological denial, the event will not be reported, but at least when a doctor is prepared to face up to the reality of what he or she is seeing, there is now a central register to which the observation can be reported.

A list of symptoms that were considered acceptable as side effects of each vaccine was drawn up, and a time frame was established in which these events have to occur if they are to be accepted as related to the vaccine.[367] So as long as the reaction a child experiences involves symptoms that are on the list, and if the symptoms occur within the given time frame, and if there is some residual damage, the child is supposed to be compensated. If the vaccine causes a type of damage that is not on the list, then no compensation will be paid. DPT can cause infantile seizures, but infantile seizures are not on the list.[368]

When it was seen that paying for some of the damage done by vaccines was going to cost far too much money, they decided to decrease the length of time after vaccination in which the reactions have to occur in order for compensation to be paid.[368] So anaphylactic shock now has to occur within four hours of vaccination, encephalopathy and encephalitis from DPT vaccine has to occur within 72 hours, and encephalitis from measles vaccine has to occur within fifteen days.[368] Most cases of encephalitis and encephalopathy from DPT only begin to become apparent after about six days, and even then they are hard to recognise by people who are not on the lookout for the subtle early signs. Many cases of encephalitis from measles vaccine only begin to show up fourteen to thirty days after vaccination. With this kind of chicanery, the American medicrats succeeded in greatly reducing the number of victims who were eligible to claim for vaccine damage. A large sum of taxpayers' money was set aside for paying compensation each year, but in the first year that the system went into operation, they ran out of money in March.[369] Despite the fact that not all cases get reported under this system, they were still getting far more cases than they had expected.

The parents consumer group called DPT has changed its name to *National Vaccination Information Center (NVIC)*. When a doctor refuses to report a reaction, NVIC can submit the report on behalf of the parent, that is, if the parent is fortunate enough to know that NVIC exists. VAERS claims that when it receives reports, "All reports received are entered into the database."[370] NVIC used the Freedom of Information Act to obtain a copy of the data about vaccine reactions that the FDA had in their computer. Despite the court order, the FDA tried to avoid complying. When NVIC finally obtained the data, they discovered that it was not accurate. Some of the cases they had assisted in getting reported were not even there, and others had the details wrong.[371]

The medicrats have built in an escape chute so that they do not have to take too much notice of the reports that do end up being typed into the computer. "Submission of a report does not necessarily denote that the vaccine caused the adverse event."[367] Any reports they do not like can simply be quashed by saying that the doctor's judgment was wrong.

The vaccine industry does not like the term "vaccine reactions." They are conducting a worldwide push to substitute it with "adverse events." New Zealand has the Adverse Event Reporting Committee that is based in Dunedin. Doctors can report reactions to them if they feel so inclined, but the bureaucrats in Dunedin are not obliged to enter the report into their computer. IAS does not know what percentage of reports are simply thrown away instead of being entered into the database, but we know of some that were not entered. Any member of the public who wants to know how many reports are entered for each vaccine for each year has to pay a lot of money for the information. So we at IAS started our own collection of reports of side effects, so that at least some would be documented for posterity. One of the questions we ask on the form is whether the doctor or nurse to whom the parent reported the reaction reported it to the committee in Dunedin.

The Australian consumer group the Australian Vaccination Network (AVN) also started their own database for Australian vaccine reactions. The official body to which reports of vaccine reactions can be made in Australia is called ADRAC. The official policy is, "Any serious or unexpected adverse event should be reported."[372] No limits have been put on the type of reactions which can be reported, and the cutoff time within which reactions have to occur has been lifted, "as some adverse events related to vaccination could occur many years later."[372] Serious reports are supposed to be followed up and the victim is supposed to be helped if possible, but victims are neither followed up nor helped. In 1999 Meryl Dorey, the president of AVN, and two AVN members, met with ADRAC representatives in Canberra. The officials admitted that less than 10% of reactions are ever reported in Australia, and of those that are, almost none are followed up to see if there have been any long term complications, or, in fact, if the person involved has survived the reaction.[373,374] The AVN currently has more than 700 cases of severe reactions on its own adverse reactions database. None of them have been reported to ADRAC by the vaccinator nor by any health professional who has been consulted about the vaccine damage.

In 1997, when there were only 200 cases on the AVN database, Meryl sent the reports, with names and addresses, stating which of them had already died from the reaction, to the Minister of Health, and asked him to investigate them all and add them to the official statistics. After 6 months of evasive action, the Minister finally said that he would neither investigate the reactions nor add them to the statistics as they had not been reported by doctors.

When the MMR vaccine was introduced, reactions were monitored for 3 weeks after injection in Britain and Finland. This method was of course not able to detect possible chronic side effects like autism and leukemia.

The MMR vaccine was not tested in Australia for safety and effectiveness before being introduced into the schedule. Four years after it was introduced into the Australian schedule, a mass vaccination campaign was conducted in schools to kick off the introduction of a second dose. The medical authorities have the temerity to claim that this was their "safety and efficacy trial." The way that they collected data about side effects during the mass vaccination campaign was by doing the vaccinations at school, and then sitting back while allowing parents to report a reaction to a doctor in private practice, and allowing the doctor to report the reaction to ADRAC if he or she felt like it.

Media reports about bad side effects erode public confidence in vaccination.[375] Therefore the World Health Organisation has commissioned the Department of Pharmacology at the University of Cape Town to design a system which each country can use for monitoring and responding to adverse reactions.[375] The system they have designed for monitoring the incidence relies on passive reporting for collecting data, but it does encourage reporting, and it has a lot of good features. If human beings were honest creatures, it would result in the collection of accurate data on vaccine side effects, the rapid withdrawal of hot lots, truthful communications to the public via the media, and all companies which produce unsafe vaccines going out of business. One of the recommendations is that when patients go to a medical outlet to report a reaction, "the supervisor and the health care worker concerned [should] ... comfort the patients and their parents."[375] Wouldn't that be nice.

Another recommendation is that an ethos of risk-benefit awareness should be created in which the public and the press should be educated about "the impressive performance record" of vaccines.[375] They have no right to claim that vaccination has a good record when no records have been kept. Vaccination has a good reputation, but it does not have a good record. My expectation is that bureaucrats in some countries will set up a system which makes it look as though they are monitoring side effects, so that they can be more credible in their claim that vaccines cause few side effects. I am not optimistic that the culture of denial that pervades the field of vaccination is about to disappear.

The World Health Organisation has started running international courses in Cape Town based on the system devised at the university. One of the things they teach people is how to handle the media when the public complains about a cluster of bad reactions. I would like to be a fly on the wall during those lectures. My experience in the field of vaccination leads me to expect that this course trains people to go through the motions of pretending to monitor vaccine reactions. I do not anticipate a fundamental change in attitude. Even though there are individual doctors and nurses who want to do the right thing, they know that they would put their jobs in jeopardy if they told the truth.

Early in 1988 I had an encounter which highlights the typical attitude of keen vaccinationists. It was with a high ranking doctor from Groote Schuur Hospital in Cape Town. My second child, Kenneth, was born at home in a small town south of Cape Town on the Cape Peninsula. When he was two months old the local public health nurse telephoned me, and I told her that he was not going to be vaccinated. A few weeks later two women suddenly turned up on my doorstep. One was the public health nurse, the other was the doctor from Groote Schuur Hospital. Ever since Chris Barnard did the world's first heart transplant at Groote Schuur Hospital, anyone associated with the hospital has bathed in reflected glory. The public health nurse thought that this doctor would be able to intimidate me. I invited them to sit down, and a lively discussion ensued between myself and the doctor. I had people living with me at the time and they gathered around to watch. The public health nurse switched off her ears and got that same glazed look in her eyes which white South Africans used to get when you told them that apartheid should be abolished. I was quite taken aback by the doctor's ignorance about the immune system, but I was amused by the expression on her face when she found out that I knew that the polio vaccine was no longer compulsory. No member of the public was supposed to know that.

I gave a number of reasons for not vaccinating Kenneth. She told me that she knew that measles vaccine has no side effects because they had just done a mass vaccination campaign against measles in Khayelitsha, and, "They would be turning up in droves at the hospital if there was any problem." What she was saying was that every child who reacted to the vaccine would present itself at the hospital.

I replied, "They'll be turning up in droves in ten years' time, and you won't know that its because of the vaccine." Khayelitsha was a slum on the eastern side of Cape Town that attracted people who faced starvation in the Ciskei and Transkei "bantustans." This doctor knew what conditions were like in Khayelitsha. She had been there and she knew that the people lived in tents or self-built shacks, and that there was no public transport, there were no telephones, the people had no money, and while the ambulance drivers did their best to get every dangerously ill person to hospital, the ambulance service was hopelessly under-funded and over-stretched. According to her method of assessing side effects, a child who suffered a severe immediate reaction was supposed to make it to hospital 30 miles away despite these difficulties.

I tried to impress on this doctor that a reaction might only show up some time after the vaccination, in the form of chronic disease, but her mind was absolutely closed to the idea. Even if a child who had suffered a severe immediate reaction made it to the hospital alive, there would have been little chance of the case being recorded as a vaccine reaction.

When it was time for the two ladies to leave, the public health nurse snapped back into consciousness and said to me, "When you bring him down to the clinic I will leave out the whooping cough part of the vaccine." She had not heard a word I had said. With all the sickness and misery that prevailed in Cape Town it is amazing that a doctor from Groote Schuur had nothing better to do with five hours than travel to the home of a white person in order to try and achieve compliance. At least she was friendly and non-aggressive.

An "evaluation" of the mass vaccination campaign in Khayelitsha was published in the *South African Medical Journal*.[376] The article evaluates how successful they were at reaching the target population, and does not even mention side effects. I am not optimistic that attitudes towards acknowledging side effects will be changed by the World Health Organisation's training course in Cape Town. The presentation of the issue is all that is likely to change.

Any country that does make a serious effort to evaluate side effects is in for a shock. When the measles vaccine was introduced, East Germany was under communist rule. The government made measles vaccine compulsory, and passed a law that every person who suffered vaccine damage must be compensated.[178] Once the claims for compensation started rolling in, the government was shocked to discover how very common severe long term side effects are.[377]

The three most serious problems in regard to the recording of side effects are those of pathological denial at the patient/provider interface, pernicious dishonesty among medical bureaucrats, and financial relationships between vaccine manufacturers and some of the highest ranking officials. An American mother whose child was killed by DPT vaccine failed to get acknowledgment of the cause of death despite going to a lot of effort to get it. During a telephone conversation with a CDC official, she was told by the official that he knew that DPT was the cause of death, but he did not dare say that to anyone else.[378]

We have to rely on anecdotal reports for information on vaccine side effects. When hepatitis B vaccine was introduced to New Zealand in 1988, everyone up to the age of 16 was targeted. I noticed that mothers were talking about an unusual type of platelet disorder that was cropping up quite frequently, and I wondered if it was related to the vaccine. It is impossible to know for sure, because the incidence of platelet disorders is not recorded, so there would be no way of seeing whether there is an increase after a certain vaccine is introduced. But the incidence of diabetes was already being recorded in New Zealand before the hepatitis B vaccine was introduced. An American doctor, Dr. J. Barthelow Classen, noticed that there was a 60% increase in diabetes after hepatitis B vaccine was introduced to New Zealand in 1988.[379,380] The vaccine bureaucracy throws its energy into denying and trivialising parents' reports about side effects, and denigrating doctors like Dr. Classen, instead of looking at epidemiological trends. Dr. Classen has also shown that Hib vaccine causes diabetes.[381]

Anecdotal reports do not tell us how often each side effect happens. Hepatitis B vaccine is documented as causing Guillain-Barre syndrome (a type of paralysis), optic neuritis, transverse myelitis, demyelinating lesions in the brain, and progressive demyelination.[382,383,384] It also causes death, which is documented on the internet[385] and in consumer group publications. IAS and AVN know of deaths in newborn babies from hepatitis B vaccine, and one death in a seven year old girl. But what proportion of recipients suffer these consequences? We do know that even if this vaccine did work, it would not be necessary to give it to children or babies. Children do not catch hepatitis B from other children,[19,20] and the hysteria about the carrier state causing cancer is just hype to promote the vaccine.[386]

Two scientists in Seattle found an explanation for how viruses and vaccines can cause auto-immune disease by a process of demyelination.[387] The myelin sheath is the insulating coat that surrounds every nerve in the body. When this insulating coat disappears for some reason, the nerve cannot function properly. The type of disease that results from the loss of the myelin sheath depends upon which nerve has lost its protection. Auto-immune diseases are ones in which the immune system itself attacks a part of the body. In the case of auto-immune demyelination, the person's own immune system attacks the myelin sheath and destroys it. Some cases of multiple sclerosis are auto-immune diseases. It is documented that vaccination causes some cases of multiple sclerosis,[388,389,390,391] but no studies have been done to asses the frequency of this side effect.

The scientists in Seattle found that a number of viruses have protein chains which are similar to the protein chains in the myelin sheath. Some people make a massive amount of antibodies after vaccination, and these antibodies can "recognise" the similar protein chains in the myelin sheath, and they set about breaking up the myelin sheath.[387] The research does not explain why it happens in some individuals and not in others, but it does give a clue as to why vaccination causes so many auto-immune diseases. It is not surprising that all types of auto-immune disease are on the increase. It has now become common for pet dogs to have auto-immune diseases like type 1 diabetes because of dog vaccinations.

The human immune system does not restrict itself to making antibodies to the germ that is contained in the vaccine. The immune system also makes antibodies to all the other ingredients in the vaccine, like mercury, formaldehyde, antibiotics, animal flesh, human flesh, vegetable matter and aluminium. Some people who suffered paralysis from a rabies vaccine that was made of brain were found to have developed anti-brain antibodies.[392] When brain is injected into someone's blood, his or her immune system automatically manufactures anti-brain antibodies. While these antibodies float around in the bloodstream they have the potential to attack the person's brain. If someone were to offer to inject me with brain, I would say, "No thank you. I don't want to have anti-brain antibodies circulating in my blood stream." Recipients of vaccines that contain brain are not told that the vaccine contains brain.

Although detecting changing trends and recording anecdotal accounts are important ways of assessing side effects of vaccination, (because they are all we have at present,) they do not give us an accurate picture of the type nor the incidence of side effects. As I have said in vaccine myth number two, the way to properly assess side effects is to compare the incidence of chronic diseases in the vaccinated and the unvaccinated. That is how the London doctors found out that measles vaccine causes Crohn's disease,[12] and how Dr. Odent's group found out that DPT vaccine causes asthma.[5,6,7,8] Of course the vaccine industry does not want comparative studies to be done, but it is the responsibility of governments to do them.

Each government that recommends vaccination should set up an extensive database to discover all the side effects of vaccination which have a delayed appearance. Some countries are setting up databases to record who is vaccinated and who is not. Their intention in recording this information is to make it easier for them to persecute the families who do not vaccinate. They have no intention of using it to evaluate side effects and effectiveness of vaccines, but it is possible that in the future these databases will be used, by people who are concerned about the welfare of children, to assess the facts and figures which up until now government agencies have so assiduously avoided collecting.

IGNORING CONTRA-INDICATIONS

In 1953 a Swiss paediatrician published an article which related his personal experience of the factors that make a baby vulnerable to suffering brain damage from whooping cough vaccine, and what he had found on the topic in the medical literature.[393] He listed five factors that greatly increase the risk of a baby suffering brain damage from the vaccine.[393] The medical establishment as a whole acknowledged that the presence of these and some other factors meant that a child should not be vaccinated with whooping cough vaccine, nor with any other type of vaccine. Every English speaking country adopted the official policy that vaccination should be withheld from children with contra-indications to vaccination. A British study published in 1974 confirmed that a child is more vulnerable to neurological damage from DPT if he or she has a history of fits, or a family history of fits in first-degree relatives, if he or she has had a reaction to a previous jab, has had a recent infection, or has neurodevelopmental defects.[394]

But contra-indications have become unpopular with the vaccine industry. In 1989 the American Immunization Practices Advisory Committee announced that some contra-indications were not really contra-indications to vaccination.[395] I wrote and asked this committee for evidence to support their stance, and they sent me 18 references. Some of these references were non-existent, some were smoke-screens, and some were just off the point. However, it was interesting that one of the references said that a hypotonic hyporesponsive episode (staring episode) after vaccination is a contra-indication to further doses.[396] These American bureaucrats have persuaded health departments around the world to ignore contra-indications, and to vaccinate babies who are known to be at risk of suffering bad side effects.

An example of the callous irresponsibility of modern medical officials is that they recommend that premature babies should be vaccinated according to their date of birth, not according to their gestational age. A proper study was eventually done in 2001, and it found that premature babies are very susceptible to suffering from serious vaccine reactions.[397] The authors of the study point out that the research on which the modern British policy of vaccinating premature babies is based is inadequate, and they call on the British Department of Health to change their policy.[397]

At about 8 pm one night I got a phone call from a woman who wanted me to give her the name of a homoeopath who would be prepared to go to Auckland hospital and treat her niece. She said the girl had reacted violently to MMR vaccination at school that day, and was "getting worse by the hour." She told me that the doctors at the hospital were saying that it had happened because the girl had been vaccinated when she had a cold, and there was nothing wrong with the vaccine. When they want to peddle the vaccine they say that it is perfectly safe to vaccinate someone who has a cold. However, when they want to protect the reputation of a vaccine, they do an about-face and say it is wrong to vaccinate someone who has a cold.

In New Zealand, the medicrats are using a variety of aggressive methods to try and increase the uptake of vaccines. Parents of vaccine damaged children are repeatedly telephoned and harassed to accept another dose. The government has instructed doctors to make their receptionists do this. Hospital staff have been instructed to ask about the vaccination status of all children who come into hospital, and to persuade the parents to "get the shots up to date." The questions are asked when the child is admitted to hospital, but the jabbing is not done until the child is discharged. Because of government cutbacks, patients are usually discharged before they are fully recovered. So children are being jabbed when they are in poor health, and then sent away instead of being observed. If the parents later have a story to relate about a reaction, there is no need to believe them because no medically trained staff saw the reaction.

Most cases of vaccine damage result in symptoms that are there all the time. For instance the child cannot walk or it has inflamed ears or it is continually violent. A strange thing is that some children get symptoms that come and go at regular intervals. It could be once a month, or every six weeks. The child has a health crisis for a few days, and then appears normal until the health crisis returns. Sometimes the crisis is so intense and frightening that the parents rush the child to hospital. Upon entry they are aggressively asked if the child's vaccinations are up to date. When the parents aggressively reply that it is vaccination that has caused the problem in the first place, the hospital staff usually look shocked and shut up. But you get some really hard cases who still carry on badgering the parents to have another dose of vaccine, while telling them that they are quite wrong in thinking that vaccination can cause such drastic and peculiar symptoms.

A package insert that accompanies one brand of DPT vaccine lists the following contra-indications;

-Acute infectious diseases.
-Currently evoluting diseases (acute or chronic).
-Because of the pertussis valency, a personal medical history of neuro-
 logical problems (convulsions, encephalitis, encephalopathy).

-A second or third DPT injection should not be given to a child who has suffered a severe adverse reaction to a previous dose. The pertussis component should be omitted and diphtheria and tetanus immunization completed.

By mentioning the last two contra-indications the company that manufactures the vaccine protects itself from litigation, but many bureaucrats, who are immune to litigation, deny that the last two contra-indications exist. There are other factors that increase the risk of an adverse reaction, and DPT vaccine is not the only vaccine which does more harm with each dose. However, if all doctors took heed of the contra-indications that are mentioned on package inserts, there would be a much smaller incidence of vaccine damage.

The same package insert says that if the baby is given "salicyles, barbiturates or antihistamines" in association with the vaccine, that will help the reaction to be "benign and transient," and reduce the risk of convulsions, brain inflammation and brain damage. I wrote to the drug company and asked them how they know that giving these drugs will prevent brain damage. They did not reply. They cannot have any evidence to support the claim, because giving these drugs on the same day as vaccination does not prevent brain damage. It is outrageous that a drug company can make a claim like that on a package insert. What is worse is that these drugs actually make a baby more vulnerable to damage from the vaccine.

A study was done looking at the effect of paracetamol (acetaminophen) during the first 24 hours after vaccination.[398] With paracetamol there was less fever, less pain at the injection site, and less fussiness. Paracetamol was voted a huge success by the authors of the study, some of whom have been publicly exposed as being on the payroll of drug companies. Another study looked at the effect of paracetamol in the first 48 hours after vaccination.[399] Babies with contra-indications to vaccination were excluded from this study. This really infuriates me, because it shows that they know that contra-indications increase the risk of a severe reaction, and they do not want to have that affecting the results of their study. But they do not exclude babies with contra-indications from vaccination in the real world outside of their study, because they would lose dollars for each child not vaccinated. This study also found that paracetamol reduced fever and pain at the site of injection. But this second study also looked at the symptom of drowsiness, and it found that the drug made no difference to drowsiness.

We have seen earlier how fever protects the body. Fever suppressing drugs make the baby's brain more vulnerable to attack by the germs, as well as to the genetic proteins and the toxins that are in the vaccine. At the same time they mask any acute reaction which might show up during the period shortly after vaccination, so that parents are less likely to be successful at suing the drug company for long term damage. It is significant that the drug did not mask the symptom of drowsiness. Drowsiness after vaccination has sinister long term implications regarding brain damage.

Prescribing paracetamol to prevent brain damage from vaccination is as unscientific as the claim of 200 years ago that taking mercury would protect people from a bad reaction to smallpox vaccination. Science is not the issue. Compliance is the issue. The latter study concluded with the statement, "Use of acetaminophen (paracetamol) may thereby relieve parental anxiety and improve compliance with recommended vaccination programs."[399] Achieving compliance, not preventing side effects, is what it is all about. The finding of this study was reported in a magazine for doctors with the title in large print, "Paracetamol Increases Immunisation Compliance."[400]

Sometimes the ingredients of a vaccine damage the brain without the person's body having been able to muster up a fever in order to defend itself, even in the absence of fever suppressing drugs. The child's initial reaction is something else, like staring episodes or somnolence, not fever. A Swedish study from the 1960s found that there was no fever in 35% of cerebral reactions, and no fever in 55% of cases of shock from DPT.[401]

Teething at the time of vaccination also increases the risk of vaccine damage, but that one was never officially acknowledged, so it has not been discarded. Separating jabs by 7 days, 14 days, or 21 days also increases the risk. Tell that to a keen vaccinator, and observe scorn spread over their face. People who want to separate MMR into M, M and R are making a terrible mistake.

Thankfully there are still doctors who have enough common sense to observe contra-indications, and therefore they do not jab children who are obviously at high risk. Unfortunately, while contra-indications increase the risk, the absence of contra-indications does not mean there is no risk. A baby who is perfectly healthy and belongs to a family of sturdy individuals can tragically suffer serious damage from vaccination. The *British Medical Journal* documents the case of a boy who came from a family with no history of anything, and who was perfectly healthy until his first dose of DPT at eight months caused profound brain damage.[402]

"SCIENTIFIC RESEARCH HAS PROVEN THAT VACCINATION DOES NOT INCREASE THE RISK OF SIDS"

Vaccine Myth number Thirteen: Some parents believe that their child died from vaccination just because it died after vaccination, but a temporal association does not mean that the vaccine was the cause. Scientific studies have shown that vaccination does not cause SIDS.

The worst thing that can happen to a parent is to lose a child, and when the child dies without explanation, or disappears without trace, the loss is almost unbearable. SIDS stands for Sudden Infant Death Syndrome, a phenomenon that claims the lives of thousands of apparently healthy babies every year. In a true case of SIDS, there is no warning that death is about to occur, and an autopsy is done which finds no explanation for the death. It is called "crib death" in the Americas and "cot death" in other English speaking regions.

It is mysterious why a baby who seems to be perfectly all right can suddenly stop being alive. Some of these babies die because they stop breathing. Others stop breathing because they die. These unexplained deaths have been happening since long before vaccination was invented.[403] Until such time as the natural causes of this phenomenon can be understood, it is important to find out which external factors increase the risk of it occurring.

217

Some studies have been done, and it has emerged that smoking during pregnancy, a lack of breast feeding, wrapping up the baby too warmly, and making the baby sleep on its tummy increases the risk. Characteristics and behaviour patterns of the parents, like the age and marital status of the mother, have been studied, but medical researchers steer away from looking at whether practices and customs of the medical establishment contribute to SIDS. When I pointed this out to a doctor at Auckland university who studies SIDS, he panicked and said it can *definitely* only be parental behaviour that affects SIDS. Unpopular topics for research include the use of prescription drugs during pregnancy, the habit of pulling on the baby's head during birth (which causes cervical subluxations), and the injection of vaccines into the baby. A study that compares the rate of cot death in babies who have been vaccinated with the rate in those who have not been vaccinated has never been done.

The practice of placing babies on their tummies was actually introduced by doctors, but the medical establishment suffers corporate amnesia about that. It did not become a parental behaviour pattern until doctors told parents to do it. In the middle of the 20th century doctors started telling mothers to put *all* babies down on their tummies, because it had been observed that *premature* babies fared better that way.[404,405] Until then all cultures in the world had put babies down on their sides or on their backs, or carried them upright in a carry pack. Chiropractors warned that being face down impedes the functioning of a baby's autonomic nervous system, but they were ignored. The medics finally got around to doing some research on the matter, and the practice is now discouraged.

A CONVENIENT ESCAPE CHUTE

One of the scandalous features of cot death is that many infant deaths that are quite obviously vaccine related, end up being described as SIDS on the death certificate. Doctors do this deliberately to hide the fact that a vaccine caused the death. When dramatic symptoms have been present before the baby dies, the death cannot accurately be labelled as SIDS. Symptoms like a weird and nasty rash, prolonged high fever, lack of colour or blueness in the face, inability to move properly, violent black diarrhoea, inability to open the mouth, convulsions and high pitched screaming are all indications that something is wrong. SIDS is a death that happens when there has been no indication that anything is wrong.

When a doctor decides to write "SIDS" on the death certificate, and does not mention serious symptoms that were present before the baby's death on the report to the coroner, the coroner can only come to the conclusion that it was a case of SIDS. Parents I have spoken with had begged their doctors to tell the coroners about serious symptoms that were present before the baby died, but their doctors refused. Coroners cannot make a correct judgement when information is being withheld from them by the doctors. A death has also not been a case of SIDS when the baby has been exhibiting the quiet symptoms of vaccine damage, like excessive sleeping, drowsiness, unresponsiveness, refusing food, petit mal epilepsy, or waving the arms in a strange way.

These cover-ups of vaccine deaths are obviously not restricted to those I was involved with in New Zealand. When Barbara Loe Fisher looked into the FDA records, she found, among other scandalous things, that deaths of babies who screamed and shrieked uncontrollably for hours and hours every day from the day of vaccination to the day of death were labelled as "SIDS."[406]

SHAM STUDIES

While many "cot deaths" are not really cases of SIDS, we are still left with those which really are mysterious and inexplicable, and it would be ideal to know all the factors that increase the risk of a cot death happening. Vaccination has of course been suspected of being a factor that increases the risk of a cot death happening, and the vaccine establishment has produced a number of studies to try and persuade parents to believe that vaccination does not carry that risk. One of the studies which is frequently cited as "proof" that vaccination does not cause SIDS was done in the American state of Tennessee.[407] A typical statement about this study is,

An American study of 129,834 babies looked at the possible risk factor between sudden infant death syndrome and immunisation against diphtheria, tetanus and pertussis. A total of 109 deaths in the ten-year period were classified as due to SIDS. The study published in 1988, concluded that there was no increase in the risk of SIDS after immunisation with the DTP vaccine.[408]

This sounds very impressive, but when you get to the library and read the study, you find that it is not at all impressive. No comparison is made between vaccinated and unvaccinated babies, and the method used is dubious. At the start of the study the researchers excluded the 1.9% of babies whose vaccination record said they had been vaccinated before the age of 29 days or given another dose less than 25 days after a previous dose, and they also excluded the 9% for whom there was no vaccination record and the 14% who were known to be unvaccinated. After doing this they were left with 109 babies who had been vaccinated according to the schedule, and had died of SIDS. They then measured the amount of time that had passed between the date of last vaccination and the date of death. They should instead have compared the number of deaths in the vaccinated group with the number of deaths in the 14% who were known to be unvaccinated.

The researchers state quite clearly at the beginning of the article that the aim of the study was to find out whether *recent* immunisation with DPT increases the risk. By *recent* they mean 7 days. They divided the time period after vaccination into five intervals; 0-3 days, 4-7 days, 8-14 days, 15-30 days, and 31 or more days. There is absolutely no scientific basis for these time intervals, they were just arbitrarily chosen. Pseudo-scientists who merely want to promote a particular point of view make baseless assumptions all the time. For the purposes of this exercise they made the assumption that if DPT can precipitate SIDS, it will do so within seven days. There is no scientific reason to assume that the side effects of DPT vaccine, or any other vaccine, will have worn off after seven days. The length of time it takes for DPT to depress the immune system has not been researched.

The study found that the number of deaths in the first seven days after vaccination was not higher than the mathematically expected number of deaths. Here we have yet another flaw in the study - the "mathematically expected" number of deaths which they used was derived from a society where DPT is used, instead of being derived from a group of vaccine free babies. In the 8-30 day period after vaccination, the number of deaths was found to be higher than what they considered to be mathematically expected.

The authors say that the study "concluded that there was no increase in the risk of SIDS after immunisation with the DPT vaccine." The data they provide does not support that conclusion. The Tennessee study was supported by the FDA and the CDC, partially funded by the NCHSR, and two of the four doctors in the study were Burroughs Wellcome Scholars in pharmacoepidemiology. Burroughs Wellcome is a drug company which makes DPT vaccine.

In an effort to keep up the vaccination rate, a high ranking medical bigwig in New Zealand issued a printed handout to be given to parents to persuade them that vaccination does not cause SIDS. He listed some studies, and next to this one he wrote that it showed that "there was no increase in SIDS deaths among vaccinated vs unvaccinated children." This is a peculiar thing to say when the study did not compare vaccinated and unvaccinated children. It makes one wonder if medical bigwigs read anything while they are being paid large salaries by the taxpayer.

Earlier I mentioned that when there is a virulent polio virus in the environment, vaccination against other diseases suppresses the immune system, so that people who would otherwise not have caught polio, do catch it. I also mentioned a study of polio in Britain in 1949 which found that most cases of polio that are provoked by vaccination, start 8 to 17 days after vaccination.[224] Another study, covering 1951 to 1953, and done by the Medical Research Council in Britain, found that the greatest number of provocation cases started from 8 to 14 days after vaccination, with the next highest number of cases starting 15 to 21 days after.[409] In Bavaria, bad reactions to smallpox vaccination peaked 8 to 13 days after.[261] From all of this we can see that if DPT vaccine can cause SIDS by depressing the immune system, the deaths would peak after the first week. The Tennessee study found that the number of deaths in the period after the first week was greater than the mathematically expected number of deaths. So this study, done by the vaccinationists, has ended up supporting the view that DPT vaccine does cause SIDS.

Leif Karlsson invented a microprocessor-based breathing monitor which can record and print out information on a baby's breathing, both while the baby is awake and asleep. He and Dr. Viera Scheibner used the monitor to investigate which factors place a baby's breathing under stress. They found that exposure to tobacco smoke, teething, and a cold which is brewing, but has not yet produced any symptoms, are among the things which place a baby's breathing under stress. Two babies they recorded had non-stressed breathing before DPT vaccination, but their breathing became stressed after vaccination, with excessive stress on days 2, 5, 6, and 16. The amount of stress was much higher in the one baby than in the other, but the days on which the stress rose and fell was the same. Viera ties this in with a number of studies done to investigate the day by day distribution of deaths after DPT vaccination.[410]

Another study[411] that is often presented as proof that DPT does not increase the risk of cot death began with the data concerning 838 babies who had died of SIDS in selected parts of the USA. 46 babies were then dropped from the study because they had not really died of SIDS. Each remaining baby was matched with two babies who were still alive. The vaccination history of the babies that had died was then compared with the vaccination histories of the two babies that had not died. This type of study is called a case-control study. It is a back to front way of looking at things, because babies who are susceptible to potentially harmful things in their environment are compared with babies who have strong constitutions. The tobacco industry compares smokers who die with smokers who do not die, in order to prove that cigarette smoking does not increase the risk of fatal diseases. Only 25% of people who smoke cigarettes die from tobacco related diseases. Researchers in the pay of the tobacco industry compare the number of cigarettes smoked by the ones who died, with the number smoked by a matched person who is still alive and well. Some people are made of such strong stuff that they can smoke 60 cigarettes a day for 55 years, and still remain healthy. Therefore, if you compare smokers who die with smokers who do not die, you can merrily say that smoking does not cause lung cancer, emphysema and heart disease. Naturally the tobacco industry likes studies that compare smokers with smokers. However, if you compare smokers with non-smokers, you get a very clear indication that smoking causes lung cancer, emphysema and heart disease.

Case-control studies can be useful if you take all the confounding factors into account, but in the case of DPT susceptibility, no-one knows what the confounding factors are. Controlling for factors that are known to increase the risk of SIDS does not necessarily mean you are controlling for factors that increase the risk of SIDS from DPT. Before a valid case-control study can be done, the factors that make a baby susceptible to dying from DPT need to be discovered. Some doctors advise parents that the start of vaccination should be delayed for frail babies, even though the vaccine manufacturers have made most countries adopt an official policy of not acknowledging contra-indications. So in a case-control study, a baby who died at 5 months after having had only one dose of DPT would be compared with a 5-month-old who was still alive after 3 doses of DPT. This would be interpreted as showing that vaccination protects against cot death, when what it might actually show is that the frail baby was pushed over the edge by his or her first dose of DPT, while the strong baby was able to cope with 3 doses. Most babies do not die from the recommended vaccination schedule, but that does not mean that all babies can cope with it. Case-control studies obscure the susceptibility of certain babies.

The only way to do a study that would truly show whether or not vaccination increases the risk of SIDS would be to select all the babies born in a large area during a certain time span, and compare the rate of cot death in the vaccinated and the unvaccinated. A large number of babies would have to be studied to get a valid result, and the study authors would need to be people who can be trusted not to tamper with the raw data. If the rate of SIDS in a huge cross section of vaccinated and unvaccinated babies were compared, both groups would include tough babies who can easily cope with DPT, as well as ones that are susceptible to DPT. So it would make a useful comparison - too useful for the vaccinationists to risk.

This particular case-control study was done by a government department in the USA. The study authors themselves do not claim that their study proves that DPT never causes SIDS, they say it shows that DPT is "not a significant factor in the occurrence of SIDS."[411] The study began with the data concerning all of the babies who had died of SIDS in the selected geographical areas, but more than one in twenty of the babies were discarded from the study because their deaths were not really cases of SIDS. Back in the real world the babies' death certificates still said "SIDS," and the parents were still left with the impression that their children had died of SIDS. 39.8% of the remaining babies had been injected with DPT, while 53.2% of the babies who were used as controls had been injected with DPT. The difference in the figures does not mean that none of the deceased babies would be alive today if they had not been injected with DPT, nor does it mean that DPT is not a significant cause of SIDS.

Another study[412] which is in the armoury of the vaccinationists was also done in Tennessee. This one is outrageously unscientific. It compares the number of SIDS deaths that occurred in a geographical region during the time that a certain batch of DPT vaccine was in use, with the number of deaths that occurred in the same area when the previous batch of DPT was in use. Because there was a similar number of deaths in the two time periods, the authors conclude that DPT vaccine does not increase the risk of SIDS. This is totally illogical. The fact that one batch of DPT is not shown to cause more deaths than another batch, does not prove that DPT vaccine cannot cause death.

Yet another study which is presented as proof that vaccination does not increase the risk of cot death[413] is silly, to say the least. The study doctors surveyed the breathing patterns of "at risk" babies for twelve hours after injection with DPT. They found that there was no increase in abnormal breathing during this time frame. This study is meaningless as a review of whether or not DPT increases the risk of SIDS. The twelve hour cut off time is ridiculous, and periodic breathing is not an indicator of SIDS. Most babies who die of SIDS do not have a history of apnoea,[414,415] and in most cases asphyxiation is not the primary cause of death. Out of 629 autopsy reports on SIDS cases in New Zealand, only 4.9% showed evidence of oxygen deprivation.[416]

There are a handful of other studies that are presented by vaccine defenders as "proof" that vaccination does not increase the risk of SIDS. Upon examination, they are all found to lack a scientific approach to resolving the question. This is a situation that will prevail until resources for large-scale research falls into the hands of individuals or groups who do not have a vested interest in defending the reputation of vaccination.

If vaccination causes SIDS indirectly by suppressing the immune system, or by interfering with any other mechanism, then it would still be accurate to say that vaccination caused the death. Low blood sugar is associated with sudden infant death.[416,417,418,419,420] In New Zealand the law does not require an autopsy to be done after a baby dies without explanation.

When an autopsy is done, it is up to the autopsy doctor to decide what to investigate. During a three year period in New Zealand the blood sugar level of 84 babies who had died inexplicably was measured at autopsy, and in 81 of them the level was found to be below the normal range.[416] DPT vaccine causes low blood sugar by stimulating insulin production.[188,421] The drop in the level of sugar in the blood starts about 8 days after injection, it peaks about 12 days after injection, and ends about 24 days after.[422] When a person dies from low blood sugar they just lie there and quietly die. It is not obvious to an onlooker why the person has died. When a baby dies from low blood sugar, the symptoms fit the criteria of SIDS. The fact that whooping cough vaccine stimulates the production of insulin is possibly the most important factor in SIDS, but it is a line of inquiry that does not arouse the interest of the medical establishment.

Two things need to happen. Firstly, procedures need to be introduced to prevent deaths which do not fit the criteria for SIDS being officially recorded as SIDS. Secondly, governments should keep a record of who gets vaccinated with what, so that long term research on the effects of vaccination can begin. Some governments are currently introducing central registers to record who gets vaccinated, but they are not doing it so that they can discover the consequences of vaccination. They are doing it so that they can exclude unvaccinated children from school, and withhold social welfare from their families. In the long term these registers might end up being used to do retrospective studies of vaccine side effects.

CIRCUMSTANTIAL EVIDENCE

In 1988 New Zealand had the highest cot death rate in the world. DPT vaccine was given at the tender age of six weeks, together with hepatitis B vaccine, and Maori and Polynesian babies were also given BCG vaccine at birth. At that time the cot death rate in New Zealand was ten times higher than in Sweden. The vaccine schedules of the two countries had significant differences. Sweden omitted the whooping cough component of DPT, so that it became DT vaccine. They did not use hepatitis B vaccine at all, and they started the first dose of DT at 3 months.

At that same time, the cot death rate in New Zealand was four times higher than in Britain. In Britain they did include the P component of DPT, but they started at three and a half months, and they did not use hepatitis B. The differences in vaccine schedules was not only reflected in the number of babies that died, it also affected the age at which they died. In Britain when DPT was started at 3.5 months, cot deaths peaked during the fourth month. In New Zealand when DPT was started at 6 weeks, cot deaths peaked during the second month. The medical establishment claims that cot deaths happen at the age when vaccinations are being done because that is the "natural age" for cot deaths. If there were such a thing as a "typical pattern for cot deaths," the age at which cot deaths peaked would have been the same in New Zealand as it was in Britain.

CRIME, AUTISM AND LEARNING DISABILITIES

Attention deficit disorders and minimal brain dysfunction are far more common in boys than in girls.[423] In many cases these behaviour problems are caused by mild brain damage,[355] which in turn can be caused by vaccination.[355] Male babies are more susceptible to severe brain damage from DPT than female babies.[424,425,188] This latter fact has been known since 1948,[425] but instead of informing doctors of this, the vaccine industry has buried that knowledge under tons of promotional literature. It is fairly obvious that if boys are more susceptible than girls to severe brain damage from DPT, they are probably also going to be more susceptible to mild brain damage from vaccination. Australian paediatrician Dr. Gordon Serfontein wrote a book to help parents of children with attention deficit disorders. In it he says,

> It is not widely known that this condition is a very common disorder and the incidence ratings vary from five percent to twenty percent of all boys. It is mainly a male condition and approximately ninety percent of all children with this problem are boys.[423]

In Byers and Molls' landmark study, published in 1948, they found that 80% of DPT victims were male.[425] Recent discoveries about differences in development between male and female infant brains[426] lend some clues as to why male infants are more vulnerable than female infants to suffering brain damage from vaccines. Dr. Serfontein goes on to say that if a non-identical twin has the condition, there is only a small chance that the other twin will have it, whereas when an identical twin has the condition, the other twin always has it. Identical twins are of the same gender and have the same

226

genetic make-up. Therefore they have the same susceptibility to DPT. Dr. Gordon Serfontein says,

> Developmental disabilities in learning and behaviour are not widely accepted. This is obviously political and economical. The prevalence of this condition is very widespread. Should the existence of this condition be acknowledged by governments or other authorities, it would then be immediately incumbent upon those authorities to provide the necessary assistance for these children. That would involve enormous sums of money which may or may not be feasible. However, in a developed country such as Australia, it is beyond my comprehension that we are unable to finance the assistance of a large body of our children who would grow up to be significant contributors to the society as a whole. There would be the added benefit of reduction in the costs of crime prevention, as a large proportion of these children with these difficulties develop into juvenile delinquents and young criminal offenders. Certainly the prevention of such an outcome would be economically more rewarding.[427]

Governments would be far better off if they just abolished the main cause of learning disabilities and behaviour disorders - vaccination. Dr. Serfontein says,

> The first question that we ask ourselves is, "What causes this common difficulty?" As is usual with problems relating to children, our initial instincts are to look to the pregnancy and the birth of the child. At first, it was thought that problems relating to pregnancy and birth were the causes of these developmental difficulties. However, research has shown that there is no greater incidence of ADD in children who had prejudicial birth histories compared to children who had no abnormalities during their birth. In other words, birth problems were not a cause of this condition.[428]

It is not what happens at birth, it is what happens after birth. There would not have been a huge upsurge of behaviour problems in children in recent decades if it were solely an inherited condition. While some people probably do inherit the condition, it is also probable that other people inherit the potential to be damaged by vaccination. So their father and their grandfather might have had the potential to be mildly brain damaged by DPT vaccine, but it did not happen to them because the vaccine was not used on them. The current batch of fathers belongs to a generation which was a target for DPT, and there is anecdotal evidence that families that have to endure ADD in more than one generation are becoming more common. Any vaccine that is intended to prevent a disease that can cause brain damage is capable of causing brain damage itself. Genetic alteration of the germ in the vaccine does not mean that the vaccine cannot cause brain damage. The new Hib vaccines and meningitis vaccines are as dangerous as the whole cell DPT vaccine. The Australian government publishes a propaganda booklet for parents called *Understanding Childhood Immunisations*. One of the untrue statements in this booklet is, "serious reactions to Hib vaccines have not been reported."[469] Yet ADRAC, the Australian government body that receives reports, has received and acknowledged 1161 reports of serious reactions to Hib vaccine, 293 of which are symptoms of brain damage.[470]

In myth number two I mentioned the researchers in Florida who found that six out of seven children who were brain damaged by DPT had a particular tissue typing antigen, and then were refused funding to research the matter any further, because the medical establishment does not want the truth about DPT to be investigated. There will come a time when science triumphs over commerce, and researchers will be able to try and find out whether some people carry a genetic code which makes them susceptible to damage from the vaccines that are capable of causing brain damage.

The emotional disturbances that often accompany attention deficit disorders are usually assumed to result from frustration at not being able to read, or to communicate easily with other people. However, they themselves sometimes can also exist as a direct result of the brain damage. As I will demonstrate, criminal behaviour is one of the side effects of vaccination.

In 1990 a young girl from London was murdered at a tourist resort in New Zealand a few days before she was due to return to London. This caused a shock wave to pass through New Zealand, because in those affluent days the crime rate was still very low. A second shock wave went through the country when a young man who had grown up in an affluent home with caring, supportive, responsible parents was arrested for the murder. The nation asked itself, "Why has he done this terrible thing?" In mitigation, the defence presented evidence that the boy had been normal until he was injected with the measles vaccine as a toddler, which had caused a personality change, and ongoing criminal behaviour. He had been found guilty of sexual offences before, but that poor girl was his first rape/murder. The judge accepted that the measles vaccine was a mitigating factor, but he said he had to give the young man a life sentence for the sake of public safety.

Many parents have told me of personality changes in their toddler after measles vaccine or MMR vaccine. It is normal for the parents of a toddler to have to endure difficult behaviour from their child, because the child's self will is developing at that age. However, the bad behaviour that results from a reaction to a vaccine is quite different. The victims of measles vaccine I hear about were all toddlers when they were vaccinated. Their behaviour had been obstreperous, just like that of most normal toddlers, but they changed and became vicious and malicious, with uncontrollable violent outbursts. It is stressful for parents when they feel it is inevitable that their child will one day harm another person.

When hepatitis B vaccine was introduced to New Zealand, it was used on preschoolers who were older than toddlers, so the behavioural changes were quite easy to see. Many such reactions were seen, but they were just dismissed by the medical establishment. Thousands of babies were given that vaccine on the day they were born. If any of them suffered the type of encephalopathy which causes this problem, it would be impossible for their mothers to perceive a personality change.

A hard blow to the head can also cause the type of brain damage that leads to criminality. For instance, there was a normal and likeable young man in Auckland, who sustained a serious blow on the head when he collided with a train on his motor bike. His personality changed so that his friends stopped liking him, and he took to killing young girls. He finally shot himself after shooting at a group of girls in a high school playground.

In Lionel Dole's book, *The Blood Poisoners,* published in 1962, he makes a remark about encephalitis from smallpox vaccine.

> The worst examples of its results are seldom kept alive in the public mind, such as that of incurable and progressive insanity leading to violence, even murder, sometimes several murders - as in the case of the wretched man of whom one of the BBC brains-trusters said that he should have been hanged for strangling three little girls. We do not consider it fair to hang a man merely because his family believed in vaccination.[429]

How many violent crimes are committed because of vaccination? Once again it needs a large-scale study, which can only be done by criminologists and sociologists who have access to information about confounding factors like poverty and parental neglect or abuse. A more practical solution is to acknowledge that vaccination causes criminal behaviour, and seeing as it is not responsible for the lack of dangerous infectious diseases, to abolish vaccination.

Psychologists are endeavouring to define the parameters of all autistic syndromes which have been identified, like Kanner's autism, Asperger syndrome, and others.[430] They are also exploring ways of helping the sufferers acquire learned behaviour which would help them get along in life. While psychologists are working on the problem, the vaccine industry is creating more autistic people for them to study. Autism can be caused by an inherited faulty gene, a bang on the head, or encephalitis, which in turn can be caused by a natural infection, or by a vaccine. Sometimes vaccination causes other mental and physical handicaps at the same time as causing autism. It depends on which part, or parts, of the brain are damaged by the vaccine. Some unfortunate victims become mentally retarded, spastic, autistic and epileptic, all from one injection.

The English speaking world first became aware of autism in 1943, when it was described in the medical literature by an American psychiatrist, Professor Leo Kanner.[431] He subsequently wrote a lot more about this phenomenon. "Prof Kanner at first thought that autism always began from birth but later he described some children who developed autistic behaviour after a period of apparently normal development."[432] Nowadays they say that the age at which MMR vaccine is given is the "natural" age for autism to start.

In the 1940s, autism only occurred in the children of well educated or intellectual parents.[433] In the 1930s and early forties it was not common for women to become well educated, yet both the mothers and the fathers of autistic children were well educated, and most had tertiary education.[433] This led some people to believe that autism resulted from emotional neglect, because the mothers were allegedly not devoted to mothering. There were others who tried to find genetic factors which caused upper middle class people to produce autistic children.[433] Among these well educated parents there was a preponderance of medical training or medical connections.[434] At this same time DPT vaccine was available only to affluent parents who chose to pay for it, but when DPT vaccine became available to all and sundry, autism began to occur in all ethnic and socioeconomic groups.[435]

When MMR vaccine causes autism, the excuse is made that 18 months is the natural age for autism to develop, and the parents are just blaming the vaccine in retrospect. But in some cases the vaccine reaction is quite obvious. A child has already reached a lot of milestones by this age and the retrogression is sudden and shocking. Some families have video footage of their dear little toddler walking and talking and making eye contact. After the acute symptoms of the vaccine reaction fade away, the child is not talking and is disconnected from other people. But even these cases are said to be "just a coincidence" by the medical establishment.

Mercury in the vaccines has been suspected of being the ingredient that triggers autism. Some consumer groups campaigned for the removal of mercury, in the belief that without mercury, vaccination would become a safe procedure. At first vaccine promoters denied that the mercury could be harmful, but then some manufacturers declared that they were going to start producing vaccines that do not contain mercury. Governments around the world proudly announced that they had switched to using vaccines that do not contain mercury. However, some brands of vaccine were being dishonestly labelled. An American health advocacy group raised funds to pay a laboratory to analyse two brands of vaccine which the manufacturers claimed were completely free of mercury, and it was found that they did contain mercury.[439] Mercury can interfere with brain function in vulnerable people, but it is dangerous to assume that mercury is the only ingredient in vaccines that can harm the brain. Some doctors are achieving improvements in autistic children by putting them on mercury detoxification regimes, but that does not convince me that if the vaccine industry ever does start producing mercury free vaccines, the recipients will be safe.

As yet there has been no study that compares the rate of autism in the vaccinated and the unvaccinated. A few studies have been done which suggest that there is a link between the vaccine and autism, but they are not decisive.

Parents in Britain started resisting MMR vaccine after there was publicity about vaccine induced cases of autism. The government responded by spending two million pounds of the taxpayer's money on pamphlets claiming that MMR vaccine is safe. The money should rather have been spent on comparing the incidence of autism in vaccinated and unvaccinated children. Measles vaccine is anecdotally associated with many serious chronic diseases, but there is no discussion of its relationship to these other diseases in the media. The British media has permitted discussion of the theory that MMR can cause autism because it was a medical doctor who raised the issue. Unlike most medical doctors, Dr. Andrew Wakefield, who is a British gastroenterologist, has the courage to speak up about what he has observed. Dr. Wakefield pursued the issue of autism when he realised that some of his patients had developed disintegrative disorders from MMR. The club of 100 have launched an attack on him and his colleagues (Barbara Loe Fisher calls it a pre-emptive strike)[436] for having the temerity to talk about the issue and to do research.

Some workers in the vaccine industry have called for research into the connection between MMR and autism to be terminated.[437] Dr. Wakefield's response is, "Clearly there are some things that may end-up being terminated as a consequence of these events: research into the possible link between MMR, autism, and bowel disease is not one of them."[438] He has been kicked out of the health department in Britain, but he is continuing his research in the USA.

A Melbourne reporter who has a gripe against anti-vaccinationists joined in the damage control campaign to counteract Dr. Wakefield's work, saying that not vaccinating against measles has, "potentially lethal or tragic consequences." He indulges in the usual scare mongering claptrap about measles, while ignoring the fact that vaccinated children can also die of measles. Then he continues,

> Sir Gustav Nossal, one of the world's leading authorities on childhood vaccinations, is a key player in the WHO's campaign to eradicate the measles virus from our planet by the end of the decade, as was successfully done with the smallpox virus in the '70s. Sir Gustav says the medical research establishment must investigate such claims, no matter how improbable, but said of the British MMR study: "When it was rigorously checked, its methodology was found to be deeply flawed. Researchers have done the hard yards to check it. They sought out a large number of children who had never received the MMR vaccine, and found that the incidence of autism was identical in children who had been vaccinated." Of the hypothetical MMR autism link, Sir Gustav said: "It does not exist. The issue is stone dead."[440]

The methodology of the British study to which he refers is not deeply flawed, it is just suggestive without being conclusive. But the study that Dr. Nossal claims "sought out a large number of children," has never been done. I wrote to Dr. Nossal and asked him for the reference to the study that compared vaccinated children with unvaccinated, but of course he could not supply me with it, as it does not exist. I then wrote to the journalist and to Dr. Nossal and advised them both to put the record straight in the newspaper. I received no response from either. They have all the power and I am just a mother who knows the facts. My children and future grandchildren are safe from the vaccine industry no matter how unlevel the playing field remains, but unfortunately there are plenty of potential victims of vaccination who believe that the information published in newspapers is factual.

Dr. Nossal made the mistake of thinking that a study which compares vaccinated against unvaccinated children had been done, because it would have been the logical way to find out whether or not MMR causes autism. If such a study were ever to be done, two potential problems could prevent the results from reflecting the truth. One is that if the study authors had the wrong credentials, the published results might be fraudulent. The other problem is that autism is caused by many things, and measles vaccine only causes a small proportion of cases. A comparative study is likely to find that there is a slightly higher number of cases of autism in the vaccinated group, and the vaccinationists would be able to say that this higher number is "not statistically significant." They would then go on to claim that the study had proven conclusively that no cases of autism are caused by measles vaccine. If someone were to make a sincere effort to find out whether or not MMR causes autism, the study would need to be very carefully designed.

A year after I wrote the above, a study was published which *almost* compared vaccinated and unvaccinated Danish children.[467] The incidence of autism was assessed according to vaccinated or unvaccinated "person-years." The time between a child's first birthday and the date he or she was vaccinated was included in the "unvaccinated person-years" column. By using this method they biased the results in favour of finding that MMR does cause autism. Strange. They found one case of autism in every 6264 vaccinated person-years, and one case of autism in every 9101 unvaccinated person-years. So there was 50% more autism in the vaccinated person-years than in the unvaccinated person-years, yet the vaccine establishment is managing to present the study as proof that MMR vaccine does not cause autism. My interpretation of the study is that it supports the hypothesis that the majority of cases of autism are not caused by MMR, while some are.

A condescending, pro-MMR article published in a British newspaper says that this study, "compared 440,000 children who had MMR with 97,000 children who didn't. The children who had MMR were no more likely to develop autism than the children who didn't."[468] That is a misleading misrepresentation of what the study did. Perhaps the writer did not read the study. Or perhaps he is not capable of recognising bad science.

The attack on Dr. Wakefield has intensified, but he is standing his ground. The vaccinators have not succeeded in silencing the debate about MMR and autism, but the media is still favouring the vaccine industry. Some items in the media have tried to besmirch Dr. Wakefield's reputation by implying that his research was unethically funded. The real scandal lies in the fact that the British government did not fund his research, when they should have provided the money to fund it. Instead of trying to find out whether or not MMR causes serious long term side effects, the British government is trying to create fear that the drop in measles vaccination is going to cause a health disaster. Dr. Richard Halvorsen was able to get his opinion published in *The Observer*. His letter said in part,

> "...the real health disaster is the epidemic of autism. The numbers of autistic children have risen 10-fold since the introduction of the MMR in 1988. ... The only way to discover the true impact of the MMR vaccine on the incidence of autism in this country is to conduct a prospective study following children up for many years. If

that had been instigated by the Department of Health when Dr Wakefield first shared his concerns in confidence with them in 1997 we would by now have the answer."[471]

The behaviour of the bureaucrats strongly suggests that they do not want to know the answer.

MEDICAL MALICE

Some doctors take revenge on parents who say that their child is vaccine damaged by accusing them of Munchausen's syndrome by proxy, or other forms of bad parenting. In some countries the accusation makes it possible for the damaged child and its siblings to be taken away from the parents. Viera Scheibner says,

An epidemic of accusations against parents and baby sitters of shaken baby syndrome is sweeping the developed world. The United States and the United Kingdom are in the forefront of such a questionable practice. Brain (mainly subdural, less often subarachnoid) and retinal haemorrhages, retinal detachments, and rib and other bone 'fractures' are considered pathognomonic. However, the reality of these injuries is very different and well documented: the vast majority occur after the administration of childhood vaccines and a minority of cases are due to documented birth injuries and pre-eclamptic and eclamptic states of the mothers. ... It does not reflect well on the justice and medical systems in the developed world which are, sadly, characterised by blindness to the most obvious and victimisation of the innocent. Those who inject babies with great numbers of vaccines within short periods of time in the first months of life, often ignoring the observed serious reactions to the previous lots of vaccines, are not only the accusers of innocent carers, but are not prosecuted or brought to justice; quite to the contrary, they continue injecting babies with toxic cocktails of vaccines and creating further innumerable cases of grievous bodily harm and death. [441]

The situation is complicated by the fact that adults do sometimes shake a baby and cause internal damage which leads to death or mental retardation. Ignorance about vaccination on the part of judges and jurors contributes to the problem. The father of an American baby who was killed by vaccination has posted a letter on the internet which says in part,

> My son Alan was vaccinated despite several contra-indications. He was a premature baby weighing only 5lb 9oz at birth. My wife's pregnancy was complicated with maternal gestational diabetes, and group B streptococcal infection (which in itself poses a high risk of infant death). My son suffered in his short life from pneumonia, respiratory distress syndrome, and hyper-bilirubinemia. Despite all of this he was given a cocktail of vaccines at eight weeks of age. The day after he was vaccinated, my baby developed a fever and started to fuss. Ten days later he elicited a high pitched scream. We were told to expect this and not to worry. A couple of days later he stopped breathing. I rushed my baby to the hospital where he died after several severe iatrogenics took place (iatrogenic diseases are those caused by physicians). Because we could not explain his injuries, and because I was the last adult alone with him, I was charged with aggravated child abuse and first degree murder. We could not afford counsel; our lawyers were public defenders.
>
> If that wasn't enough, our four-year-old daughter was taken by the authorities to 'protect her' from I - the accused who was in a maximum security facility without bond. She was used by the police and authorities to threaten and blackmail my wife to help them fabricate evidence and testify against me. My wife adamantly refused to do this. She was charged as an accessory to murder and our daughter was placed in extended custody. Here, she was sexually battered and molested when her 'protectors' left her unsupervised with two boys who had a history of deviant behaviour. My wife's charges were dismissed after great effort and cost and our daughter was returned. They both fight every day to bring our family together and have been fighting since 1997.
>
> More recently, we discovered that one of the vaccines given to my son - DTAP - was from a batch of vaccines that stands as the number one ranking in deaths, the number one ranking in non-recoveries, and the fourth ranking in total events reported. DTAP 7H81507, which was given to my baby was a Hot Lot. I am serving a life sentence in Florida without the possibility of parole. I did not kill my son. His death was the result of the medical treatment he

received and a fatal reaction to his childhood immunisations. Since my conviction, I have rallied the support of an armada of scientists, doctors, and organisations which support my innocence. Doctors and scientists from 15 countries, including the US, have stood up to support us; some of these are listed overleaf. We have numerous reports from experts whom after record review, have declared my innocence. Many are up in arms at the iatrogenic implications shown in the records.[442]

150 doctors from around the world are preparing to testify that it was the vaccine that killed the baby, not the father. Success in this court case would set a precedent which would make it more difficult for parents of vaccine damaged or vaccine killed children to be blamed or persecuted.[442]

[After spending six years in prison this father was released on 27 August 2004, thanks to the testimony of doctors who are willing to speak the truth. These doctors and their supporters are now directing their energy towards helping other parents who are imprisoned because a vaccine killed their baby. Some of these parents are on death row.]

THE ORIGIN OF AIDS

There are many theories on how the HIV virus suddenly infected a million people in Central Africa. Here are some of them;

* The virus flew in from outer space.

* A monkey in Central Africa acquired a taste for human blood, and went around biting millions of people in the space of one year.

* An American homosexual had sex with a monkey in Africa, and then went back to California and had sex with thousands of people.

* Some scientists created the virus in a laboratory because they wanted to reduce the world's population.

* The CIA manufactured a virus which they knew would destroy part of the immune system, and then went and poured it in the Congo river in an attempt to wipe out the African resistance movement which was endeavouring to liberate the region from Belgian colonial rule.

* Some Africans became infected with the virus by eating monkeys.

* The vaccine stock that was used by the World Health Organisation in its "smallpox elimination" campaign in Zaire was contaminated with a bovine virus that mutated into the HIV virus, and that is why a million people came down with AIDS in the space of one year.

*   An American vaccine manufacturer trialled a polio vaccine in Central Africa in 1957, not realising that the vaccine was contaminated with the AIDS virus. A small number of people were thus infected, and later the virus was spread from person to person by the smallpox vaccinators, who did not sterilise the needles between recipients.

Thanks to Blaine Elswood, Tom Curtis and Ed Hooper, the sad and horrible truth about how this virus was transferred from animals to humans has been exposed. Central Africa has two countries called "Congo." The larger one of the two is the one in which the HIV virus was transmitted from chimpanzees (not from monkeys) to human beings. In 1885 the European powers declared that King Leopold II of Belgium could "have" this huge geographical area, with all its tribes, and a bite out of the Zambian copperbelt, which is why Zambia ended up being such a strange shape. King Leopold's region was called *The Belgian Congo* until 1971, when it was renamed *Zaire*. Then in 1997 it was changed again to *Democratic Republic of the Congo*.

In 1986 the World Health Organisation employed an outside consultant to go to Central Africa and find out what had caused AIDS to appear there. This researcher realised that the explosion of AIDS cases had followed the intensive smallpox vaccination campaign that the World Health Organisation had conducted in Zaire, Uganda, Tanzania, Zambia, Malawi, Rwanda and Burundi. The World Health Organisation's brag book about the vaccination campaign says, "In the African Region, Zaire strategically had the highest priority for the allocation of WHO resources."[443]

The outside consultant deduced that the vaccination campaign had sparked AIDS. When he reported his findings to the World Health Organisation, they fired him. So he went to the London Times with his story. On the 11th May 1987 the London Times carried a front page article entitled *Smallpox vaccine 'triggered Aids virus'*. It told how the countries in which smallpox vaccination was done were the countries in which a million cases of AIDS suddenly appeared, and how the researcher had been fired by the World Health Organisation for making that discovery.

At this point the plot thickens. It is normal procedure for any news item that appears in the British press to be networked to the USA on the same day, so that when the sun comes up in the Americas, the morning papers have already printed the story. But this story was intercepted. American readers were not going to be allowed to be exposed to this piece of information. Jon Rappaport investigated the blackout, and found that the news had been cut off in London, so that it never reached the news distributors at Associated Press, Reuters nor United Press International.[444]

The obvious connection between the smallpox vaccination campaign and the sudden appearance of AIDS led to the theory that the HIV virus may have been in the smallpox vaccine. But the earliest evidence of HIV in a human being was found in a blood sample taken in the Belgian Congo in 1959.[445,446,447] Blood samples were taken from 818 people in South Africa and the Belgian Congo in 1959 to do genetic studies, and one from Kinshasa in the Belgian Congo was infected with HIV.[445] This means that the HIV virus was already in humans in Central Africa before the smallpox vaccination campaign started in 1967.

An independent medical researcher, Blaine Elswood, developed suspicions that the HIV virus got into humans through a polio vaccination campaign conducted by an American company in the Belgian Congo from 1957 to 1960. The company had been hoping that after their vaccine had been used in Africa, the American government would accept it for use in the USA. The vaccinators travelled by car through Central Africa, stopping at distribution points, to which the natives were called by drums. Drum language was understood by all Africans, no matter which tongue they spoke.

In those days polio vaccines were usually made by growing the polio virus on monkey kidneys, and then putting a bit of monkey kidney into each vial of vaccine. Any germs that happened to be living on the monkey kidney before the scientists got hold of it were therefore also put into the vial of vaccine. When people are injected with vaccine made from monkey kidney, or when they swallow oral vaccine made from uncooked monkey kidney, they take into their bodies any viruses that are unintentionally included in the vaccine, along with the polio virus. There are a group of viruses called SIV that live in the bodies of monkeys without killing the monkeys. When these viruses get into human beings they cause disease because human beings have not yet adapted to them. The SIV viruses are similar in structure to the HIV virus. Blaine Elswood asked an investigative journalist, Tom Curtis, to follow up the leads he had, to see if AIDS had started from this vaccination campaign in Central Africa.

Tom Curtis found strong circumstantial evidence associating the polio vaccination campaign with the beginning of AIDS. He published the evidence in the music magazine, *Rolling Stone*.[448] Part of this evidence came from a map that the vaccinators themselves had published in the *British Medical Journal*.[449] The map showed the region that the vaccination campaign had covered. This area, the eastern Congo, Rwanda and Burundi, had the highest incidence of AIDS in the world by 1988. The first cases of AIDS had appeared in that region in 1962. The *Rolling Stone* article provoked debate and denials, and a law suit which cost *Rolling Stone* half a million dollars in defence costs before the suit was dropped.[450] Using law suits to silence their critics is a time honoured tactic of the drug companies. They aim to make editors and publishers frightened of publishing anything that could make the public aware of issues which threaten drug company profits.

Representatives of the vaccine industry said that the virus could not have come from a vaccine because the SIV viruses that are found in monkeys are not the same as the HIV virus; only viruses found in chimpanzees are the same as the HIV virus. Another argument was that a sailor from Manchester in England, who had left the Congo before the polio vaccination campaign started, had died of AIDS.

Ed Hooper investigated all the theories about the origin of AIDS very thoroughly. Some theories led to dead ends, but the leads to the polio vaccination campaign kept getting warmer. In 1999 he published the story of his search for the truth in a book entitled *The River: A journey to the source of HIV and AIDS*.[451] Among other things he unearthed the facts that the Manchester sailor did not die of AIDS, and that some batches of the polio vaccine were made using chimpanzee kidneys, not monkey kidneys. A compound had been specially built out in the wilds in the Belgian Congo, and chimpanzees had been caught locally and kept in cages until they were killed. More than one million doses of vaccine were administered between 1957 and 1960, and unfortunately some of the chimp kidneys had contained the HIV virus.

The vaccinators had used two strongly built cars and had travelled on dirt roads to the collection points at which people had gathered. The African people had walked from their far flung huts to the gathering places. What a sinister message was carried on the wind when those drums called the people to bring their children to be "protected" by white man's medicine.

The method of assessing side effects was the usual one of permitting passive reporting. "Medical authorities were asked to report any occurrence of illness which could be attributed to vaccination, but none was reported."[449] Ed Hooper interviewed the only doctor still living who had done some of the vaccinations in Africa, and he confirmed that seeking information about side effects had been done in this way.[452] In industrialised countries this method might be useful if doctors had any inclination towards reporting side effects. But it is absurd to even pretend to have an interest in determining side effects when using this method in the wilds of Africa, where people live far apart with no means of mechanical transport, and where there are very few medical doctors.

So the polio vaccination campaign created a pool of HIV infected Africans, and later the World Health Organisation started its mass vaccination campaign against smallpox in Central Africa using jet injectors. Jet injectors do not need to be sterilised after each vaccination, because they can shoot smallpox pus through the skin, without making contact with the skin. Only the pus goes through the skin, and the jet injector does not become contaminated with the recipient's blood. However, the jet injectors kept on breaking down, so in 1968 they changed to using the bifurcated needle. A bifurcated needle has two prongs at the tip, with a U shaped gap between them. A clump of pus hangs in the gap, clinging to the prongs. When the prongs are stabbed into the flesh of the recipient, some of the pus goes through the person's skin, and some of the person's blood in turn clings to the prongs. They did not sterilise the needle between vaccinations, so small amounts of blood from people who already carried the HIV virus got into millions of people. The bifurcated needle takes 20 minutes to sterilise between recipients.

> The bifurcated needle was developed by Wyeth Laboratories, Philadelphia, which allowed the eradication program to use it without patent costs. It became a basic tool in the program, and enabled a vaccinator to give up to 1,500 vaccinations a day.[453]

Ed Hooper interviewed a doctor who had "personally witnessed smallpox vaccinations being conducted in the Ruzizi Valley with no attempt being made to sterilize the needles between jabs."[454] In 1982 I overheard doctors in Johannesburg talking about the unhygienic way in which the smallpox vaccinations had been done in Central Africa.

So an overview of what happened is that a million people were given polio vaccine in Central Africa between 1957 and 1959, and some batches of vaccine were made with chimpanzee kidney instead of the usual monkey kidney. The vaccinators did not know that the chimpanzee kidney contained a virus that can survive for a long time in the human body, and eventually destroys the immune system of the person it has entered. At least fifty people became infected with this virus, and they infected other people through sexual contact. More than a decade later the World Health Organisation conducted a smallpox vaccination campaign in the region, and they did not clean the needles they used to scratch the vaccine into each person's flesh in between vaccinations. This meant that blood was taken from person to person on the tip of the needle, and a million people became infected with the chimpanzee virus. The virus was later called HIV, and the disease that it caused was called AIDS.

This is by no means the first time that vaccination has caused an unwanted germ to get into the recipients. Thousands of people have contracted hepatitis B from contaminated vaccines. On one occasion 50,000 people got hepatitis B from yellow fever vaccine.[386] Smallpox vaccine was often contaminated with syphilis.[455] In one incident in 1884, 1,773 babies died because the vaccine with which they were scratched contained human syphilis germs.[456] There is a type of SIV virus called SV40 which only lives in Asian monkeys, not in African monkeys. It causes cancer in humans. When it was discovered in the 1950s that American polio vaccine contained the SV40 virus, the manufacturers started getting their monkeys from Africa instead of from Asia, to avoid the virus. They sold all remaining stocks of contaminated vaccine to other countries. New Zealand and Australia bought stocks of this vaccine, knowing that it was contaminated, because it was going cheap. Some cancers from this source were acknowledged, but the general hushing up of the matter has been very effective.

A geneticist who is investigating a stealth virus that is associated with chronic fatigue syndrome has found that the virus is more closely related to a monkey virus than to a human virus.[457,458] The implication that polio vaccine may have caused the current epidemic of chronic fatigue syndrome has thrown the vaccine industry into damage control/research suppression mode.

Vaccines that are grown on animal flesh are inevitably contaminated with bacteria and viruses. In the World Health Organisation's book on their mass vaccination campaign, they discuss what level of bacterial contamination is acceptable. Yuk! They do not discuss what level of viruses is acceptable. One of the reasons that the vaccine industry is increasingly moving towards manufacturing vaccines on aborted human foetuses is that the flesh is not likely to be contaminated with animal viruses. However, the main reason is that it is much cheaper to buy the bodies of aborted babies than to breed monkeys or other animals, or to obtain animals from the wild. Organs that have been stolen from babies who have died of cot death are not suitable for manufacturing vaccines, because when babies have lived out in the world for a while, they have germs and antibodies in their tissue.

Polio vaccine made on aborted babies was already being used in 1962.[459] Some people have religious objections to eating aborted human babies. These include Hindus, Buddhists, Moslems, Christians and religious Jews, and they constitute most of the world's population. Naturally the vaccine industry does not want most of its customer base to know that they and their children are being fed with or injected with cells from an aborted baby, which is why there is no discussion of the matter in the mainstream media.

Ed Hooper's book generated still more denials. All the people still living who worked on the Congo vaccine have closed ranks and come up with a coherent story denying that any stocks were made with chimpanzee kidneys. But it is too late. Their earlier statements about procedures have been documented for posterity. Every person who works for the vaccine industry has their own motives for wanting the truth about the origin of AIDS to be suppressed. In fact everyone who works for any part of the medical establishment has good reason to want the public not to know about this. If your local library does not hold a copy of Ed Hooper's book, ask them to buy it. If your friends do not want to read it, show them the cover, and the photos between pages 686 and 687.

The HIV virus kills helper T cells, which means it can disable the human immune system. This makes the victim very vulnerable to other germs and to cancer. Most people who are infected with the HIV virus are heterosexuals. 21 million people have died so far, and 45 million more are infected. 10% of South African children are born infected. A catastrophe of this magnitude became inevitable when Edward Jenner and Louis Pasteur started moving animal matter into the bodies of human beings. Pasteur's cruelty to rabbits, monkeys and dogs was later extended to mice, chimpanzees, armadillos and other species. It was not a question of *whether* a catastrophe like AIDS was going to happen, but *when* it was going to happen.

INTIMIDATION AND THE LAW

The USA is the only English speaking country that makes vaccination compulsory under some circumstances. The American constitution protects religious freedom, but it does not protect life and limb from the vaccine industry. Bureaucrats can require vaccination for school entry or summer camp attendance. Each state in the USA makes its own laws about the matter. Some states do not make vaccination compulsory, some make it compulsory but permit conscientious objection or religious objection, while other states only permit religious objection. In the latter states parents can refuse vaccination on the grounds that they believe it to be a spiritually harmful procedure, but they cannot refuse on the grounds that they believe it to be a physically harmful procedure. More than a million children in the USA are home-schooled, and therefore cannot be targeted by school entry laws. This irks the vaccinationists. Hillary Clinton tried to introduce draconian laws to catch home-schooling parents in the vaccination net, but she failed.

The law making vaccination compulsory for school entry in Canada was repealed in 1884, yet many Canadian parents are still not aware that vaccination is optional. Hesitant parents are often intimidated into vaccinating by threats of legal action,[460] even though no legal action can be taken against them.

The concept of civil rights originated in Britain with the signing of the Magna Carta by King John in 1215 AD. Vaccine mongering bureaucrats in Britain are willing to besmirch this proud heritage. A shocking event happened to Nita and Albrecht Bastian, who live in Northern Ireland. Their first child suffered a severe reaction to the hepatitis B vaccine, so they did not want their second child to have the injection. While Nita was pregnant,

Albrecht wrote a letter to the authorities explaining their reasons for declining, and the letter he received in reply was quite chilling. They planned a home birth to keep the baby out of the clutches of the medical fraternity. A few hours after Cecilia Bastian was born, seven adults dressed in official uniforms arrived at the door. They forcibly removed Cecilia from her home and took her to the local hospital, where she was injected with the filthy stuff.

Some countries have adopted a system that was initially called "mandatory choice." The term "mandatory choice" has been dropped, but the system remains in use in New Zealand, some states in Australia, and some European countries. Policy makers say that the purpose of mandatory choice is to catch the parents who do not vaccinate because they are too lazy or too ignorant, while giving conscientious objectors the right to refuse as long as they fill in some paperwork. But included in the legislation is a punishment for the parents who make a decision not to vaccinate. In primary school and kindergarten years, their children can be excluded from school during outbreaks of certain infectious diseases.

This legislation paves the way for much lying. In Australia it is misrepresented to nearly every new mother. Sometimes when the baby is only a few weeks old she is told that if she does not vaccinate, her child will not be able to attend school at all. I know people who did not want to vaccinate, but they were so frightened by the thought of their child not getting an education that they gave in. Their children have ended up mildly vaccine damaged, and they wish that they had found out before it was too late that the doctors and nurses were lying.

The Australian state of Victoria has introduced legislation that allows children who have not been vaccinated to be kicked out of school or kindergarten for three weeks under certain circumstances. The authorities do not tell schools, kindergartens nor parents what those circumstances are, with the result that children are often illegally excluded. Soon after we moved to Victoria in Australia, Kenneth came home from school with some propaganda promoting MMR vaccine. This had been compiled by the Victorian Health Department, and it said that children could be excluded from school if they are not vaccinated against mumps. That was not true. Soon after that my neighbour's child was thrown out of kindergarten because a vaccinated child at the kindergarten had whooping cough. That was illegal. Since then the law in Victoria has been changed so that it now is legal to kick a vaccine free child out of kindergarten or school when a vaccinated child gets whooping cough. These wicked laws aim at hurting the parents for being non-compliant. In many instances they do succeed in causing emotional, financial and physical harm.

The law requires every school and kindergarten to keep a list of the vaccination status of each child. During the 2001 measles epidemic in Melbourne I received a number of phone calls from parents who had received a letter from their child's school saying that they either had to remove their child from the school, or have them vaccinated against measles. I told these parents that it was illegal for the schools to send out these letters, because an official in the Department of Health is the only person empowered to do that. I suggested that they just ignore the letters, but promised them that if they did get a similar letter from the Department of Health, I would intervene on their behalf. They did ignore the letters, and no further action was taken against them.

Britain and Australia have adopted a system of bribes for doctors to increase the vaccination rate. General practitioners are paid extra money by the government for persuading patients to accept vaccination. In Australia a doctor gets paid $18.50 for filling in a form that tells the Health Insurance Commission that the patient has completed one of 6 levels of the vaccine schedule.[14] But doctors get paid nothing for signing a form that enables a vaccine free family to obtain social welfare, and nothing for reporting an adverse reaction.[14]

For Australian doctors there is also the "outcomes payment," which means that he or she will be paid $12 per patient per year if 80% or more of his or her child patients are vaccinated. If more than 90% of the child patients are vaccinated, he or she gets $14 per patient per year. Even if the injections are given by the council clinic, the doctor gets the payment for having the patient on his or her books. A patient who makes only one visit to a doctor is not regarded as belonging to that doctor, but a second visit by the patient means that he or she will enter the calculations. Doctors do not have to register to get these payments if they do not want them.[14] So if a doctor has 80 child patients whose parents do vaccinate, and 20 child patients whose parents do not vaccinate, he or she gets $960 per year. But if one more vaccine free child enters the practice, the doctor gets nothing. So it is not surprising that so many vaccine free families are being told by doctors that they are not wanted in the practice.

In Britain general practitioners only have to reach a target of 70% to get the first outcomes payment, and the amount they get paid for each child goes up when 90% of the children on their books are vaccinated.

In Australia it is made to appear that vaccination is a pre-requisite for receiving welfare payments, but the constitution actually forbids that. In 1946, after a referendum, social welfare was added to the Australian constitution. Section 51 xxiii A protects recipients of social welfare from losing any financial benefits if they do not vaccinate. Someone in 1946 must have known that inevitably some politicians would want to use social welfare as a means of controlling society. Such a batch of politicians are in parliament in Australia at present, and they are faced with the fact that they cannot tie welfare payments to vaccination because of the constitution.

So they have used two techniques to try and defeat the constitution. They have passed laws which make it extremely difficult for a vaccine free family to obtain the welfare payments to which they are entitled, and secondly, they lie to parents about their right to obtain social welfare without vaccination.

The lies are told in welfare publications, on welfare application forms, and by individuals behind the counter in welfare offices. Two types of welfare payment are affected by the legislation; the final maternity payment at 18 months, and the child care subsidy for working mothers. If a parent chooses not to vaccinate, these payments can only be obtained by filling in a form and then getting it signed by a doctor or council nurse. That sounds simple enough, but they make it really hard for parents by not telling them that the form exists, then not telling them where they can get a form, then discouraging doctors and nurses from signing it. Of course it would make no sense for the vaccinationists to introduce coercive legislation which is aimed at bullying parents into accepting a medical intervention, and then inform the parents that they can avoid the intervention by getting a doctor or nurse to sign a form.

When the new law stating that non-vaccinating parents can only obtain the final instalment of maternity allowance if they sign a conscientious objection form was brought in, the magazine which is sent to all recipients of welfare said three times on page 3 that the payment would not be made unless the baby was immunised.[461] Meryl Dorey, the president of the Australian Vaccination Network, managed to make telephone contact with an assistant to the Minister of Social Welfare, and she complained to him about these printed lies. She managed to get him to promise that the truth would be told in future issues of the magazine, but he refused to inform the recipients of that issue that it had contained wrong information.[462] The next issue of the magazine told the truth, but in subsequent editions the text has been cleverly worded so that it misrepresents the truth without blatantly lying.

Often parents have to spend considerable time and money on finding a doctor or nurse who will sign the form. Some mothers contact me after having taken the conscientious objection form to four doctors, and each one has refused to sign it. Some of the doctors are abusive to the mother, raising their voices and accusing her of bad character. Council nurses also sometimes refuse to sign it. The mother has to take a toddler with her on these excursions, and toddlers get bored and fractious waiting for up to an hour in a doctor's waiting room. Schlepping the child on busses or in the car adds to the stress, and the mother also has to pay for the transport used getting to and from all these doctors and nurses. The cost of getting the form signed can put a considerable dent into the value of the one-off maternity payment. Those who are hurt the most by this heinous legislation are the poor families who struggle to pay for the cost of a young child. In telephone conversations with various officials I have often encountered the attitude that poor people deserve to be hurt if they choose not to vaccinate, but the officials never let that attitude show in their letters. When the application is for a child-care subsidy, the mother has to take days off work to get the form filled in.

One of the aims of all this legislation is to cause stress, in the hope that the mother will just give up and vaccinate. It is all very clever because the way that the legislation is written does not infringe the constitution, but the de facto way it is applied defeats the aims of the constitution.

In the 1980s a group of paediatricians developed plans to make vaccination compulsory in New Zealand, but their scheme was foiled when Geoffrey Palmer gave New Zealand a Bill of Rights. Before Jenny Shipley came to power in New Zealand, she said she intended tying welfare payments to immunisation. She received some letters from individuals asking her who was going to pay for the process involved in getting exemption, and she found herself unable to answer the question satisfactorily. I do not know exactly what it was that made her drop the idea of tying welfare payments to vaccination, but I strongly suspect that making her aware of that issue played a part.

Anti-discrimination legislation was introduced into New Zealand by a medically trained politician who was a keen vaccinationist. The legislation was worded to make it illegal for anyone to discriminate against a person who has a germ that is known to cause disease in his or her body, but to make it legal to discriminate against a person who refuses to have a germ that is known to cause disease injected into his or her body. The first part is good because it means that people who are HIV positive cannot be persecuted, but the second part leaves the way open for the persecution of people who refuse to have aborted baby injected into their bodies.

COPING WITH DISAPPROVAL

If you decide to keep your child vaccine free, you not only have to contend with irate officials, you also have to deal with relatives and friends who voice their disapproval, and try and make you conform. This can cause emotional stress, and drain the energy of new parents. Before you decide how to handle your critics, consider their reasons for condemning you. Be careful to differentiate between people who want to persuade you to "immunise" because they are genuinely concerned about the welfare of the baby, and those who are just angry with you because you threaten their belief in the sacred cow of modern medicine.

There is no point in trying to defend your decision to someone who is not interested in knowing your reasons. This kind of person will stop bothering you sooner than the ones who are genuinely concerned about your baby, but they will be more stressful to cope with while they are still harassing you. It is no fun having accusations flung at you, and then not being given a chance to explain. With this kind of person it is best to try and distance yourself from the emotional baggage that is being thrown at you, and pretend you are a psychologist who is trying to work out why he or she feels so threatened.

When someone is genuinely concerned that you are exposing your baby to dangerous diseases by not vaccinating, then you owe them an explanation for your decision. That does not mean they will necessarily listen, but give them a chance. It is not easy for people to come to terms with the issue when their own children have been vaccinated, but many do. You will find that elderly people who had their children before the vaccine industry went rampant are less likely to condemn you.

The people who condemn you the most are the ones who are the least likely to be prepared to look at scientific information about vaccination. If you offer them literature and documentation to read, and they refuse, then you have grounds for telling them that they are not to mention the subject again until they have read what you are offering.

No matter what evidence you present to some people, they will continue to cling to the myths of vaccination. I employed a student to go to a medical library and photocopy some articles on BCG side effects. There are a lot of articles and even photos on this topic in medical journals because BCG has been used to make tumours shrink, with gruesome and sometimes fatal side effects. The student read some of the articles, and was horrified to learn what the BCG vaccine can do to a human body. She told her sister-in-law, who is a medical technologist, about what she had been reading, and a heated argument resulted. The sister-in-law refused to read any of the photocopies, even though they all came from orthodox medical journals, and they were right there in front of her. She would not read them because she was afraid she might learn something that would make her have to change her world view.

What some people want most from life is to avoid having to think. They do not want to take responsibility for making a decision, so they prefer to let a bureaucracy make decisions about their children's health. My husband offered a business colleague some information about vaccination, and the latter displayed unusual honesty when refusing to read it. He said, "If I don't immunise my children and they get sick, it would be my fault. If I do immunise them and they get sick, then the doctor is to blame. So it's better to have it done."

Some people get angry with you for "endangering" their children. They believe that vaccines prevent disease, and they have had vaccines injected into their children, so they should believe that their children are "safe" from the germs allegedly brewing in your children. Although you know that they are being illogical, their attacks on you can still cause you a lot of stress.

When a breast feeding mother is subjected to emotional stress the volume of milk production decreases. If you are being harassed by people telling you to stop breast feeding, or to start supplementing, or that you are a bad person because you are not "protecting" your baby with vaccination, you would find it helpful to talk with other vaccine free families. The network of support groups does not yet reach all regions, so some of you will have to be pioneers.

TREATING VACCINE DAMAGE

Some of the damage caused by vaccination can be undone, but unfortunately not every victim responds. Homoeopaths have been treating vaccine damage ever since Edward Jenner started creating vaccine damage. Some homoeopaths go straight to antidoting the vaccine with the potentised form of the vaccine, while others prefer to use constitutional remedies.

A potentised vaccine usually brings about some degree of improvement in the condition. Sometimes the improvement is dramatic and total, but usually it does not go that far. The potentised form of DPT vaccine is often effective at curing chronic ear problems and asthma in vaccinated children, but it does not fix brain damage. Potentised BCG usually helps the lymph system recover from BCG.

The harm done by a vaccine can be lessened long after the vaccine has been administered. Even 50 years afterwards is not too late. The results of giving a potentised vaccine seem all the more amazing when the condition has been present for a long time. It is sensible to antidote vaccines one at a time, in the reverse order to which they were administered. Enough time should be allowed to lapse between each antidote, so that all the symptoms associated with that vaccine can work their way out of the body.

Sometimes when a potentised vaccine is used to antidote the symptoms that are known to have arisen as a result of that particular vaccine, other symptoms unexpectedly clear up too. With hindsight it makes the victim or the victim's mother realise that those symptoms arose soon after vaccination, and that they must have also been caused by the vaccine.

When a vaccine is potentised, the "other ingredients," like aluminium, formaldehyde, mercury, animal flesh, animal blood, human flesh, human blood and antibiotics are also potentised. The contaminating germs that were in the vaccine cannot be antidoted unless the remedy is made from a vial of the same batch of the vaccine. So, for instance, if a person has a condition like chronic fatigue syndrome or myelagic encephalopathy which was caused by measles vaccine, the extra viruses in the vaccine mixture could be contributing to the slow but relentless attack on the muscle controlling enzymes. Antidoting the measles vaccine with homoeopathically potentised measles vaccine from another batch might only solve half the problem, if there was a contaminating virus in the original vaccine.

The MMR antidote worked very well in a little boy whose reaction started two days after vaccination. From the time he woke up he was hyperactive. "Off his head," was the phrase his mother used. He also had a weird rash. He hardly slept that night. By the next day he had changed to being listless and floppy, rubbing his head as if it hurt, and sometimes seeming semiconscious. A fever developed during that day, and in the afternoon he had a major convulsion. An ambulance took him to hospital, where they gave him paracetamol. One of the doctors told the parents that vaccine reactions do not start until 3 or 4 days after vaccination, so this could not be one. (When the reaction does start 3 or 4 days after, they tell parents that it is not a vaccine reaction, because it did not start straight after the injection.) Blood tests and X rays found nothing, and the toddler was much improved the next day, so they went home. There were no more convulsions, and the mother thought he was better because the weird rash had gone, and he was neither wreaking havoc in the house, nor flopping into an immobile state.

The doctor who administered the vaccine refused to report the incident to the Adverse Reactions Committee. The mother contacted me to express her fury about what had happened to her boy, and she was especially angry that she had not been warned of the possibility of a convulsion before she agreed to vaccination. "If I had known that this could happen, I wouldn't have had him vaccinated," she said.

"That's why they didn't tell you," I replied. She wanted to warn other parents through the media. Television New Zealand has a documentary programme after the news on Channel 1 which prides itself on exposing the wrongs of the world. The mother thought this would be a suitable platform for her to warn other mothers. A junior journalist from the programme team was keen to do the story, and she was optimistic that it would be permitted. I warned them that the producer of the program is an ardent supporter of vaccination. They persevered in their attempts to get the story aired, but to no avail.

During my first conversation with the mother, I asked tactful but pointed questions about the child's condition. Her feeling at that time was one of great relief that it was all over, but I knew that there was no certainty that it really was all over. As is often the case, the subtle early symptoms of long term brain damage were present, but she had not recognised them. The toddler was clumsy, and unco-ordinated, and he was not alert. He was troubled and listless, and unable to settle. I was placed in the position of having to recommend homoeopathic treatment for those symptoms, without wanting to scare her. She was an intelligent lady, and my guarded comments did scare her.

I gave her the phone number of her nearest homoeopathic chemist, and she ordered six doses of *MMR 30*. After only one dose he reverted back to being the same little boy he had been before the vaccination. His clumsy unco-ordination just evaporated, he went back to sleeping through the night, and he began to play again. It was only when she saw the dramatic change brought about by the remedy that she fully realised how changed he had been. I spoke to her again three days after he had had the potentised MMR. "He's pottering and playing again. I hadn't noticed that he had stopped playing. The difference is quite remarkable. It's lovely having him play again. I can do things." Whew. The mother had learned enough during her crash course on vaccine damage to realise that the change brought about by the remedy meant that the insidious progress of brain damage had been halted, and their family had had a very close shave.

Perhaps one of the reasons why the antidote was so effective in this case was that it was made from the same brand of vaccine as had been injected into the boy, so that it contained the same type of egg yolk, the same toxic metals and so on as had been in the vaccine. Another factor would be the timing. The vibration of the remedy cut off the deterioration of the central nervous system before it had become irreparable.

Even years after central nervous system damage has occurred, constitutional homoeopathy can bring about amazing improvements. Unfortunately I have never yet heard of a case where the person recovers completely from brain damage when the treatment starts a long time after the damage occurred.

The Peto Institute in Hungary has a form of treatment which undoes a lot of the brain damage problems caused by vaccination. Occupational therapists in New Zealand have brought about great improvements in children who are brain damaged by vaccination, as well as by birth trauma.

I do not understand how cranial osteopathy can undo damage done by toxins and foreign proteins, but it does. Pharmaceutical medicine adheres to the medieval belief that the bones of the skull are fused to one another, forming a solid plate. This is not so. The separate bones can move out of their correct position, and when this happens, it has a negative impact on the rest of the body. Sometimes a baby's skull bones do not get back into the right position after moulding for birth. A mild blow on the head of an adult can move a bone out of position, and a variety of health problems, including migraines, can result. Cranial osteopaths can move the bones of the skull back into their correct alignment. It is logical that this would ease pressure on the brain, and thus fix certain problems, but why it helps with neurological problems from vaccination will remain a matter for speculation until research provides the answer. Perhaps the bones get pushed out of alignment by inflammation during the acute reaction.

Some babies who react to DPT vaccine suffer from persistent high-pitched screaming while they are in the acute phase of the reaction. I know of one case where a two-year-old girl who had reacted to DPT vaccine as a baby let out a long high-pitched scream when a cranial osteopath released a particular band of tension through her head. Her mother was shaken because it sounded just like that terrible scream she had heard in the days after DPT. After the treatment the child was able to co-ordinate in ways she had not been doing before the treatment. Cranial osteopathy is a post-graduate diploma for qualified osteopaths. In some countries it is legal for a non-osteopath to take a short course on skulls, and then call themselves a "cranial osteopath" - so beware.

THE *THUJA* MYTH

A myth has arisen that the homoeopathic remedy called *thuja* antidotes all vaccines. It is such a compelling myth that some parents think that if they give *thuja* minutes after vaccination, adverse reactions will not be possible. *Thuja* is often, but not always, the correct remedy to antidote smallpox vaccination.

The possible origin of the myth is a little book from the 1880s, called *Vaccinosis*, by J. Comptom Burnett MD.[463] This little book describes how the author cured many people who had been suffering from serious long term effects of smallpox vaccination. The case histories are fascinating, but nowhere does the author suggest that a century later, parents will be able to protect their babies from the cocktail of DPTHibOPHepB by giving them a dose of *thuja* as they walk out of the clinic.

One of the stories he tells is of a little girl with ringworm that was complicated by residual immune system disturbance from smallpox vaccine. The ringworm did not respond to the usual remedy for ringworm, but when *thuja* was given, the scabby nature of the ringworm changed, and *bacillinum 30* was then able to cure the ringworm. This principle still applies today - get the vaccine damage out of the way, and the door opens for other remedies.

One of his patients was a 19-year-old girl who had been vaccinated as a baby, vaccinated again at the age of seven years, caught smallpox at the age of nine years, and was vaccinated again at the age of 14 years. She was suffering from severe headaches twice a week, an enlarged liver, occasional boils, and what is now called chronic fatigue syndrome. He used a constitutional remedy, and a month later she was a little better. He then gave her low potency *thuja* every day for a month, and she only had one headache in that time, and her energy level improved a lot. Then he gave her a higher potency of *thuja*, and she developed nausea and fever, and broke out in smallpox pustules. Her mother said the pustules looked exactly like the ones she had when she had smallpox. They lasted five days before turning yellow and then fading away. After that she was completely cured. This course of events strongly suggests that she had been suffering residual problems from the smallpox as well as from the vaccinations.

He also tells of a baby who became very ill from drinking the milk of a wet nurse who had been vaccinated for smallpox. The wet nurse only had a sore arm and a pusty eruption at the site of vaccination, but the baby was in dire straits. The baby and the wet nurse were treated with *thuja*, and both recovered rapidly.

When I had smallpox vaccine antidoted, the homoeopath decided to use the nosode of the vaccine, not *thuja*. Nosode is just a fancy word for a potentised remedy made from yukkie disease matter. I had had ten smallpox vaccinations, and nine of them were done with the vaccine gunk manufactured in Johannesburg. The other vaccination was done at Heathrow Airport, so I do not know in which country the vaccine was manufactured. (Britain stopped manufacturing smallpox vaccine in 1932 because of the cruelty to cows, but still purchased vaccine manufactured on foreign cows. The product was made in bulk by slicing long slits along the flank of cows, and rubbing pus into the wounds. The cows' heads were braced to stop them licking it off. The pus then foamed and grew in volume, and was harvested and scratched into humans.) The nosode that the homoeopath used to fix me was made from Johannesburg vaccine. I only had one dose, (I do not know in what potency,) and it caused a radical improvement in my state of health. This happened six months after I had departed from the clutches of pharmaceutical medicine and had started becoming healthy under homoeopathy. So I was already on the upward path to good health, but the effect of that potentised smallpox vaccine was like jumping up a cliff on the path.

"HOMOEOPATHIC VACCINATION CAN BE USED AS A SUBSTITUTE FOR BIOLOGICAL VACCINATION"

Vaccine Myth number Fourteen: By giving a baby the homoeopathic remedy which would be used to cure an infectious disease, we can ensure that the child will never catch the disease.

Society has been seduced by the concept of artificial immunisation, so some people fall into the trap of believing that a homoeopathic "shot" will protect their child from infectious disease. Homoeopaths have become polarised about the issue of "homoeopathic immunisation." Those who oppose the practice and those who support it can become quite heated when arguing with one another. I believe that homoeopathic remedies should not be given to a person who has no symptoms, both because the procedure does not stimulate immunity to germs, and because it causes insidious long term side effects.

The people who promote homoeopathic vaccination say that giving a baby 1, 2 or 3 doses of a potentised germ, or giving it one of the potentised remedies which can be used to treat a particular disease, will make the baby immune for life. But no properly controlled studies have been done to assess effectiveness over time. Combining common sense with knowledge of how homoeopathic remedies work leads to the conclusion that treating a disease in advance is both unsafe and ineffective.

The claim that "homoeopathic immunisation" is an effective procedure rests mainly on anecdotal reports of people not contracting the disease after being administered with a remedy. The typical approach is, "Jimmy Bloggs had *morbillinum 30* as a baby, and now he is 15 years old and has still not had measles, so this must be because of the *morbillinum 30*." This is just as unscientific as the sweeping claims made for biological vaccination. An absurd but oft quoted claim for effectiveness is that the potentised remedy *diphtherium* was able to make people immune to diphtheria, because it made them react positively to the Schick test. The Schick test has been discarded by the medical establishment, but even before it was discarded it was an unscientific, inaccurate skin test for immunity against diphtheria. If a potentised remedy could make a person "Schick positive," (which I very much doubt it can do,) it would be of no consequence anyway.

Can a medicine which contains nothing more than a vibration alter the state of a person's vital energy in a way that would make the person unable to contract a specific disease for the rest of his or her life? Firstly, there is the problem that a remedy is being chosen for a person who has no symptoms. When a polio epidemic breaks out, the homoeopaths have to take a look at each patient who is suffering from polio, before they can choose the right remedy to cure that individual patient. Each epidemic has a slightly different virus, which causes slightly different symptoms, and each victim reacts slightly differently to each virus. So how can you be sure you are choosing the right remedy 10 years before the epidemic breaks out? To give a baby three doses of *sativa 30* or *gelsemium 30* and tell the parents that no polio virus will ever be able to harm the child is outrageously irresponsible. The homoeopaths who are doing this at present are getting away with it because there is no virulent polio virus in the environment. If the polio virus became virulent again, parental complacency about the danger could have tragic results.

If a potentised version of the polio vaccine were used, it would contain the vibration of the three main strains of polio virus. This is one of the remedies to consider when treating a patient with polio, or with paralysis caused by polio vaccine. But to give it to a baby and claim it will alter the vital force for the rest of the baby's life is absurd. Even if an introduced vibration could last that long in the body, it would only do so if the person never eats roast mutton with mint sauce, never brushes their teeth with ordinary toothpaste, never picks the leaf of a eucalyptus tree and crushes it in their fingers, never catches a whiff of mosquito repellent, never has an X ray taken, and never uses one of a thousand other homoeopathic remedies which can de-activate the polio vibration. Even if the introduced vibration could last for decades in the body, it would be totally impractical in the real world.

Some homoeopaths who support the practice do not go so far as to claim that a potentised remedy can make a person immune for life. They say that it can make a difference for a few weeks, and therefore should be used during epidemics. They do not restrict this advice to trying to prevent undesirable infectious diseases, but also recommend that parents attempt to prevent the beneficial childhood illnesses.

If an epidemic of polio broke out, and I knew my children were being exposed to a virulent polio virus, I would not give them a potentised remedy. Nutrition is of prime importance in preventing polio, and sufficient rest comes second. Providing children with wholesome substances to eat requires far more effort than making them suck a sweet tasting little white homoeopathic pill, but no effort should be spared in trying to prevent polio. Caring for a child who has been damaged by the polio virus would require far more effort. Of course if my efforts failed and one of them did actually contract polio, I would not hesitate to use homoeopathy to cure the disease.

Hundreds of studies which confirm that homoeopathy is an effective method of curing disease have been done. A few of them have even made it into medical journals. If ever any large-scale, long term, properly controlled studies which show that "homoeopathic immunisation" is effective were to be done, I would reconsider my standpoint on effectiveness. However, I would still want solid scientific evidence that giving a potentised remedy to someone with no symptoms does not cause side effects.

When the homoeopath gave me potentised smallpox vaccine I was showing symptoms of chronic poisoning from the 10 vaccinations to which I had been subjected. The use of nosodes is another issue that strongly divides homoeopaths. Some homoeopaths maintain that giving a non-indicated nosode can cause profound negative changes in the body, and I find that believable. It is possible that introducing the vibration of potentised viruses and bacteria can disrupt a baby's electromagnetic field, without the effects of the disruption being immediately obvious. It is easy to overlook the subtle long term side effects of crude vaccines if you are not watching out for them. How much easier it would be to miss any subtle, insidious, long term side effects of a potentised virus. When the subject of side effects is broached, promoters of homoeopathic vaccination respond by saying that no-one has reported any side effects to them.

I am particularly unhappy that the potentised Epstein Barr virus is sometimes given to babies with the promise that it will prevent glandular fever (infectious mononucleosis). This is a very nasty virus which can cause diverse things like chronic fatigue syndrome and cancer. I believe that introducing the vibration of the Epstein Barr virus into the bodies of very young babies will harm those who do not have a strong vital force.

Dr. Dorothy Shepherd argues very eloquently against the injection of cells and chemicals into the body on the grounds that they can cause physical disease by changing the vibration of the body's cells.[464] But her arguments can be used equally strongly against the introduction of non-indicated homoeopathic vibrations. All living cells have a vibration.[465] Germs are living cells, and if a species of germ vibrates at a frequency which is incompatible with the natural frequency of human cells, then potentising the germ and giving it to a person with no symptoms makes no sense, unless you are trying the make the person sick for research purposes.

If you throw a stone into a still pool of water, rings of waves will move out from where the stone hits the surface. If you throw two stones into a pool at the same time, their waves will alter each other when they meet. This is what happens continuously inside the body, but most of the alterations are not detrimental. Each type of cell has a set of metabolic oscillations which are characteristic of its type.[465] When healthy tissue becomes malignant, the oscillation of the cells changes.[466] It does not strike me as wise to introduce a homoeopathically potentised virus into the body of a tiny baby, even if the baby is perfectly healthy at the time. Too little is known about oscillations and electromagnetic fields in a baby's body to start introducing unnecessary waves and frequencies.

CONCLUSION

At the time that my first child was born I was living in a police state in which vaccination was compulsory. I was aware that some vaccines cause serious side effects that are not acknowledged by the medical establishment, and as I intended refusing some of the vaccines that were on the schedule, I thought I had better look up some statistics in case I found myself appearing in court. My investigations led me to discover that there is a much greater problem with vaccination than the fact that a few vaccines cause serious side effects. I discovered that vaccination is responsible for a wide range of chronic diseases, and that it is not the reason why diseases like diphtheria and whooping cough have declined. I also discovered that it is not a good idea to try and prevent childhood illnesses, and that the infectious diseases that are not a normal part of childhood can be prevented by methods that are far more reliable than vaccination. I had heard it said that it was wrong to suppress fever, and I was surprised to discover that there is solid scientific evidence to support that view. Later I learned that suppressing fever is one of the most dangerous things that modern medicine does. By delving into the history of vaccination, I discovered that it is a procedure based on falsehood, cruelty and supposition. The vaccine industry is still not accountable for its actions.

Every child on the planet is now a target for vaccination, and the result is that we already see epidemics of chronic diseases that are far more serious than the diseases they are trying to prevent. The vaccinationists pursue their goals with religious fervour, and they do not stop and take stock of their actions. In democratic countries the bureaucrats pay lip service to the idea that a parent has a right to make an informed choice, while at the same time withholding information. When democratic countries started introducing iniquitous laws to make life difficult for non-compliant parents, I felt motivated to share what I had learned with other parents. Our children are our most precious asset, and every parent needs to make a responsible decision about what will and will not be put into their bodies.

REFERENCES

1. Miller, D.L., Frequency of Complications of Measles, 1963 - Report on a National Inquiry by the Public Health Laboratory Service in Collaboration with the Society of Medical Officers of Health. *Brit Med J* July 11 1964;75-78.
2. Dyer, C., Families win support for vaccine compensation claim. *Brit Med J* September 24 1994;309:759.
3. Cockburn, A., Ridgeway J., Scientist J. Anthony Morris - He Fought the Flu Shots And the US Fired Him. *Washington Post*, 13 March 1977. At this time the Washington Post still had the same editor as the one who permitted the Watergate journalists to publish what they had discovered.
4. Researcher Denied Funds to Study DPT. *NVIC News* October 1991;1(3):3.
5. Long-term effects of early vaccinations. *Primal Health Research* 1994;1(4):3-7.
6. Odent, M., Culpin, E., Kimmel, T., Pertussis Vaccination and Asthma: Is there a link? *JAMA* 1994;272(8):592-593.
7. Odent, M., Culpin, E., Kimmel, T., Atopic Eczema. *Lancet July 9* 1994;344:140.
8. Whooping cough vaccination and asthma in childhood: is there a link? *Primal Health Research* 1997;4(4):3-6. To subscribe to the Primal Health Research newsletter write to 72 Savernake Rd, London, NW3 2JR, UK. Residents of Canada and the USA can subscribe via Birth Works, Inc., P O Box 2045, Medford, NJ 08055, USA. Donations towards unbiased research on infant health should be sent to the London address. British taxpayers can get a tax deduction by using the registered charity number 328090.
9. Wakefield, A.J., et al., Evidence of Persistent Measles Virus Infection in Crohn's Disease. *J Med Virol* 1993;39:345-353.
10. Lewin, J., et al., Persistent measles virus infection of the intestine: confirmation by immunogold electron microscopy. *Gut* 1995;36:564-569.
11. Barton, J.R., et al., Incidence of inflammatory bowel disease in Scottish children between 1968 and 1983: marginal fall in ulcerative colitis, three fold rise in Crohn's disease. *Gut* 1989;30:618-622.
12. Thompson, N.P., Montgomery, S.M., Pounder, R.E., Wakefield, A.J., Is measles vaccination a risk factor for inflammatory bowel disease? *Lancet* April 29 1995;345:1071-1074.

13. Morrs, D.L., Montgomery, S.M., et al., Measles Vaccination and Inflammatory Bowel Disease: A National British Cohort Study. *Am J Gastroenterol* 2000;95(12):3507-3512.

14. Health Insurance Commission, Health and Family Services, *An Outline of the Practice Incentives Program*, 1998.

15. Benjamin, C.M., Chew, G.C., Silman, A.J., Joint and limb symptoms in children after immunisation with measles, mumps, and rubella vaccine. *Brit Med J* April 25 1992;304:1075-1078.

16. Weibel, R.E., Benor, D.E., Chronic arthropathy and musculoskeletal symptoms associated with rubella vaccines. A review of 124 claims submitted to the National Vaccine Injury Compensation Program. *Arthritis Rheum* 1996;39(9):1529-1534.

17. Cooper, L.Z., Ziring, P.R., et al., Transient Arthritis After Rubella Vaccination. *Amer J Dis Child* 1969;118:218-225.

18. Hedrich, A.W., Monthly estimates of the child population "susceptible" to measles, 1900-1931, Baltimore, MD. *Amer J Hyg* 1933;17:613-636.

19. Kids don't spread hepatitis B. *Australian Doctor Weekly* 6 November 1992.

20. Burgess, M.A., McIntosh, E.D.G., et al., Hepatitis B in urban Australian schoolchildren - No evidence of horizontal transmission between high-risk and low-risk groups. *Med J Aust* 5 September 1993;159:315-319.

21. Stanton, A.N., Scott, D.J., Downham, M.A., Is overheating a factor in some unexpected infant deaths? *Lancet* May 17 1980;1:1054-1057.

22. Fleming, P.J., Gilbert, R., et al., Interaction between bedding and sleeping position in the sudden infant death syndrome: a population based case-control study. *Brit Med J* July 14 1990;301:85-89.

23. Ponsonby, A.L., Dwyer, T., et al., Thermal environment and sudden infant death syndrome: case-control study. *Brit Med J* February 1 1992;304:277-282.

24. Kluger, M.J., Fever. *Pediatrics* 1980;66(5):720-724.

25. Hanson, D.F., Fever, Temperature and the Immune Response. *Ann NY Acad Sci* 1997;813:453-464.

26. Nahas, G.G., Tannieres, M.L., Lennon, J.F., Direct measurement of leukocyte motility: effects of pH and temperature. *Proc Soc Exp Biol Med* 1971;138:350-352.

27. Bernheim, H.A., Bodel, P.T., et al., Effects of Fever on Host Defence Mechanisms after Infection in the Lizard Diposaurus Dorsalis. *Br J Exp Pathol* 1978;59:76-84.

28. Ellingson, H.V., Clark, P.F., The Influence of Artificial Fever on Mechanisms of Resistance. *J Immunol* 1942;43:65-83.

29. Bodel, P., Atkins, E., Release of Endogenous Pyrogen by Human Monocytes. *New Engl J Med* 1967;276(18):1002.

30. Cranston, W.I., Goodale, F., Snell, E.S., Wendt, F., The Role of Leukocytes in the Initial Action of Bacterial Pyrogens in Man. *Clin Sci* 1956;15:219-226.
31. Weinberg, E.D., Iron and Infection. *Microbiol Rev* 1978;42:45-66.
32. Bullen, J.J., The Significance of Iron in Infection. *Rev Infect Dis* 1981;3(6):1127-1138.
33. Kluger, M.J., Rothenburg, B.A., Fever and Reduced Iron: Their Interaction as a Host Defense Response to Bacterial Infection. *Science* 1979;203:374-376.
34. Ballantyne, G.H., Rapid Drop in Serum Iron Concentration as a Host Defense Mechanism. *Amer Surg* 1984;5(8):405-411.
35. Kluger, M.J., Fever: Role of Pyrogens and Cryogens. *Physiol Rev* 1991;71(1):93-127.
36. Rager-Zisman, B., Bloom, B.R., Interferons and Natural Killer Cells. *Brit Med Bull* 1985;41(1):22-27.
37. Heron, I., Berg, K., The actions of interferon are potentiated at elevated temperature. *Nature* 1978;274:508-510.
38. Roberts, N.J., Temperature and Host Defense. *Microbiol Rev* 1979;43(2):241-259.
39. Manzella, J.P., Roberts, N.J., Human Macrophage and Lymphocyte Responses to Mitogen Stimulation after exposure to influenza virus, ascorbic acid, and hyperthermia. *J Immunol* 1979;123(5):1940-1944.
40. Smith, J.B., Knowlton, R.P., Agarwal, S.S., Human Lymphocyte responses are enhanced by culture at 40° C. *J Immunol* 1978;121(2):691-694.
41. Roberts, N.J., Sandberg, K., Hyperthermia and Human Leukocyte Function: II. Enhanced Production of and Response to Leukocyte Migration Inhibition Factor (LIF). *J Immunol* 1979;122(5):1990-1993.
42. Duff, G.W., Durum, S.K., The pyrogenic and mitogenic actions of inerleukin -1 are related. *Nature* 1983;304:449-451.
43. Duff, G.W., Atkins, E., Fever and immunoregulation: hyperthermia, interleukins 1 and 2, and T cell proliferation. *Yale J Biol Med* 1982;55:437-442.
44. Hanson, D.F., Murphy, P.A., Silican, R., Shin, H.S., The effect of temperature on the activation of thymocytes by interleukins I and II. *J Immunol* 1983;130:216-221.
45. Mackowiak, P.A., Marling-Cason, M., Cohen, R.L., Effects of Temperature on Antimicrobal Susceptibility of Bacteria. *J Infect Dis* 1982;145(4):550-553.
46. Sande, M.A., Sande, E.R., et al., The Influence of Fever on the Development of Experimental Streptococcus Pneumoniae Meningitis. *J Infect Dis* 1987;156(5):849-850.

47. Kluger, J.M., Ringler, D.H., Anver, M.R., Fever and Survival. *Science* 1975;188:166-168.
48. Carmichael, L.E., Barnes, F.D., Percy, D.H., Temperature as a Factor in Resistance of Young Puppies to Canine Herpesvirus. *J Infect Dis* 1969;120(6):669-678.
49. Bernheim, H.A., Kluger, M.J., Fever: Effect of Drug-Induced Antipyresis on Survival. *Science* 1976;193:237-239.
50. Vaughn, L.K., Veale, W.L., Cooper, K.E., Antipyresis: Its effect on mortality rate of bacterially infected rabbits. *Brain Res Bull* 1980;5:69-73.
51. Hoefs, J., Sapico, F.L., et al., The Relationship of White Blood Cell (WBC) and Pyrogenic Response to Survival in Spontaneous Bacterial Peritonitis (SBP). *Gastroenterology* 1980;78(5)Part 2:1308.
52. Weinstein, M.P., Iannini, P.B., et al., Spontaneous bacterial peritonitis. A review of 28 cases with emphasis on improved survival and factors influencing prognosis. *Am J Med* 1978;64:592-598. "The presence of fever with temperatures greater than 38° was associated with significantly diminished mortality (P=0.0240)."
53. Bryant, R.E., Hood, A.F., et al., Factors Affecting Mortality of Gram-Negative Rod Bacteremia. *Arch Intern Med* 1971;127:120-128. In this study 71% of humans without fever died, while 27% of those with fever died.
54. Mackowiak, P.A., Browne, R.H., et al., Polymicrobial Sepsis: An Analysis of 184 Cases Using Log Linear Models. *Am J Med Sci* 1980;280:73-80. In this study the association of fever with survival was stronger when the patient did not have an underlying terminal illness.
55. Poston, R.N., *Nutrition and Immunity,* in, Jarrett, R.J., (ed), *Nutrition and Disease.* Croom Helm, London, 1979, 199.
56. Scrimshaw, N.S., Béhar, M., Malnutrition in Underdeveloped Countries. *New Engl J Med* 1965;272(4):193-198.
57. Ebrahim, G.J., *The Problems of Undernutrition,* in, Jarrett, R.J., (ed), *Nutrition and Disease.* Croom Helm, London, 1979, 85-86.
58. Doran, T.F., De Angelis, C., et al., Acetaminophen: More harm than good for chickenpox? *J Ped* 1989;114(6):1045-1048. (Acetaminophen and paracetamol are the same thing.)
59. Stuart, J., and Malcolm, D.McK., (eds), *The Diary of Henry Francis Fynn.* Shuter and Shooter, Pietermaritzburg, 1969, 42-43. There was international distribution of a TV mini series called *Shaka Zulu,* which was claimed to have been based on the diaries of Dr. Fynn, but was actually a racist corruption of Fynn's diary. Made by the Botha regime in 1986, it was based on a Stalinesque "history" penned during the

Verwoerd era. Not to be confused with the films called *Zulu, Zulu Dawn* nor *Shaka.*
60. Arnold, Nell, *Rye - A book of Memories.* Rye - Tootagarook Area Committee, 1989, 17.
61. Spock, Benjamin, *Baby and Child Care.* W. H. Allen and Co, London, 1983, 497-502.
62. Nelson, K.B., Ellenberg, J.H., Prognosis in Children with Febrile Seizures. *Pediatrics* 1978;61(5):720-727.
63. Verity, C.M., Greenwood, R., Golding, J., Long-term Intellectual and Behavioral Outcomes of Children with Febrile Convulsions. *N Eng J Med* 1998;338(24):1723-1728.
64. Annergers, J.H., Hauser, W.A., et al., The risk of epilepsy following febrile convulsions. *Neurology* 1979;29:297-303.
65. Camfield, P., Camfield, C., et al., What types of epilepsy are preceded by febrile seizures? A population based study of children. *Dev Med Child Neurol* 1994;36:887-892.
66. Sofijanov, N., Sadikario, A., Dukovski, M., Kuturee, M., Febrile Convulsions and Later Development of Epilepsy. *Am J Dis Child* 1983;137:123-126.
67. Verity, C.M., Golding, J., Risk of epilepsy after febrile convulsions; a national cohort study. *Brit Med J* November 30 1991;303:1373-1376.
68. Knüdsen, F.U., Paerregaard, A., et al., Long term outcome of prophylaxis for febrile convulsions. *Arch Dis Child* 1996;74:13-18.
69. Hirtz, D.G., Febrile Seizures. *Pediatr in Rev* 1997;18(1):5-8.
70. West, R., Epidemiologic study of malignancies of the ovaries. *Cancer* 1966;19:1001-1007.
71. Newhouse, M.L., Pearson, R.M., et al., A case control study of carcinoma of the ovary. *Brit J Prev Soc Med* 1977;31:148-153.
72. Pasquinucci, G., Possible Effect of Measles on Leukaemia. *Lancet* January 16 1971;136.
73. Gross, S., Measles and Leukaemia. *Lancet* February 20 1971;397-398.
74. Hutchins, G., Observations on the relationship of measles and remissions in the nephrotic syndrome. *Am J Dis Child* 1947;73:242-243.
75. Blumberg, R.W., Cassady, H.A., Effect of Measles on the Nephrotic Syndrome. *Am J Dis Child* 1947;73:151-166.
76. Bluming, A.Z., Ziegler, J.L., Regression of Burkitt's Lymphoma in association with measles infection. *Lancet* July 10 1971;105-106.
77. Burnet, F.M., Measles as an Index of Immunological Function. *Lancet* September 14 1968; 610-613.

78. Olding-Stenkvist, E., Bjorvatn, B., Rapid Detection of Measles Virus in Skin Rashes by Immunoflourescence. *J Infect Dis* 1976;134(5):463-469.
79. Dossetor, J., Whittle, H.C., Greenwood, B.M., Persistent measles infection in malnourished children. *Brit Med J* June 25 1977;1633-1635.
80. Pharmacy Guild of New Zealand (Inc.), *Your Health Update*, Issue No. 3. Undated.
81. Cantacuzène, J., *Ann Inst Pasteur*, 1898, 12: Paris, 273, cited in Silverstein, A.M., *A History of Immunology*, Academic Press Inc., San Diego, 1989, 49.
82. Morely, D., Severe Measles in the Tropics. - I. *Brit Med J* February 1 1969;297-300.
83. Hardy, I.R.B., Lennon, D.R., Mitchell, E.A., Measles epidemic in Auckland 1984-85. *NZ Med J* 13 May 1987;273-275.
84. Lydall, W., Scaremongering about measles. *Soil and Health* 1992;51(1):55.
85. Kalokerinos, Archie, *Every Second Child*. Keats Publishing, Inc., New Canaan, Connecticut, 1981.
86. Kalokerinos, Archie, *Science Friction*. International Symposium, The Vaccination Dilemma, Auckland, 1992.
87. Kalokerinos, Archie, *Experience with Immunisation Reactions*. International Symposium, The Vaccination Dilemma II, Auckland, 1995.
88. Zahorsky, J., Roseola Infantum. *JAMA* October 18 1913;61(16):1446-1450.
89. Koplik, H., The Diagnosis of the Invasion of Measles from a Study of the Exanthema as it Appears on the Buccal Membrane. *Arch Pediatr* 1896;12:918-922.
90. Beckford, A.P., Kaschula, R.O., Stephen, C., Factors associated with fatal cases of measles. A retrospective autopsy study. *S Afr Med J* 1985;68(12):858-863.
91. Griffin, D.E., Ward, B.J., et al., Natural killer cell activity during measles. *Clin Exp Immunol* 1990;81:218-224.
92. Cole, T.J., Relating Growth Rate to Environmental Factors - Methodological Problems in the Study of Growth-Infection Interaction. *Acta Paediatr Suppl* 1989;350:14-20.
93. Ebrahim, G.J., *The Problems of Undernutrition*, in, Jarrett, R.J., (ed), *Nutrition and Disease*. Croom Helm, London, 1979, 60 & 74.
94. Harris, H.F., A Case of Diabetes Mellitus Quickly Following Mumps. *Boston Med Surg J* 1899;140(20):465-469.

95. Swartout, H.O., *Modern Medical Counsellor.* Signs Publishing Company, Warburton, Australia, 1958, 715.
96. Das, B.D., Lakhani, P., et al., Congenital rubella after previous maternal immunity. *Arch Dis Child* 190;65:545-546.
97. Partridge, J.W., et al., Congenital rubella affecting an infant whose mother had rubella antibodies before conception. *Brit Med J* January 17 1981;187-188.
98. Bott, L.M., Eizenberg, D.H., Congenital rubella after successful vaccination. *Med J Aust* 12 June 1982;514-515.
99. Strannegård, Ö., Holm, S.E., et al., Case of Apparent Reinfection with Rubella. *Lancet* January 31 1970;240-241.
100. Ushida, M., Katow, S., Furukawa, S., Congenital Rubella Syndrome due to Infection after Maternal Antibody Conversion with Vaccine. *Jpn J Infect Dis* 2003;56:68-69.
101. Numazaki, K., Fujikawa, T., Intracranial calcification with congenital rubella syndrome in a mother with serologic immunity. *J Child Neurol* 2003;18(4):296-297.
102. American College of Obstetricians and Gynecologists, ACOG Committee Opinion: number 281, December 2002. Rubella vaccination. *Obstet Gynecol* 2002;100(6):1417.
103. Tingle, A.J., Mitchell, L.A., et al., Randomised double-blind placebo-controlled study on adverse effects of rubella immunisation in seronegative women. *Lancet* May 3 1997;349:1277-1281.
104. Geier, D.A., Geier, M.R., A one year followup of chronic arthritis following rubella and hepatitis B vaccination based upon analysis of the Vaccine Adverse Events Reporting System (VAERS) database. *Clin Exp Rheumatol* 2002;20(6):767-771.
105. Plotkin, S.A., Cornfeld, D., Ingalls, T.H., Studies of Immunization With Living Rubella Virus. *Amer J Dis Child* 1965;110:381-389.
106. Plotkin, S.A., Farquhar, J.D., et al., Attenuation of RA 27/3 Rubella Virus in WI-38 Human Diploid Cells. *Amer J Dis Child* 1969;118:178-185.
107. Bell, J.A., Pittman, M., Olson, B.J., Pertussis and aureomycin. *Public Health Rep* 1949;64:589-598.
108. Silver, H.K., Kempe, C.H., Bruyn, H.B., *Handbook of Pediatrics,* 14th Edition. Lange Medical Publications, Los Altos, California, 1977, 507.
109. Mullan, B., *The Enid Blyton Story.* Boxtree Ltd., London, 1987, 15.
110. Centers for Disease Control, Pertussis Surveillance - United States, 1986 - 1988. *MMWR Morb Mortal Wkly Rep* February 2 1990;39(4):57-66.
111. Taranger, J., Mild Clinical Course of Pertussis in Swedish Infants of Today. *Lancet* June 12 1982;1360.

112. Pollock, T.M., Miller, E., Lobb, J., Severity of whooping cough in England before and after the decline in pertussis immunisation. *Arch Dis Child* 1984;59:162-165.

113. Takahashi, M., Okuno, Y., et al., Development of a Live Attenuated Varicella Vaccine. *Biken J* 1975;18:25-33.

114. Takahashi, M., Development and Characterization of a Live Varicella Vaccine (Oka strain). *Biken J* 1984;27:31-36.

115. Barbara Loe Fisher, *NVIC Press Release*, April 1995. (1.4 deaths per 100,000 cases in healthy children, and 31 deaths per 100,000 cases in adults.)

116. Centers for Disease Control, Recommendations of the Immunization Practices Advisory Committee (ACIP) Varicella-Zoster Immune Globulin for the Prevention of Chickenpox. *MMWR Morb Mortal Wkly Rep* February 24 1984;33(7):84-90. "Although less than 2% of reported cases occur among individuals 20 years of age or older, almost a quarter of all the mortality is reported in this age group."

117. Ronne, T., Measles virus infection without rash in childhood is related to disease in adult life. *Lancet* January 5 1985;1-5.

118. Rolfe, M., Measles immunization in the Zambian Copperbelt: cause for concern. *Trans Royal Soc Trop Med Hyg* 1982;76(4):529-530.

119. Poland, G.A., Jacobson, R.M., Failure to Reach the Goal of Measles Elimination. *Arch Intern Med* 1994;154:1815-1820.

120. Hartley, P., Tulloch, W.J., et al., *A Study of Diphtheria in Two Areas of Great Britain*. Medical Research Council, Special Report Series No 272, His Majesty's Stationary Office, London, 1950, 4.

121. The official statistics collected for England and Wales from 1866 record the ages of victims.

122. Immunisation against Diphtheria and Scarlet Fever. *Lancet* March 14 1931;589.

123. Joint Committee on Vaccination and Immunisation, *Immunisation against Infectious Disease.* Her Majesty's Stationary Office, London, 1988, 19.

124. Hartley, P., Tulloch, W.J., et al., *A Study of Diphtheria in Two Areas of Great Britain*. Medical Research Council, Special Report Series No 272, His Majesty's Stationary Office, London, 1950.

125. Linklater, A., *An Unhusbanded Life, Charlotte Despard, Suffragette, Socialist and Sinn Feiner*. Hutchinson, London, 1980.

126. Ibid., 98-99.

127. Ibid., 99.

128. Douglas Hume, Ethel, *Béchamp or Pasteur? A Lost Chapter in the History of Biology*. C. W. Daniel, Ashingdon, Rochford, Essex, Fourth Edition, 1963, 217-218.

129. Moskowitz, R., Immunizations: The Other Side. *Mothering* #31, Spring 1984, 33-38.
130. Douglas Hume, Ethel, *Béchamp or Pasteur? A Lost Chapter in the History of Biology.* C. W. Daniel, Ashingdon, Rochford, Essex, Fourth Edition, 1963, 207.
131. Centers for Disease Control, Diphtheria Outbreak - Russian Federation, 1990 - 1993. *MMWR Morb Mortal Wkly Rep* November 5 1993;42(43):840-841 & 847.
132. Centers for Disease Control, Diphtheria Epidemic - New Independent States of the Former Soviet Union, 1990-1994. *MMWR Morb Mortal Wkly Rep* March 17 1995;44(10):177-181.
133. Fisher, P., The World's Most Famous Homoeopathic Hospital. *Homoeopathy Today*, 1989;2(12):6.

Bibliography re bubonic plague and cholera;

Philip Ziegler, *The Black Death.* Collins, London, 1969.
Arthur M. Silverstein, *A History of Immunology.* Academic Press, Inc., San Diego, 1989.
Stanley L. Robbins, M.D., *The Pathologic Basis of Disease.* W. B. Saunders Company, Philadelphia, 1974.
Folke Henschen, *The History of Disease.* Longmans Green and Co. Ltd., London, 1966.
Norman Longmate, *King Cholera.* Hamish Hamilton, London, 1966.
George Deaux, *The Black Death.* Hamish Hamilton, London, 1969.
Charles E. Rosenberg, *The Cholera Years.* University of Chicago Press, Chicago, 1962.

134. Cherry, J.D., The 'New' Epidemiology of Measles and Rubella. *Hospital Practice*, July 1980;49-57. With regard to herd immunity, Cherry not only twists the sense of the research finding, he also changes the percentage to 68%. "He (Hedrich) reported that when 68% of the children less than 15 years of age were immune to measles, epidemics did not develop." What Hedrich actually reported is that when measles epidemics die out, the percentage of children who are immune is never higher than 53%. The research done by Hedrich shows that the number of immune people in a community has absolutely nothing to do with the decline in virulence of the measles virus when an outbreak comes to an end. The figures collected by Hedrich show that the concept of herd immunity is fundamentally flawed.
135. Fine, P.E.M., Herd Immunity: History, Theory, Practice. *Epidemiol Rev* 1993;15(2):265-302.

136. Centers for Disease Control, Measles Outbreak among Vaccinated High School Students - Illinois. *MMWR Morb Mortal Wkly Rep* June 22 1984;33(24):349-351.

137. Hull, H.F., Montes, J.M., et al., Risk factors for measles vaccine failure among immunized students. *Pediatrics* 1985;76:518-523.

138. Davis, R.M., Whitman, E.D., et al., A persistent outbreak of measles despite appropriate prevention and control measures. *Am J Epidemiol* 1987;126:438-449.

139. Gustavson, T.L., Brunell, P.A., et al., Measles outbreak in a 'fully immunized' secondary school population. *New Eng J Med* 1987;316:771-774.

140. Nkowane, B.M., Bart, S.W., et al., Measles outbreak in a vaccinated school population: epidemiology, chains of transmission and the role of vaccine failures. *Am J Pub Health* 1987;77:434-438.

141. Chen, R.T., Goldbaum, G.M., et al., An explosive point-source measles outbreak in a highly vaccinated population: modes of transmission and risk factors for disease. *Am J Epidemiol* 1989;129:173-182.

142. Hersh, B.S., Markowitz, L.E., et al., A measles outbreak at a college with a prematriculation immunization requirement. *Am J Pub Health* 1991;81:360-564.

143. Centers for Disease Control, Measles in an immunized school-aged population - New Mexico. *MMWR Morb Mortal Wkly Rep* 1985;34:52-54, 59.

144. Anderson, R.M., May, R. M., Immunisation and herd immunity. *Lancet* March 17 1990;641-645.

145. Centers for Disease Control, International Notes: Measles - Hungary. *MMWR Morb Mortal Wkly Rep* October 6 1989;38(39):665-668.

146. Williams, P.J., and Hull, H.F., Status of Measles in the Gambia, 1981. *Rev Infect Dis* 1983;5(3):460-462.

147. Lamb, W.H., Epidemic Measles in a Highly Immunized Rural West African (Gambian) Village. *Rev Infect Dis* 1988;10(2):457-462.

148. Norby, E., The Paradigms of Measles Vaccinology. *Curr Top Microbiol Immunol* 1993;191:117.

149. Markowitz, L.E., Preblud, S.R., et al., Patterns of Transmission in Measles Outbreaks in the United States, 1985 - 1986. *New Engl J Med* 1989;320(2):75-81.

150. Cogger, H.G., *Reptiles and Amphibians of Australia*, 5th Edition. Reed Books of Australia, 1996, 121-122.

151. Gay, N.J., Eliminating measles - no quick fix. *Bull WHO* 2000;78(8):949.

152. World Health Organisation, Global Eradication of Poliomyelitis by the Year 2000. *Wkly Epidemiol Rec* 1988;63:161-162.

153. Personal communication, Ministry of Health, Fiji.

154. Samuel, R., Balraj, V., John, T.J., Persisting poliomyelitis after high coverage with oral polio vaccine. *Lancet* April 3 1993;903.

155. Sutter, R.W., Patriarca, P.A., et al., Outbreak of paralytic poliomyelitis in Oman: evidence for widespread transmission among fully vaccinated children. *Lancet* September 21 1991;338:715-720.

156. Williams, G.D., Matthews, N.T., et al., Infant pertussis deaths in New South Wales 1996-1997. *Med J Aust* 16 March 1998;168:281-283.

157. Fine, P.E.M., Clarkson, J.A., The recurrence of whooping cough: possible implications for assessment of vaccine efficacy. *Lancet* March 20 1982;666-669. The writers state, "Since epidemic frequency is a function of the rate of influx of susceptibles, it is surprising that the inter-epidemic period did not decrease after the 1974 fall in vaccine uptake." Epidemic frequency is not a function of the rate of influx of susceptibles. This delusion is absolute nonsense.

158. Stewart, G.T., Whooping cough and pertussis vaccine: A comparison of risks and benefits in Britain during the period 1968 - 83. *Dev Biol Stand* 1985;61:395-405.

159. Stewart, G.T., Whooping cough and whooping cough vaccine: the risks and benefit debate. *Am J Epidemiol* 1984;119(1):135-137.

160. Miller, E., Acellular pertussis vaccines. *Arch Dis Child* 1995;73(5):390-391.

161. Nielsen, A., Larsen, S.O., Epidemiology of Pertussis in Denmark: The Impact of Herd Immunity. *Int J Epidemiol* 1994;23(6):1300-1307.

162. Mortimer, E.A., Immunization Against Infectious Disease. *Science* 26 May 1978;200:902-907.

163. *What Doctors Don't Tell You*, 4(4):10. 4 Wallace Rd, London N1 2PG, UK.

164. van Rensburg, J.W.J., Whooping Cough in Cape Town. *Epidemiological Comments* April 1992;19(4):69-75.

165. The historical details of this story are based on chapter 3 of Silverstein, A.M., *A History of Immunology,* Academic Press Inc., San Diego, 1989, but the interpretation of the commercial significance is my own.

166. Hartley, P., Tulloch, W.J., et al., *A Study of Diphtheria in Two Areas of Great Britain.* Medical Research Council, Special Report Series No 272, His Majesty's Stationary Office, London, 1950, 1.

167. Ibid., 16.

168. Ibid., 81.

169. Ibid., 37.

170. Ibid., 39.

171. Nossal, G.J.V., *Antibodies and Immunity.* Basic Books Inc., New York, 1978.

172. Burnet, M., *The Integrity of the Human Body.* Harvard University Press, Cambridge, 1962, 42-43.
173. Good, R.A., Zak, S.J., Disturbances in Gamma Globulin Synthesis as "Experiments of Nature". *Pediatrics* 1956;18(1):109-149.
174. Ruata, C., Vaccination in Italy. *NY Med J* July 22 1899;133-134.
175. Johnson, S., Schoub, B.D., et al., Poliomyelitis outbreak in South Africa, 1982. II. Laboratory and vaccine aspects. *Trans Royal Soc Trop Med Hyg* 1984;78:26-31.
176. Paunio, M., Peltola, H., et al., Explosive school-based measles outbreak: intense exposure may have resulted in high risk, even among revaccinees. *Am J Epidemiol* 1998;148(11):1103-1110.
177. Measles Striking More Under Age 1. *Washington Post*, November 22, 1992;a17.
178. Albonico, H., Klein, P., Grob, Ch., Pewsner, D., Vaccination against measles, mumps and rubella. A constraining project for a dubious future? *IAS Newsletter* December 1991;4(3):4.
179. Douglas Hume, Ethel, *Béchamp or Pasteur? A Lost Chapter in the History of Biology.* C. W. Daniel, Ashingdon, Rochford, Essex, Fourth Edition, 1963, 198.
180. Campos-Outcalt, D., Measles Outbreak in an Immunized School Population. *New Engl J Med* 1987;317(13):834-835.
181. Dew, Kevin, *The Measles Vaccination Campaigns In New Zealand, 1985 and 1991: The Issues Behind the Panic.* Department of Sociology and Social Policy, Working Papers No 10, 1995, Victoria University of Wellington.
182. *Measles end Nikki's hopes for Olympics.* North Shore Times Advertiser, September 12 1991; 1.
183. Galloway, Y., Stehr-Green, P., Measles in New Zealand, 1991. *CDNZ: communicable disease New Zealand* December 1991;91(12):107-109.
184. Markowitz, L.E., Preblud, S.R., et al., Duration of live measles vaccine-induced immunity. *Ped Infect Dis J* 1990;9(2):101-110.
185. Lambert, S., Lynch, P., Measles Outbreak - Young Adults at High Risk. *Victorian Infectious Diseases Bulletin* May 1999;2(2):21-22.
186. Another Measles Outbreak in Young Adults in Melbourne. *Victorian Infectious Diseases Bulletin* December 2001;4(4):52.
187. Guidelines for the control of measles outbreaks in Australia. *Communicable Diseases Intelligence* Technical Report Series No. 5, 2000, 10.
188. Stewart, G.T., Vaccination against whooping-cough. Efficacy versus risks. *Lancet* January 29 1977;234-237.

189. Mansoor, O., and Durham, G., Does Control of Pertussis Need Rethinking? *CDNZ: communicable disease New Zealand* April 1991;91(4):43-45,48.

190. Centers for Disease Control, Pertussis Outbreak - Oklahoma. *MMWR Morb Mortal Wkly Rep* January 13 1984;33(1):2-10.

191. Centers for Disease Control, Pertussis Outbreaks - Massachusetts and Maryland, 1992. *MMWR Morb Mortal Wkly Rep* 1993;42(11):197-200.

192. Keitel, W.A., Edwards, K.M., Acellular Pertussis Vaccines in Adults. *Infectious Dis Clin North Am* 1999;13(1):83-94.

193. Department of National Health and Population Development - Pretoria, Poliomyelitis Epidemic in Natal and Kwazulu. *Epidemiological Comments* March 1988;15(3):28-29.

194. Slater, P.E., Orenstein, W.A., et al., Poliomyelitis outbreak in Israel in 1988: a report with two commentaries. *Lancet* May 19 1990;1192-1198.

195. Douglas Hume, Ethel, *Béchamp or Pasteur? A Lost Chapter in the History of Biology.* C. W. Daniel, Ashingdon, Rochford, Essex, Fourth Edition, 1963, 198 & 201.

196. Ibid., 201.

197. Wilson, Graham S., *The Hazards of Immunization.* The Athlone Press, London, 1967, 180.

198. Douglas Hume, Ethel, *Béchamp or Pasteur? A Lost Chapter in the History of Biology.* C. W. Daniel, Ashingdon, Rochford, Essex, Fourth Edition, 1963, 202.

199. D'Arcy Hart, P., et al., *B.C.G. and Vole Bacillus Vaccines in the Prevention of Tuberculosis in Adolescence and Early Adult Life.* Third Report to the Medical Research Council by their Tuberculosis Vaccines Clinical Trials Committee, Fisher, Knight and Co, Ltd., Gainsborough Press, St Albans, undated.

200. James, E.F., B.C.G. and Vole Bacillus Vaccines. *Brit Med J* October 6 1956;826-827.

201. Tuberculosis Prevention Trial, Madras. Trial of BCG vaccines in South India for tuberculosis prevention. *Indian J Med Res* 1979;70:349-363.

202. Tuberculosis Prevention Trial, Madras. Trial of BCG vaccines in South India for tuberculosis prevention. *Indian J Med Res* 1980;72:suppl.,1-74.

203. Editorial, BCG: Bad News from India. *Lancet* January 12 1980;73-74.

204. Editorial, BCG Vaccination after the Madras Study. *Lancet* February 7 1981;309-310.

205. Editorial, Is BCG Vaccination Effective? *Tubercle* 1981;62:219-221.

206. Böttiger, M., Romanus, V., et al., Osteitis and Other Complications Caused by Generalised BCG-itis: Experiences in Sweden. *Acta Paediatr Scand* 1982;71(3):471-478.

207. The information about how Hahnemann discovered homoeopathy comes from; Cook, T.M., *Samuel Hahnemann, The Founder of Homoeopathic Medicine.* Thorsons Publishers Ltd., Wellingborough, Northamptonshire, 1981. Another book on Hahnemann's life (in two volumes) is Haehl, Richard, *Samuel Hahnemann: His Life and Work.* London, Homoeopathic Publishing Co., 1922.

208. Hahnemann, Samuel, *Organon of Medicine*, 6th edition. 10, J P Tarcher, Inc., 9110 Sunset Blvd, Los Angeles, CA 90069, USA, 1982.

209. Pauling, Linus, *Vitamin C, the Common Cold and the Flu.* Berkley Books, New York, 1983, 167-168.

210. Stone, Irwin, *The Healing Factor, Vitamin C against Disease.* Grosset and Dunlap, New York, 1972.

211. Cheraskin, E., Ringsdorf, W.M., Sisley, E.L., *The Vitamin C Connection: Getting well and staying well with Vitamin C.* Thorsons, Wellingborough, Northamptonshire, 1983.

212. Chan, R.C., Penney, D.J., et al., Hepatitis and death following vaccination with 17D-204 yellow fever vaccine. *Lancet* July 14 2001;121-122.

213. Ayvazian, L.F., Risks of Repeated Immunization. *Annals of Internal Medicine* 1975;82(4):589.

214. Tshabalala, R.T., Anaphylactic Reactions to BCG in Swaziland. *Lancet* March 19 1983;653.

215. Davis, Adelle, *Let's Get Well.* Unwin Paperbacks, London, 1979, 102-112.

216. Ibid., 34-55.

217. Davis, Adelle, *Let's Eat Right to Keep Fit.* Unwin Paperbacks, London, 1984, 97-102.

218. Beukes, V., *The Killer Foods of the 20th Century (and How to Avoid Them).* Perskor Publishers, Johannesburg, 1982, 8-15.

219. Churchill, Allen, *The Roosevelts.* Frederick Muller Limited, London, 1966.

220. Lloyd Aycock, W., Tonsillectomy and poliomyelitis. *Medicine* 1942;21(65):65-94.

221. Southcott, R.V., Studies on a long range association between bulbar poliomyelitis and previous tonsillectomy. *Med J Aust* 22 August 1953;2(8):281-298.

222. Wright, A.E., The Changes Effected by Anti-typhoid Inoculation in the Bactericidal Power of the Blood: with Remarks on the Probable Significance of These Changes. *Lancet* September 14 1901;715-723.

223. Wilson, Graham S., *The Hazards of Immunization.* The Athlone Press, London, 1967, 265.

224. Bradford Hill, A., Knowelden, J., Inoculation and Poliomyelitis: A statistical investigation in England and Wales in 1949. *Brit Med J* July 1 1950;1-6.

225. Shelton, H.N., *Serums and Polio*, Dr Shelton's Hygienic Review, August 1951, reprinted in McBean, E., *The Poisoned Needle.* Health Research, 1974, 164.

226. Shepherd, Dorothy, *Homoeopathy in Epidemic Diseases.* Health Science Press, Rustington, Sussex, 1967, 76.

227. Shelton, H.N., *Serums and Polio*, Dr Shelton's Hygienic Review, August 1951, reprinted in McBean, E., *The Poisoned Needle.* Health Research, 1974, 165.

228. Wilson, Graham S., *The Hazards of Immunization.* The Athlone Press, London, 1967, 273.

229. Sutter, R.W., Patriarca, P.A., et al., Attributable Risk of DPT (Diphtheria and Tetanus Toxoids and Pertussis Vaccine) Injection in Provoking Paralytic Poliomyelitis during a Large Outbreak in Oman. *J Infect Dis* 1992;165:444-449.

230. Shepherd, Dorothy, *Homoeopathy in Epidemic Diseases.* Health Science Press, Rustington, Sussex, 1967, 76-78.

231. Honorof, I., McBean, E., *Vaccination the Silent Killer: A Clear and Present Danger.* Honor Publications, Sherman Oaks, California, 1977, 32-33.

232. Pauling, Linus, *Vitamin C and the Common Cold and the Flu.* Berkley Books, New York, 1983, 52. Linus Pauling gives 11 references to Klenner's documentation of the treatment in medical journals.

233. Davis, Adelle, *Let's Eat Right to Keep Fit.* Unwin Paperbacks, London, 1984, 111-112.

234. Oppewal, S.R., Sister Elizabeth Kenny, an Australian nurse, and treatment of poliomyelitis victims. *Image J Nurs Sch* 1997;29:83-84.

235. Pauling, Linus, *Vitamin C, the common cold and the flu.* Berkley Books, New York, 55.

236. Jahan, K., Ahmad, K., Ali, M.A., Effect of Ascorbic Acid in the Treatment of Tetanus. *Bangladesh Med Res Counc Bull* June 1984;24-28.

237. Douglas Hume, Ethel, *Béchamp or Pasteur? A Lost Chapter in the History of Biology.* C. W. Daniel, Ashingdon, Rochford, Essex, Fourth Edition, 1963, 232.

238. Cook, T.M., *Samuel Hahnemann, The Founder of Homoeopathic Medicine.* Thorsons Publishers Ltd., Wellingborough, Northamptonshire, 1981, 146.

239. Blackie, Margery G., *The Patient, Not The Cure.* Macdonald and Jane's, London, 1976, 32.

240. Ibid., 1976, 31.
241. Cook, T.M., *Samuel Hahnemann, The Founder of Homoeopathic Medicine.* Thorsons Publishers Ltd., Wellingborough, Northamptonshire, 1981, 148.
242. Blackie, Margery G., *The Patient, Not The Cure.* Macdonald and Jane's, London, 1976, 34.
243. Clarke, John Henry, *Dictionary of Materia Medica.* Health Science Press, Bradford, Holsworthy, Devon, 1977, 736. (First printed in 1901.)
244. Douglas Hume, Ethel, *Béchamp or Pasteur? A Lost Chapter in the History of Biology.* C. W. Daniel, Ashingdon, Rochford, Essex, Fourth Edition, 1963, 222.
245. Ibid., 224.
246. Martin, C.J., Upjohn, W.G.D., The distribution of typhoid and paratyphoid infections amongst enteric fevers at Mudros. *Brit Med J* September 2 1916;313-316.
247. Thucydides, *The Peloponnesian War*, in, *Herodotus, The History.* Great Books of the Western World, Encyclopaedia Britannica Inc., 1952;349-593.
248. Cook, T.M., *Samuel Hahnemann, The Founder of Homoeopathic Medicine.* Thorson's Publishers, 1981, 103-104.
249. Control of Rickettsial Infections. *Lancet* May 5 1945;563-564.
250. Lagget, M., Rizetto, M., Current pharmacotherapy for the treatment of chronic hepatitis B. *Expert Opin Pharmacother* 2003;4:1821-1827.
251. Davis, Adelle, *Let's Get Well.* Unwin Paperbacks, London, 1979, 157-158.
252. Swartout, H.O., *Modern Medical Counsellor.* Signs Publishing Company, Warburton, Victoria, Australia. 1958, 763.
253. Clarke, John Henry, *Dictionary of Materia Medica.* Health Science Press, Bradford, Holsworthy, Devon, 1977, 211. (First printed in 1901.)
254. Blackie, Margery G., *The Patient, Not the Cure.* MacDonald and Jane's, London, 1976, 39 & 81-82.
255. Carmichael, A.E., Silverstein, A.M., *J Hist Med Allied Sci* 1987;42:147-168.
256. *Vaccination Tracts: Opinions of Statesmen, Politicians, Publicists, Statisticians, and Sanitarians*. No 1. Second Edition. William Young, London, 1879.
257. Wilson, Graham S., *The Hazards of Immunization.* The Athlone Press, London, 1967, 256.
258. Fenner, F., Henderson, D.A., et al., *Smallpox and its Eradication.* World Health Organization, Geneva, 1988, 302.

259. Lane, J.M., Ruben, F.L., Neff, J.M., Millar, J.D., Complications of Smallpox Vaccination, 1968: Results of Ten Statewide Surveys. *J Infect Dis* 1970;122(4):303-309.

260. Crookshank, E.M., *History and Pathology of Vaccination.* Vol 1. H. K. Lewis, 1889, 74.

261. Stickl, H., Die Nichtenzephalitischen Erkrankungen nach der Pockenschutzimpfung. *Deutsche Medizinische Wochenschrift* 1968;93:511-517.

262. Wolfe, R.M., Sharp, L.K., Anti-vaccinationists past and present. *Brit Med J* August 24 2002;325:430-432.

263. The manuscript of the article which Jenner submitted to the Royal Society in the hopes that they would publish it in their *Transactions of the Royal Society* was just left lying in a drawer until it was shown to E.M. Crookshank by the librarian at the Royal College of Surgeons in January 1888. E.M. Crookshank ensured "that it has been carefully preserved, and entered in the catalogue of the Library, and may be consulted by anyone desiring to do so." Crookshank, E.M., *History and Pathology of Vaccination.* Vol 1. H. K. Lewis, 1889, page viii. It was later published in the Lancet of 20th January 1923, on pages 137-141.

264. Jenner, Edward, *An Inquiry into the Causes and Effects of the Variolae Vaccinae, a disease discovered in some of the western counties of England, particularly Gloucestershire, and known by the name of the Cow Pox.* Sampson Low, London, 1798. Facsimile Reprint, An Inquiry into the Causes and Effects of the Variolae Vaccinae. Dawsons of Pall Mall, London, 1966.

265. Douglas Hume, Ethel, *Béchamp or Pasteur? A Lost Chapter in the History of Biology.* C. W. Daniel, Ashingdon, Rochford, Essex, Fourth Edition, 1963, 171.

266. Jenner, Edward, *An Inquiry into the Causes and Effects of the Variolae Vaccinae, a disease discovered in some of the western counties of England, particularly Gloucestershire, and known by the name of the Cow Pox.* Sampson Low, London, 1798. Facsimile Reprint, An Inquiry into the Causes and Effects of the Variolae Vaccinae. Dawsons of Pall Mall, London, 1966, 37.

267. Crookshank, E.M., *History and Pathology of Vaccination.* H. K. Lewis, 1889, 1:270.

268. Ibid., 269-273.

269. Further Observations on the Variole Vaccinae, or Cow Pox. Edward Jenner, M.D., F.R.S., &c, in Crookshank, E.M., *History and Pathology of Vaccination.* Vol 1. H. K. Lewis, 1889, 2:155-190. Page 169 is where the death is mentioned.

270. Fenner, F., Henderson, D.A., et al., *Smallpox and its Eradication.* World Health Organization, Geneva, 1988.

271. Jenner, Edward, *An Inquiry into the Causes and Effects of the Variolae Vaccinae, a disease discovered in some of the western counties of England, particularly Gloucestershire, and known by the name of the Cow Pox.* Sampson Low, London, 1798. Facsimile Reprint, An Inquiry into the Causes and Effects of the Variolae Vaccinae. Dawsons of Pall Mall, London, 1966, 6.

272. Jenner, E., *Facts, for the most part unobserved, or not duly noticed, respecting variolous contagion.* S. Gosnell, London, 1808. There is an original copy of this in Melbourne on which Jenner has written, "A. Cooper Esq, with the best wishes of the Author."

273. Fenner, F., Henderson, D.A., et al., *Smallpox and its Eradication.* World Health Organization, Geneva, 1988, 271.

274. Ibid., 273.

275. Thagard, Paul, *How Scientists Explain Disease.* Princeton University Press, Princeton, 1999, 155-156.

276. Trusted, Jennifer, *Theories and Facts, Unit 7, The Germ Theory of Disease.* The Open University Press, Milton Keynes, 1981, 10.

277. Dobell, C., *Antony van Leewenhoek and his "Little Animals".* Russel and Russel Inc., New York, 1958.

278. Geison, G.L., *The Private Science of Louis Pasteur.* Princeton University Press, Princeton, New Jersey, 1995, 267.

279. Ibid., 267-269.

280. Douglas Hume, Ethel, *Béchamp or Pasteur? A Lost Chapter in the History of Biology.* C. W. Daniel, Ashingdon, Rochford, Essex, Fourth Edition, 1963.

281. Geison, G. L., *The Private Science of Louis Pasteur.* Princeton University Press, Princeton, New Jersey, 1995.

282. Katz Miller, S., The Daring and Devious Father of Vaccines. *New Sci* 20 February 1993;137:10.

283. Anderson, C., Pasteur Notebooks Reveal Deception. *Science* 19 February 1993;259:1117.

284. Geison, G. L., *The Private Science of Louis Pasteur.* Princeton University Press, Princeton, New Jersey, 1995, 3.

285. Douglas Hume, Ethel, *Béchamp or Pasteur? A Lost Chapter in the History of Biology.* C. W. Daniel, Ashingdon, Rochford, Essex, Fourth Edition, 1963, 38.

286. Ibid., 58.

287. Ibid., 101.

288. Ibid., 90.

289. Ibid., 92.

290. Ibid., 93.
291. The World Book Encyclopedia 1994;15:212. World Book International.
292. Geison, G. L., *The Private Science of Louis Pasteur.* Princeton University Press, Princeton, New Jersey, 1995, 145-176.
293. Douglas Hume, Ethel, *Béchamp or Pasteur? A Lost Chapter in the History of Biology.* C. W. Daniel, Ashingdon, Rochford, Essex, Fourth Edition, 1963, 185-186.
294. Ibid., 191-192.
295. Ibid., 192.
296. Nass, M., Anthrax Vaccine; Model of a Response to the Biologic Warfare Threat. *Infectious Dis Clin North Am* 1999;13(1):187-208.
297. Pearson, R.B., *Pasteur, Plagiarist, Imposter.* 1942. Reprinted by Health Research, Mokelumne Hill, California, 1964, 95.
298. Ad Hoc Group for the study of pertussis vaccines, Placebo-Controlled Trial of two acellular pertussis vaccines in Sweden - Protective Efficacy and Adverse Events. *Lancet* April 30 1988;955-960.
299. Geison, G. L., *The Private Science of Louis Pasteur.* Princeton University Press, Princeton, New Jersey, 1995, 240-245.
300. Ibid., 240.
301. Ibid., 240-241.
302. Ibid., 241.
303. Ibid., 243.
304. Ibid., 189.
305. Ibid., 191.
306. Ibid., 213.
307. Ibid., 213 -214.
308. Douglas Hume, Ethel, *Béchamp or Pasteur? A Lost Chapter in the History of Biology.* C. W. Daniel, Ashingdon, Rochford, Essex, Fourth Edition, 1963, 196.
309. Human Viral and Rickettsial Vaccines, *Wld Hlth Org Tech Rep Ser* 1966;325:31.
310. Dole, Lionel, *The Blood Poisoners.* Gateway Book Company, Croydon, Surrey, 1965, 58.
311. Douglas Hume, Ethel, *Béchamp or Pasteur? A Lost Chapter in the History of Biology.* C. W. Daniel, Ashingdon, Rochford, Essex, Fourth Edition, 1963, 195.
312. Ibid., 200.
313. Geison, G. L., *The Private Science of Louis Pasteur.* Princeton University Press, Princeton, New Jersey, 1995, 221.
314. McBean, E., *The Poisoned Needle.* Health Research, 1974, 188.

315. Plotkin, S.A., Vaccine production in human diploid cell strains. *Am J Epidemiol* 1971;94(4):303-306.

316. Koprowski, H., Laboratory techniques in rabies: vaccine for man prepared in human diploid cells. *Monogr Ser World Health Organ* 1973;(23):256-260.

317. Plotkin, S.A., Wiktor, T.J., et al., Immunization Schedules for the new human diploid cell vaccine against rabies. *Am J Epidemiol* 1976;103(1):75-80.

318. Oelofsen, M.J., Gericke, A., et al., Immunity to rabies after administration of prophylactic human diploid cell vaccine. *S Afr Med J* 17 August 1991;80:189-190.

319. Mansour, A.B., Abrous, M., Properties and potency of a rabies vaccine produced on the brain matter of young goats and inactivated by beta-propiolactone. *Dev Biol Stand* 1978;41:217-224.

320. Lin, F., Zeng, F., et al., The primary hamster kidney cell rabies vaccine: adaptation of viral strain, production of vaccine and pre- and post exposure treatment. *J Infect Dis* 1983;147(3):467-473.

321. Wasi, C., Chaiprasithikul, P., et al., Purified chick embryo cell rabies vaccine. *Lancet* January 4 1986;40.

322. van Wezel, A. L., van Steenis, G., Production of an inactivated rabies vaccine in primary dog kidney cells. *Dev Biol Stand* 1978;40:69-75.

323. Gorman, C., Drug Safety; Can Drug Firms Be Trusted? *Time*, February 10, 1992, 33.

324. Coulter, H.L., Loe Fisher, B., *DPT; A Shot in the Dark.* Warner Books, New York, March 1986, 286.

325. Braithwaite, J., *Corporate Crime in the Pharmaceutical Industry.* Routledge and Kegan Paul, London, 1984.

326. Tom Mangold, *The Halcion Nightmare.* Panorama, BBC.

327. McCarthy, M., Conflict of interest taints vaccine approval process, charges US report. *Lancet* September 2 2000;356:838.

328. *Vaccination, The Choice is Yours* 6(2):2000, 38, quoting Kathi Williams of NVIC. The congressman is Dan Burton of Indiana.

329. Coulter, H.L., Loe Fisher, B., *DPT A Shot in the Dark.* Warner Books, New York, March 1986, 314.

330. Ibid., 163.

331. Globus, J.H., Kohn, J.L., Encephalopathy Following Pertussis Vaccine Prophylaxis. *JAMA* October 22 1949;141(8):507-509.

332. Acellular pertussis vaccines: new vaccines for an old disease. *Lancet* January 27 1996;347:209-210.

333. Miller, H.G., Stanton, J.B., Neurological Sequelae of Prophylactic Inoculation. *Q J Med* 1954;23:1-27.

334. Wilson, Graham S., *The Hazards of Immunization.* The Athlone Press, London, 1967, 200.

335. Coulter, H.L., Loe Fisher, B., *DPT A Shot in the Dark.* Warner Books, New York, March 1986, 44-46.

336. Whooping Cough Immunization Committee of the Medical Research Council, Vaccination Against Whooping-Cough. *Brit Med J* August 25 1956;2:454-462.

337. Coulter, H.L., Loe Fisher, B., *DPT A Shot in the Dark.* Warner Books, New York, March 1986, 34.

338. Ibid., 32.

339. Ibid., 28-31.

340. Pittman, M., *Bordatella Pertussis - Bacterial and Host Factors in the Pathogenesis and Prevention of Whooping Cough,* in, Mudd, S., *Infectious Agents and Host Reactions,* W.B. Saunders Co, Philadelphia, 1970, 261.

341. Ibid., 259.

342. Dellepiane, N., Griffiths, E., Milstien, J.B., New Challenges in assuring vaccine quality. *Bull WHO* 2000;78(2):155.

343. Cody, C.L., Baraff, L.J., Cherry, J.D., Marcy, S.M., Manclark, C.R., Nature and Rates of Adverse Reactions Associated with DTP and DT Immunizations in Infants and Children. *Pediatrics* 1981;68(5):650-660.

344. Coulter, H.L., Loe Fisher, B., *DPT A Shot in the Dark.* Warner Books, New York, March 1986, 244.

345. DPT, *The Fresno Bee.* December 1984, 3.

346. Coulter, H.L., Loe Fisher, B., *DPT A Shot in the Dark.* Warner Books, New York, March 1986, 243-254.

347. Ibid., 248-251.

348. Aicardi, J., Chevrie, J.J., *Archives Francaises de Pediatrie,* April 1975;32(4):309-317, cited in AVN Newsletter, *Vaccination, The Choice is Yours* 3(2):1997.

349. Coulter, H.L., Loe Fisher, B., *DPT A Shot in the Dark.* Warner Books, New York, March 1986, 253.

350. Conflict of Interest Charges Leveled Against Federal Vaccine Advisors. *NVIC News,* October 1991;1(3):1.

351. Hodgekinson, N., *Mother wins 20-year battle against vaccine drug giant.* The Sunday Times, 25 April 1993.

352. Stuart-Smith, Lord Justice. Judgement, Susan Jaqueline Loveday v. Dr. GH Renton and The Wellcome Foundation Limited, 29-30 March 1988. London, Chilton Vint and Co.

353. Dyer, C., Judge "not satisfied" that whooping cough vaccine causes permanent brain damage. *Brit Med J* April 23 1988;296:1189-1190.

354. Against All Odds - Margaret's Story, BBC.

355. Coulter, H.L., Loe Fisher, B., *DPT A Shot in the Dark.* Warner Books, New York, March 1986.

356. Child vaccine may be delayed. *New Zealand Herald*, 8 September, 1992.

357. Stewart, G.T., Toxicity of pertussis vaccine: frequency and probability of reactions. *J Epidemiol Comm Health* 1979;33:150-156.

358. Fox, R., Immunisation against whooping cough (letter). *Brit Med J* February 21 1976;458-459.

359. Official Line on Vaccine Does U-turn. *New Zealand Herald*, 11 July, 1987.

360. Giarnia Thompson - An Innocent Bystander. Hilary Butler, *IAS Newsletter* April 1992;4(5):2-6.

361. Hood, A., Edwards, I. R., Meningococcal vaccine - do some children experience side effects? *NZ Med J* 1989;102(862):65-67.

362. *IAS Newsletter* August 1989;2(1):12.

363. Personal communication, Hilary Butler, after she had been speaking to the Medical Assessor.

364. Butler, H., *Introducing the New Zealand Department of Health's Meningococcal Meningitis Immunisation Campaign.* IRONI, 1987.

365. Ibid., 1987, 24.

366. President Reagan Signs Vaccine Injury Compensation and Safety Bill Into Law. *DPT News*, Spring 1987;3(1):1, 10-16.

367. Centers for Disease Control, Vaccine Adverse Events Reporting System - United States. *MMWR Morb Mortal Wkly Rep* October 19 1990;39(41):730.

368. Morris, J. Anthony, *Childhood Vaccine Injury Compensation Programme in the US; Hope Versus Reality.* International Symposium, The Vaccination Dilemma, Auckland, 1992.

369. Personal communication, Hilary Butler, after talking on the phone to Dr. Morris.

370. Annex 1, Q and A's: Vaccine Adverse Event Reporting System (VAERS).

371. NVIC/DPT Investigation Shows That Doctors And Government Fail To Report And Monitor Vaccine Death And Injury Reports. *NVIC News* August 1994;4(1).

372. National Health and Medical Research Council, *The Australian Immunisation Handbook*, 7th Edition. March 2000, 22.

373. Personal communication, Meryl Dorey.

374. Grimsey, L., Our trip to Canberra. *Vaccination, The Choice is Yours* 4(2):1998, 22.

375. Mehta, U., Milstien J.B., et al., Developing a national system for dealing with adverse events following immunization. *Bull WHO,* 2000, 78(2):170-175.

376. Kearney, M., Yach, D., et al., Evaluation of a mass measles immunisation campaign in a rapidly growing peri-urban area. *S Afr Med J* 1989;76:157-159.

377. Personal communication, Dr. J. Anthony Morris.

378. Coulter, H.L., Loe Fisher, B., *DPT; A Shot in the Dark.* Warner Books, New York, March 1986, 100.

379. Classen, J.B., Childhood immunization and diabetes mellitus. *NZ Med J* 24 May 1996;109(1022):195.

380. Classen, J.B., The diabetes epidemic and the hepatitis B vaccines. *NZ Med J* 27 September 1996;109(1030):366.

381. Classen, J.B., Classen, D.C., Association between type 1 diabetes and hib vaccine. *Brit Med J* October 23 1999;319:1133.

382. Shaw, F.E., Graham, D.J., Guess, H.A., et al., Postmarketing surveillance for neurologic adverse events reported after Hepatitis B vaccination. Experience of the first three years. *Am J Epidemiol* 1988;127(2):337-352.

383. Hepatitis B vaccines: reported reactions. *WHO Drug Inf* 1990;4(3):129.

384. Herroelen, L., De Keyser, J., Ebinger, G., Central-nervous-system demyelination after immunisation with recombinant hepatitis B vaccine. *Lancet* November 9 1991;338:1174-1175.

385. http://www.whale.to/vaccines/belkin.html

386. Seeff, L.B., Beebe, G.W., et al., A serologic follow-up of the 1942 epidemic of post-vaccination hepatitis in the United States Army. *New Engl J Med* 1987;316(16):965-970.

387. Jahnke, U., Fischer, E.H., Alvord, E.C., Sequence Homology Between Certain Viral Proteins and Proteins Related to Encephalomyelitis and Neuritis. *Science* 19 July 1985;229:282-284.

388. McAlpine, D., Acute Disseminated Encephalomyelitis: Its Sequele and its Relationship to Disseminated Sclerosis. *Lancet* April 18 1931;846-852.

389. Miller, H., Schapira, K., Aetiological Aspects of multiple sclerosis. Part I. *Brit Med J* March 21 1959;737-740.

390. Miller, H., Schapira, K., Aetiological Aspects of multiple sclerosis. Part II. *Brit Med J* March 28 1959;811-815.

391. Miller, H., Cendrowski, W., Schapira, K., Multiple Sclerosis and vaccination. *Brit Med J* April 22 1967;210-213.

392. Kaprowski, H., Lebell, I., The presence of complement-fixing antibodies against brain tissue in sera of persons who had received antirabies vaccine treatment. *Amer J Hyg* 1950;5:292-299.

393. Kong, Von E., Zur Pertussisimpfung und ihren Gegenindikationen. *Helvetica Paediatrica Acta* 1953;1:90-98. The summary is given in German, French, Italian and English.

394. Kulenkampff, M., Schwartzman, J. S., Wilson, J., Neurological complications of pertussis inoculation. *Arch Dis Child* 1974;49(1):46-49.

395. Centers for Disease Control, Recommendations of the Immunization Practices Advisory Committee (ACIP): Misconceptions Concerning Contraindications to Vaccination. *MMWR Morb Mortal Wkly Rep* April 7 1989;38(13):223-224.

396. Baraff, L.J., Cody, C.L., Cherry, J.D., DTP-Associated Reactions: An Analysis by Injection Site, Manufacturer, Prior Reactions, and Dose. *Pediatrics* 1984;73(1):31-36.

397. Sen, S., Cloete, Y., et al., Adverse events following vaccination in premature infants. *Acta Paediatr* 2001;90:916-920.

398. Lewis, K., Cherry, J. D., et al., The effect of Prophylactic Acetaminophen Administration on Reactions to DTP Vaccination. *Am J Dis Child* January 1988;142:62-65.

399. Ipp, M.M., Gold, R., et al., Acetaminophen prophylaxis of adverse reactions following vaccination of infants with diphtheria-pertussis-tetanus toxoids-polio vaccine. *Ped Infect Dis J* 1987;6(8):721-725.

400. Paracetamol Increases Immunisation Compliance. *Current Therapeutics* September 1988;29(9):12.

401. Strom J., Further Experience of Reactions, Especially of a Cerebral Nature, in Conjunction with Triple Vaccination: A Study Based on Vaccinations in Sweden 1959 - 65. *Brit Med J* November 11 1967;4:320-323.

402. Berg, J.M., Neurological Complications of Pertussis Immunization. *Brit Med J* July 5 1958;24-27.

403. Limerick, S.R., Sudden infant death in historical perspective. *J Clin Pathol* 1992;45(Suppl):3-6.

404. Stewart-Brown, S., Cot death and sleeping position. *Brit Med J* 1992;304:1508.

405. Hiley, C., Babies' sleeping position. *Brit Med J* 1992;305:115.

406. Statement to the National Vaccine Advisory Committee by Barbara Loe Fisher, Co-Founder & President National Vaccine Information Center September 26, 1994. *NVIC News* November 1994;4(2).

407. Griffin, M.R., Wayne, M.P.H., et al., Risk of Sudden Infant Death Syndrome after immunization with the diptheria-tetanus-pertussis vaccine. *New Engl J Med* 1988;319(10):618-623.

408. Editor's note in reply to letter from Wendy Baldock, *Little Treasures*, Christmas '90; 53.

409. Medical Research Council Committee on Inoculation Procedures and Neurological Lesions, Poliomyelitis and Prophylactic Inoculation Against Diphtheria, Whooping-cough and Smallpox. *Lancet* December 15 1956;1223-1231.

410. Scheibner, V., *Vaccination - 100 years of Orthodox Research shows that Vaccines Represent a Medical Assault on the Immune System.* 1993, 178 Govetts Leap Rd, Blackheath, NSW 2785, Australia.

411. Hoffman, H.J., Hunter, J.C., et al., Diphtheria-Tetanus-Pertussis Immunization and Sudden Infant Death: Results of the National Institute of Child Health and Human Development Cooperative Epidemiological Study of Sudden Infant Death Syndrome Risk Factors. *Pediatrics* April 1987;79(4):598-611.

412. Bernier, R.H., et al., Diphtheria-tetanus toxiods-pertussis vaccination and sudden infant deaths in Tennessee. *J Ped* 1982;101(3):419-421.

413. Keens, T.G., Davidson Ward, S.L., et al., Ventilatory Pattern Following Diphtheria-Tetanus-Pertussis Immunization in Infants at Risk for Sudden Infant Death Syndrome. *Am J Dis Child* 1985;139:991-994.

414. Apnoea and Unexpected Child Death. *Lancet* August 18 1979;339-340.

415. National Institutes of Health Consensus Development Conference on Infantile Apnea and Home Monitoring, Sept 29 to Oct 1, 1986. *Pediatrics* 1987;79:292-299.

416. Horvarth, C.H.G., Sudden infant death syndrome. *NZ Med J* 14 March 1990;107.

417. Hirvonen, J., Jantti, M., et al., Hyperplasia of Islets of Langerhans and Low Serum Insulin in Cot Deaths. *Forensic Sci Int* 1980;16:213-226.

418. Read, D.J.C., Williams, A.L., et al., Sudden Infant Deaths: Some Current Research Strategies. *Med J Aust* September 8 1979;2(5):236-238, 240-241, 244.

419. Aynsley-Green, A., Polak, J.M., et al., Averted Sudden Neonatal Death Due to Pancreatic Nesidioblastosis. *Lancet* March 11 1978;550-551.

420. Cox, J.N., Guelpa, G., Terrapon, M., Islet-cell Hyperplasia and Sudden Infant Death. *Lancet* October 2 1976;739-740.

421. Hannik, C.A., Cohen, H., Changes in plasma insulin concentration and temperature of infants after Pertussis vaccination. 4th International Symposium on Pertussis, Bethesda, Md. USA, IABS Special publication, 1979, 297-299, cited in Hennessen, W., Quast, U., Adverse Reactions After Pertussis Vaccination. *Dev Biol Stand* 1979;43:95-100.

422. Dhar, H.L., West, G.B., Sensitization procedures and the blood sugar concentration. *J Pharm Pharmac* 1972;24:249.

423. Serfontein, Gordon, *The Hidden Handicap: Dyslexia, Hyperactivity and Behavioural disorders in children.* David Bateman, Buderim, Qld, 1989, 17.

424. Wilson, Graham S., *The Hazards of Immunization.* The Athlone Press, London, 1967, 198.
425. Byers, R.K., and Moll, F.C., Encephalopathies following prophylactic pertussis vaccine. *Pediatrics* April 1948;1(4):437-456.
426. Biddulph, Steve, *Raising Boys.* Finch Publishing, Sydney, 2003, 51-64.
427. Serfontein, Gordon, *The Hidden Handicap: Dyslexia, Hyperactivity and Behavioural disorders in children.* David Bateman, Buderim, Qld, 1989, 12.
428. Ibid., 27.
429. Dole, Lionel, *The Blood Poisoners.* Gateway Book Company, Croydon, Surrey, 1965, 56.
430. Frith, U., (ed), *Autism and Asperger syndrome.* Cambridge University Press, 1991.
431. Coulter, H.L., *Vaccination, Social Violence and Criminality.* North Atlantic Books, Berkeley, 1990, 1.
432. Wing, Lorna, *Autistic Children.* Constable and Co., London, 1971, 8.
433. Coulter, H.L., *Vaccination, Social Violence and Criminality.* North Atlantic Books, Berkeley, 1990, 51.
434. Ibid., 51-52.
435. Ibid., 52.
436. Loe Fisher, B., (letter). *Lancet* May 2 1998;351:1357-1358.
437. Bower, H., New research demolishes link between MMR vaccine and autism. *Brit Med J* June 19 1999;318:1643.
438. Wakefield, A.J., MMR vaccination and autism (letter). *Lancet* September 11 1999;354:949-950.
439. Vaccines Not Mercury Free. Health Advocacy in the Public Interest, Press Release, August 12, 2004. http://hapihealth.com
440. O'Neill, G., Autism Linked to Diet. *Sunday Herald Sun* 1 April 2001; 50.
441. Scheibner, V., Shaken Baby Syndrome Diagnosis On Shaky Ground. *Australasian College of Nutritional and Environmental Medicine* August 2001;20(2):5-8, 15.
442. www.freeyurko.bizland.com
443. Fenner, F., Henderson, D.A., et al., *Smallpox and its Eradication.* World Health Organization, Geneva, 1988, 911.
444. Rappaport, J., News Blackout on pox vaccine link to AIDS protecting WHO (World Health Organization)? *Easy Reader*, 4 June 1987. Reprinted in *Report to the Consumer* September 1987;396:1.
445. Nahmias, A.J., Weiss, J., et al., Evidence for Human Infection with an HTLV III/LAV-Like Virus in Central Africa, 1959. *Lancet* May 31 1986;1279-1280.
446. The Sunday Times Magazine, June 21, 1987, 66.

447. Brown, P., Polio vaccine 'did not cause AIDS epidemic'. *New Sci* 31 October 1992;136:8.

448. Curtis, T., The Origin of AIDS: A Startling New Theory Attempts to Answer the Question 'Was it an Act of God or an Act of Man?', *Rolling Stone*, March 19, 1992, 626:54-60, 106, 108.

449. Courtois, G., Flack, A., et al., Preliminary Report on Mass Vaccination of man with live attenuated poliomyelitis virus in the Belgian Congo and Ruanda-Urundi. *Brit Med J* July 26 1958;187-190.

450. Cribb, J., *The White Death.* Angus and Robertson, Sydney, 1996, 187.

451. Hooper, E., *The River: A Journey to the Source of HIV and AIDS.* Little, Brown and Company, Boston, New York, London, 1999. ISBN 0-316-37261-7 (hc) In the same year it was published in Britain by Allen Lane, The Penguin Press, with the same page numbering. ISBN 0-713-99335-9.

452. Hooper, E., *The River: A Journey to the Source of HIV and AIDS.* Little, Brown and Company, Boston, New York, London, 1999, 274.

453. Technology, Determination Win Against Implacable Enemy. *Dateline:CDC* October 1979;11(10):2, 8.

454. Hooper, E., *The River: A Journey to the Source of HIV and AIDS.* Little, Brown and Company, Boston, New York, London, 1999, 307.

455. Fenner, F., Henderson, D.A., et al., *Smallpox and its Eradication.* World Health Organization, Geneva, 1988, 264 - 265.

456. Schippell, T.M., Let us Face the Facts. *Herald of Health,* August 1955. Reprinted in McBean, E., *The Poisoned Needle,* Health Research, 1974, 160.

457. Martin, W.J., Zeng, L.C., et al., Cytomegalovirus-related sequences in an atypical cytopathic virus repeatedly isolated from a patient with the chronic fatigue syndrome. *Am J Pathol* 1994;45:440-451.

458. Martin, W.J., Ahmed, K.N., et al., African green monkey origin of the atypical cytopathic stealth virus isolated from a patient with chronic fatigue syndrome. *Clin Diagn Virol* 1995;4:93-103.

459. Hooper, E., *The River: A Journey to the Source of HIV and AIDS.* Little, Brown and Company, Boston, New York, London, 1999, 329.

460. *Variance* Toronto, Ontario, Canada. (www.vran.org)

461. *You & Your Family* Centrelink, December 1997; 3.

462. *Vaccination, The choice is yours* 4(2):1998, 5.

463. Compton Burnett, J., *Vaccinosis* (reprint), 1960, Health Science Press.

464. Shepherd, D., *Homoeopathy in Epidemic Diseases.* Health Science Press, Rustington, Sussex, 1967, 92-94.

465. Gilbert, D.A., *Temporal Organisation, Reorganisation, and Disorganisation in Cells*, in, Edmunds, L.N., (ed), *Cell Cycle Clocks.* Marcel Dekker, Inc., New York and Basel, 1984.

466. Personal communication, Don Gilbert, Department of Biochemistry, University of the Witwatersrand, 20th February 1990.

467. Madsen, K.M., Hviid, A., et al., A Population-Based Study of Measles, Mumps, and Rubella Vaccination and Autism. *New Engl J Med* 2002;347(19):1477-1482.

468. Ben Goldacre, *Never mind the facts.* The Guardian, December 11, 2003.

469. Australian Government Department of Health and Ageing, *Understanding Childhood Immunisations*, Department of Health and Ageing Publications, Approval number 2387, Revised March 2004.

470. Therapeutic Goods Administration, Medicine Summary, Haemophilus Influenzae Type B Vaccine, 17 August 2004.

471. Halvorsen, Richard, (letter). *The Observer*, February 29, 2004.

Printed in the United States
62132LVS00003B/96

9 781418 450175